The Global Impact of AIDS

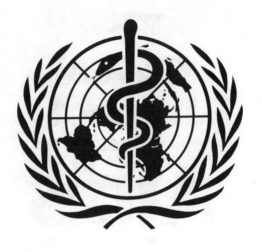

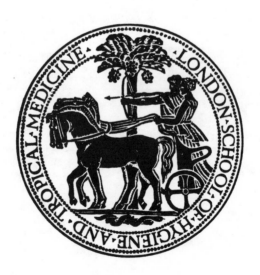

The Global Impact of AIDS

Proceedings of the First International Conference on the Global Impact
of AIDS, Co-Sponsored by the World Health Organization and the
London School of Hygiene and Tropical Medicine, Held in London,
March 8–10, 1988

Editors

Alan F. Fleming
London School of Hygiene
and Tropical Medicine
London

Manuel Carballo
Global Programme on AIDS
World Health Organization
Geneva

David W. FitzSimons
Bureau of Hygiene
and Tropical Diseases
London

Michael R. Bailey
London School of Hygiene
and Tropical Medicine
London

Jonathan Mann
Global Programme on AIDS
World Health Organization
Geneva

Alan R. Liss, Inc., New York

Address all Inquiries to the Publisher
Alan R. Liss, Inc., 41 East 11th Street, New York, NY 10003

While the authors, editors, and publisher believe that drug selection and dosage and the specifications and usage of equipment and devices, as set forth in this book, are in accord with current recommendations and practice at the time of publication, they accept no legal responsibility for any errors or omissions, and make no warranty, express or implied, with respect to material contained herein. In view of ongoing research, equipment modifications, changes in governmental regulations and the constant flow of information relating to drug therapy, drug reactions and the use of equipment and devices, the reader is urged to review and evaluate the information provided in the package insert or instructions for each drug, piece of equipment or device for, among other things, any changes in the instructions or indications of dosage or usage and for added warnings and precautions.

Library of Congress Cataloging-in-Publication Data

International Conference on the Global Impact of AIDS (1st : 1988 :
    London, England)
    The global impact of AIDS : proceedings of the First International
Conference on the Global Impact of AIDS / co-sponsored by the World
Health Organization and the London School of Hygiene and Tropical
Medicine, held in London, March 8–10, 1988 ; editors, Alan F.
Fleming . . . [et al.]
        p.   cm.
    Includes bibliographies and index.
    ISBN 0-8451-4270-4. ISBN 0-8451-4271-2 (pbk.)
    1. AIDS (Disease)—Social aspects—Congresses. I. Fleming, A.F.
II. World Health Organization. III. London School of Hygiene and
Tropical Medicine. IV. Title.
    [DNLM: 1. Acquired Immunodeficiency Syndrome—congresses. WD 308
I607g 1988]
RA644.A25I58 1988
362.1'9697'92—dc19
DNLM/DLC
for Library of Congress   88-8277
                                                           CIP

Contents

Contributors

Nick Abel, School of Development Studies and Overseas Development Group, University of East Anglia, Norwich, United Kingdom [145]

Omar B. Ahmad, Center for the Study of Population, Florida State University, Tallahassee, FL 32306-4063 [175]

R.M. Anderson, Parasite Epidemiology Research Group, Department of Pure and Applied Biology, Imperial College of Science and Technology, London University, London SW7 2BB, United Kingdom [95]

George Ankra-Badu, Department of Haematology, University of Ghana Medical School, Accra, Ghana [9]

A. Asamoah-Adu, Ministry of Health, Public Health Laboratories, Accra, Ghana [9]

Michael R. Bailey, London School of Hygiene and Tropical Medicine, London WC1E 7HT, United Kingdom [xvii]

L.S. Bakketeig, Department of Epidemiology, National Institute of Public Health, 0365 Oslo 3, Norway [53]

Tony Barnett, School of Development Studies and Overseas Development Group, University of East Anglia, Norwich, United Kingdom [145]

Paola Baudoux, Department of Pediatrics, Mama Yemo Hospital, Kinshasa 2, Zaire [167]

Christopher Beer, HelpAge International, London EC1R 0BE, United Kingdom [171]

Simon Bell, School of Development Studies and Overseas Development Group, University of East Anglia, Norwich, United Kingdom [145]

Cecilia Bentsi, Ministry of Health, Public Health Laboratories, Accra, Ghana [9]

S. Bertozzi, Global Programme on AIDS, World Health Organization, CH-1211 Geneva 27, Switzerland [123]

Piers Blaikie, School of Development Studies and Overseas Development Group, University of East Anglia, Norwich, United Kingdom [145]

E.C. Buning, Drug Department, Municipal Health Service Amsterdam, 1452 XS Amsterdam, The Netherlands [369]

M. Carael, Global Programme on AIDS, World Health Organization, CH-1211 Geneva 27, Switzerland [81]

The numbers in brackets are the opening page numbers of the contributors' articles.

ix

Manuel Carballo, Global Programme on AIDS, World Health Organization, CH-1211 Geneva 27, Switzerland [xvii, 81]

James Chin, Global Programme on AIDS, World Health Organization, CH-1211 Geneva 27, Switzerland [61,123]

Hesio Cordeiro, National Institute of Medical Care and Social Welfare, Rio de Janeiro, RJ CEP 20031, Brazil [119]

R.A. Coutinho, Public Health Department, Municipal Health Service Amsterdam, 1000 HE Amsterdam, The Netherlands [369]

Sholto Cross, School of Development Studies and Overseas Development Group, University of East Anglia, Norwich, United Kingdom [145]

James W. Curran, The Centers for Disease Control, Public Health Service, U.S. Department of Health and Human Services, Atlanta, GA 30333 [35]

Farzin Davachi, Department of Pediatrics, Mama Yemo Hospital, Kinshasa 2, Zaire [167]

Bruce Dick, Community Health Department, League of Red Cross and Red Crescent Societies, CH-1211 Geneva 19, Switzerland [271]

Timothy J. Dondero, The Centers for Disease Control, Public Health Service, U.S. Department of Health and Human Services, Atlanta, GA 30333 [35]

Françoise Dubois-Arber, University Institute for Social and Preventive Medicine, CH-1005 Lausanne, Switzerland [219]

Isaac W. Eberstein, Center for the Study of Population, Florida State University, Tallahassee, FL 32306-4063 [175]

David W. FitzSimons, Bureau of Hygiene and Tropical Diseases, London WC1E 7HT, United Kingdom [xvii]

Alan F. Fleming, London School of Hygiene and Tropical Medicine, London WC1E 7HT, United Kingdom [xvii, 357]

S. Franceschi, Epidemiology Unit, Centro di Riferimento Oncologico, 33081 Aviano (PN), Italy [43]

Ronald Frankenberg, Centre for Medical Social Anthropology, Keele University, Staffordshire, United Kingdom ST5 5BG [191]

Kazuo Fukutomi, Department of Public Health Statistics, The Institute of Public Health, Tokyo 108, Japan [251]

G. Gordon, International Planned Parenthood Federation, Regents College, London NW1 4NS, United Kingdom [289]

C.E. Gordon Smith, London School of Hygiene and Tropical Medicine, London WC1E 7HT, United Kingdom [xv]

A. Griffiths, Health Management Institute, CH-1206 Geneva, Switzerland [111]

R.N. Grose, Global Programme on AIDS, World Health Organization, CH-1211 Geneva 27, Switzerland [263]

Felix Gutzwiller, University Institute for Social and Preventive Medicine, CH-1005 Lausanne, Switzerland [219]

C. Hartgers, Public Health Department, Municipal Health Service Amsterdam, 1000 HE Amsterdam, The Netherlands [369]

Tomonori Hasegawa, Department of Environmental and Community Medicine, Teikyo University School of Medicine, Tokyo 173, Japan [251]

Dominique Hausser, University Institute for Social and Preventive Medicine, CH-1005 Lausanne, Switzerland **[219]**

Wataru Hirano, Department of Environmental and Community Medicine, Teikyo University School of Medicine, Tokyo 173, Japan **[251]**

Philip R. Hiza, Ministry of Health, Dar Es Salaam, Tanzania **[233]**

C.J. Hospedales, Caribbean Epidemiology Centre (CAREC), Port of Spain, Trinidad, West Indies **[27]**

D.C. Jayasuriya, Institute of Comparative Health Policy and Law, Nawala, Sri Lanka **[313]**

Ichiro Kai, Department of Environmental and Community Medicine, Teikyo University School of Medicine, Tokyo 173, Japan **[251]**

Lars O. Kallings, National Bacteriological Laboratory and WHO Collaborating Centre for AIDS, Stockholm 105 21, Sweden **[335]**

John L. Kilgour, HM Prison Services, London SW1P 4LN, United Kingdom **[323]**

The Hon. Justice Michael Kirby CMG, President, Court of Appeal, Supreme Court, Sydney, Australia **[317,397]**

Anthony Klouda, International Planned Parenthood Federation, Regents College, London NW1 4NS, United Kingdom **[107]**

Yasuki Kobayashi, Department of Environmental and Community Medicine, Teikyo University School of Medicine, Tokyo 173, Japan **[251]**

C. Everett Koop, Surgeon General, U.S. Public Health Service, Rockville, MD 20852 **[307]**

I.L. Kvalem, Department of Epidemiology, National Institute of Public Health, 0365 Oslo 3, Norway **[53]**

Susan M.L. Laver, Department of Community Medicine, University of Zimbabwe, Harare, Zimbabwe **[281]**

Philippe Lehmann, University Institute for Social and Preventive Medicine, CH-1005 Lausanne, Switzerland **[219]**

J. Leowski, Tuberculosis Unit, World Health Organization, CH-1211 Geneva 27, Switzerland **[21]**

Gary A. Lloyd, Institute for Training and Research in HIV Counseling, Tulane University School of Social Work, New Orleans, LA 70118 **[183]**

P. Magnus, Department of Epidemiology, National Institute of Public Health, 0365 Oslo 3, Norway **[53]**

S. Mahabir, Caribbean Epidemiology Centre (CAREC), Port of Spain, Trinidad, West Indies **[27]**

Jonathan Mann, Global Programme on AIDS, World Health Organization, CH-1211 Geneva 27, Switzerland **[xvii,xxv,3,21,167,203]**

Anthony J. Meyer, Global Programme on AIDS, World Health Organization, CH-1211 Geneva 27, Switzerland **[329]**

Michael Micklin, Center for the Study of Population, Florida State University, Tallahassee, FL 32306-4063 **[67]**

J.A.A. Mingle, Department of Microbiology, University of Ghana Medical School and Noguchi Memorial Institute for Medical Research, Legon, Accra, Ghana **[9]**

W. Meade Morgan, The Centers for Disease Control, Public Health Service, U.S. Department of Health and Human Services, Atlanta, GA 30333 **[35]**

Ndoko Kabote, Department of Pediatrics, Mama Yemo Hospital, Kinshasa 2, Zaire **[167]**

Alfred R. Neequaye, Department of Internal Medicine, University of Ghana Medical School, Accra, Ghana **[9]**

Janet E. Neequaye, Burkitt's Tumor Project and Department of Child Health, University of Ghana Medical School, Accra, Ghana **[9]**

Anthony Newton, MP, HM Minister of Health, London, United Kingdom **[xxvii]**

B. N'Galy, National AIDS Control Programme, Ministry of Health, Kinshasa, Zaire **[123,167]**

Benjamin M. Nkowane, Department of Community Medicine, University of Zambia School of Medicine, University Teaching Hospital, Lusaka, Zambia **[155]**

Gary R. Noble, The Centers for Disease Control, Public Health Service, U.S. Department of Health and Human Services, Atlanta, GA 30333 **[35]**

K. Nyamuryekung'e, National AIDS Control Programme, Tanzania **[123]**

Gen Ohi, Department of Environmental and Community Medicine, Teikyo University School of Medicine, Tokyo 173, Japan **[251]**

Philista Onyango, Department of Sociology, University of Nairobi, Nairobi, Kenya **[301]**

Lawrence Osei, Department of Community Health, University of Ghana Medical School and Noguchi Memorial Institute for Medical Research, Legon, Accra, Ghana **[9]**

M. Over, World Bank, Washington, DC **[123]**

Maria Paalman, Dutch Foundation for STD Control, NL-3511 GE Utrecht, The Netherlands **[215]**

J. Riber, Development Through Self Reliance, Harare, Zimbabwe **[289]**

Lair Guerra de Macedo Rodrigues, National Division of Sexually Transmitted Diseases and AIDS, Ministry of Health, Brasilia DF, CEP 70058, Brazil **[229]**

Ann Rose, HelpAge International, London EC1R 0BE, United Kingdom **[171]**

Timothy S. Rothermel, Division of Global and Interregional Programmes, United Nations Development Programme, New York, NY 10017 **[161]**

S. Saracchini, Department of Medical Oncology, Centro di Riferimento Oncologico, 33081 Aviano (PN), Italy **[43]**

Inon Schenker, AIDS Project, School of Public Health and Community Medicine, Faculty of Medicine, Hebrew University, Jerusalem, Israel **[341]**

Anne A. Scitovsky, Health Economics Division, Palo Alto Medical Foundation/Research Institute, Palo Alto, CA and Institute for Health Policy Studies, School of Medicine, University of California, San Francisco, CA **[137]**

D.K. Sekimpi, Occupational Health and Hygiene Department, Ministry of Labour, Kampala, Uganda **[241]**

Richard M. Selik, The Centers for Disease Control, Public Health Service, U.S. Department of Health and Human Services, Atlanta, GA 30333 **[35]**

Pramilla Senanayake, International Planned Parenthood Federation, Regents College, London NW1 4NS, United Kingdom **[107]**

William J. Serow, Center for the Study of Population, Florida State University, Tallahassee, FL 32306-4063 **[175]**

D. Serraino, Epidemiology Unit, Centro di Riferimento Oncologico, 33081 Aviano (PN), Italy **[43]**

Gary Slutkin, Global Programme on AIDS, World Health Organization, CH-1211 Geneva 27, Switzerland **[21]**

David F. Sly, Center for the Study of Population, Florida State University, Tallahassee, FL 32306-4063 **[67]**

Gracelyn J. Smallwood, Townsville, Queensland 4812, Australia **[277]**

S. Smith, Development Through Self Reliance, Inc., Columbia, MD 21045 **[289]**

Kenji Soda, Department of Public Health, Yokohama City University School of Medicine, Yokohama 236, Japan **[251]**

E. Spicer, Edwina Spicer Productions (PVT) Ltd., Harare, Zimbabwe **[289]**

Jon Martin Sundet, Department of Epidemiology, National Institute of Public Health, 0365 Oslo 3, Norway **[53]**

D. Tarantola, Global Programme on AIDS, World Health Organization, CH-1211 Geneva 27, Switzerland **[207]**

Tebebe Yemane-Berhan, Division of Medicine, All Africa Leprosy and Rehabilitation Training Centre (ALERT), WHO Collaborating Centre for Training in Leprosy, Addis Ababa, Ethiopia **[17]**

Hiroaki Terao, Department of Environmental and Community Medicine, Teikyo University School of Medicine, Tokyo 173, Japan **[251]**

U. Tirelli, Department of Medical Oncology, Centro di Riferimento Oncologico, 33081 Aviano (PN), Italy **[43]**

Ken Tout, HelpAge International, London EC1R 0BE, United Kingdom **[171]**

E. Vaccher, Department of Medical Oncology, Centro di Riferimento Oncologico, 33081 Aviano (PN), Italy **[43]**

G. van Santen, Drug Department, Municipal Health Service Amsterdam, 1452 XS Amsterdam, The Netherlands **[369]**

A.D. Verster, Public Health Department, Municipal Health Service Amsterdam, 1000 HE Amsterdam, The Netherlands **[369]**

Pervin Walji, Department of Sociology, University of Nairobi, Nairobi, Kenya **[301]**

Norman L. Webb, Gallup International, London NW3 6BL, United Kingdom **[347]**

Ian V.D. Weller, Academic Department of Genito-Urinary Medicine, University College and Middlesex School of Medicine, London W1N 8AA, United Kingdom **[385]**

Arie J. Zuckerman, Department of Medical Microbiology and World Health Organization Collaborating Centre for Reference and Research on Viral Hepatitis, London School of Hygiene and Tropical Medicine (University of London), London WC1E 7HT, United Kingdom **[375]**

FOREWORD TO THE PROCEEDINGS

C E Gordon Smith, Dean of the London School of
Hygiene and Tropical Medicine

AIDS is predominantly a sexually transmitted disease which
is at present incurable and fatal. It therefore represents a major
challenge to medical research and formidable problems of medical
care. The epidemic is international and projections of its scale are
daunting. Every country needs to develop or improve its policies
and capacities for controlling the infection and caring for the
sick.

In addition, however, AIDS has social and economic
implications which extend to the very core of our communal and
personal lives, and these increasingly important aspects have been
relatively neglected, as compared with the scientific and medical.
The London School of Hygiene and Tropical Medicine recognised
the interdisciplinary approach required to deal with the social and
economic as well as the medical and scientific problems. Its wide-
ranging teaching and research encompasses communicable
diseases, epidemiology, social, behavioural and economic sciences,
community and international health. The School was thus in the
unique position to draw together experience and expertise from
around the world to address the problems posed by HIV infections .
and AIDS in both industrialized and developing countries.

This Conference provided a forum for discussion of the
nature and extent of these issues and to encourage the
identification and development of priorities and policies for the
future. Thereby the social and economic impact of AIDS globally
may be predicted, ameliorated and controlled.

This task could not have been undertaken without the
wholehearted support of the World Health Organization, as co-

sponsors of the Conference. Nor could it have been successful without the help of the Commonwealth Secretariat, the Department of Health and Social Security, the Health Education Authority, the London School of Economics and the Overseas Development Administration. Finally nothing could have been achieved without the participation of our speakers and chairmen, and most importantly, of the delegates from around the world.

PREFACE

More than has been the case with any other epidemic, the AIDS pandemic is fast becoming associated with a wide range of social, medical, economic, demographic and political issues, whose profundity and long-term implications call for urgent consideration and action. This volume, which covers the proceedings of the **First International Conference on the Global Impact of AIDS,** London, 8-10 March 1988, reflects the wide variety of problems and concerns that were covered by an international group of experts representing both governmental and non-governmental organizations. All oral presentations have been included with the exception of a few which the authors themselves did not wish to publish. Regrettably, it has not been possible to include the posters, nor to reflect the exciting and stimulating discussions that took place in response to and around these presentations.

In organizing the Conference, care was taken to ensure that as many different disciplines as possible would be involved. Thus, the contributions in this volume concern a broad spectrum of interrelated approaches ranging from the biomedical, epidemiological, clinical, social, behavioural, economic and demographic to the political and legal. The geographic representation in the papers reflects not only the international aspect of AIDS, but more importantly, the fact that just as the epidemiology of the problem varies from one culture to another, so will the needs and the responses also vary. If comprehensive control and prevention strategies are to be developed, they will have to take into account both the current socio-epidemiological patterns and those that may emerge as the pandemic continues.

Some societies are already experiencing an increase of morbidity and mortality associated with AIDS. In some communities, it is primarily affecting young single males; in others, it is affecting men and women alike, and more and more, having an impact on infants and children. Families are being made to bear demanding burdens of care for their sick, and at the same time are losing the earnings of their productive members. There is no doubt that the ways families are being affected could have ramifications for their organization, functioning and, possibly, structure.

The fact that AIDS affects people in their most intellectually, economically and biologically productive years has implications for society in general. Especially in resource-poor countries, the impact of the loss of young minds needs to be addressed. Similarly, the potential consequences for industry and agriculture of debilitation and death associated with AIDS cannot be overlooked in assessing how best the international community and nations can take up the challenge of AIDS.

Any discussion of AIDS must take into account the fact that during the short years since the disease was first identified, tremendous progress has been made. The virus was quickly isolated and described, as were the modes of transmission. It is evident today that AIDS is preventable; indeed, it may, in principle, be one of the diseases most amenable to prevention. Translating that knowledge into action, however, remains a vital challenge. Some strategies are already emerging. Public information and education are priorities for all countries. Condom-initiatives are being taken up in selected areas of the world and for specific high-risk communities; much needs to be done to ensure that this work is extended to cover all individuals who are at risk. Strengthening of blood transfusion systems, including the systematic screening of blood donations, is underway in most countries, both developed and developing. Programmes designed for drug-injectors are being assessed; needle-exchange schemes, "needle-washing" projects and outreach activities are being increasingly considered in various cities around the world.

Underlying all these activities is the fact that the social rights of all concerned have to be respected. AIDS is bringing to the forefront the importance of legal and ethical considerations in public health. If the rights of the individual are not respected, then the rights of the many are threatened.

The Conference on the Global Impact of AIDS reviewed all these and many other themes. The proceedings document the wealth of observations, anecdotal reports, scientific findings and administrative recommendations that have already emerged. Nevertheless, much remains to be done; more research is urgently required in a variety of areas; recommendations already available need to be implemented; scientific findings must be translated into policy alternatives. The tasks call for the interaction of many disciplines and for many approaches to AIDS-control and prevention. They call for new and innovative measures that will test the creativity of researchers and administrators alike. This volume should assist in identifying some of these issues, some of the ways of approaching them, and some of the ways in which existing knowledge and experience can be built upon.

Alan F. Fleming
Manuel Carballo
David W. FitzSimons
Michael R. Bailey
Jonathan Mann

ACKNOWLEDGEMENTS

The Global Impact of AIDS Conference was co-sponsored by the World Health Organization and the London School of Hygiene and Tropical Medicine. Additional support was provided by the Commonwealth Secretariat, the Department of Health and Social Security (UK), the Health Education Authority (UK), the London School of Economics and Political Sciences and the Overseas Development Administration (UK). Delegate administration and facility organization was by EMAP Maclaren Exhibitions Ltd.

Session chairmen and summarisers managed the oral presentations and focussed discussion from the floor. The contribution of these participants to the Conference is hereby gratefully acknowledged.

Session One: HIV and AIDS Today. Chairmen: Professor M. Alder, UK and Dr. R. Ancelle, France.

Session Two: Demography of the AIDS Pandemic. Chairmen: Professor W. Brass, UK, Professor V. Pokrovsky, USSR, Professor K. Thairu, UK and Dr J. Pape, Haiti. Summariser: Dr P. Piot, Belgium.

Session Three: Economic Impact. Chairmen: Professor I. Patel, UK, Dr M. Malliori, Greece, Dr J. Sepulveda-Amor, Mexico and Dr R. Andres Medina, Spain. Summariser: Ms R. Sabatier, UK.

Session Four: Social Impact of HIV and AIDS. Chairmen: Dr H. N'jie, The Gambia, Dr B. Gredler, Austria, Emeritus Professor J. La Fontaine, UK and Dr A. Johnson, UK. Summariser: Professor H. Glennerster.

Session Five: Epidemic Control and Individual Freedom. Chairmen: Hon Justice Kirby, Australia, Dr M. Paalman, The Netherlands, Dr C. Bartholomew, Trinidad and Mr. N. Partridge, UK. Summariser: Dr S. Hagard, UK.

Session Six: National and International Policy. Chairmen: Sir Donald Acheson, UK and Dr K. Tsiquaye, UK. Closing Remarks: Sir John Reid, UK and Hon. Justice Kirby, Australia.

The editors also acknowledge with gratitude the advice of the International Consultative Committee and of the Executive Committee.

International Consultative Committee

Professor B. Abel Smith	United Kingdom
Sir Donald Acheson	United Kingdom
Professor M. Alder	United Kingdom
Professor C. Bartholemew	Trinidad
Professor F. Deinhardt	Federal Republic of Germany
Dr W. Dowdle	United States of America
Dr S. Galbraith	United Kingdom
Dr R. Gallo	United States of America
Dr J. Gallwey	United Kingdom
Dr C. Gordon Smith	United Kingdom
Professor A. Glynn	United Kingdom
Dr S. Hagard	United Kingdom
Professor L. Kallings	Sweden
Dr C.E. Koop	United States of America
Dr J. Mann	World Health Organization
Professor L. Montagnier	France
Dr E. Njelesani	Zambia
Dr B. N'galy	Zaire
Dr H. N'jie	The Gambia
Dr A. Paintal	India
Dr J. Pape	Haiti
Dr A. Pinching	United Kingdom
Dr P. Piot	Belgium
Professor V. Pokrovsky	Un. of Soviet Socialist Republic
Sir John Reid	United Kingdom
Dr R. St John	World Health Organization
Dr J. Sepulveda-Amor	Mexico
Dr T. Nakayama	Japan
Professor K. Thairu	Commonwealth Secretariat
Mr A. Whitehead	United Kingdom

Executive Committee

Professor P. Hamilton **(Chairman)**	London School of Hygiene and Tropical Medicine

Mr M. Bailey (Executive Organiser)	London School of Hygiene and Tropical Medicine
Dr M. Carballo	World Health Organization
Mr D. FitzSimons	Bureau of Hygiene and Tropical Diseases, London
Dr A. Fleming	London School of Hygiene and Tropical Medicine
Professor H. Glennerster	London School of Economics
Mr M. Guy	London School of Hygiene and Tropical Medicine
Dr A. Johnson	Middlesex Hospital Medical School, London
Dr C. MacCormack	London School of Hygiene and Tropical Medicine
Professor K. McAdam	London School of Hygiene and Tropical Medicine
Dr J. Mann	World Health Organization
Dr P. Nunn	London School of Hygiene and Tropical Medicine
Dr R. Rothman	Department of Health and Social Security, London
Ms R. Sabatier	Panos Institute, London
Dr K. Tsiquaye	London School of Hygiene and Tropical Medicine
Professor A. Zuckerman	London School of Hygiene and Tropical Medicine

Executive Secretariat

Mrs J. Conyers	London School of Hygiene and Tropical Medicine
Miss J. Hawthorne	London School of Hygiene and Tropical Medicine

We also thank the following people for their hard work and support:-

EMAP Maclaren Exhibitions Ltd.

Mrs I. Hutchins
Miss J. Mott
Mrs A. Laker
Mr P. Blinkhorn

Global Programme on AIDS, World Health Organization

Dr R. Widdus
Mr T. Netter
Mr J. Bunn
Miss C. Greasley

We also wish to thank Mr John Garbrera of the Visual Aids Unit, London School of Hygiene and Tropical Medicine, for preparing the figures for publication, Mr Anthony Pettit of Interword, 102 Dean Street, London W1, for his most careful preparation of the text for printing and Ms Dianne Fishman of the Bureau of Hygiene and Tropical Diseases for her scrupulous proof-reading.

INTRODUCTION

Jonathan Mann, Director of the Global Programme on
AIDS, World Health Organization

It is humbling to realise that in the late 1970s the human
immunodeficiency virus was spreading silently - unrecognised and
unnoticed - around the world. By 1981, when AIDS was first
described, it was already one of the most significant public health
problems the world has ever confronted. The global response,
however, has been rapid. The global AIDS strategy was designed
and adopted, and during 1987 we saw an extraordinary and
unprecedented global mobilization of resources to prevent and
control HIV infection and AIDS.

During this period it has also become increasingly clear that
AIDS goes far beyond a matter of health statistics. It has major
social, economic and demographic implications for society.
Understanding them and learning how best to reduce the personal
and social impact of this disease constitutes a major challenge.

Fortunately, the world is much better equipped today than it
would have been fifty years ago to confront the AIDS epidemic.
Fifty years ago, we would not have been able to identify the
aetiological agent, develop diagnostic tests, and proceed so
rapidly towards a treatment and vaccine.

Fifty years ago, we would not have had the support of
sophisticated social and behavioural science, nor of economic
analysis, to permit a more detailed understanding of the epidemic
and its impacts. Finally, fifty years ago, the international
community could not have reacted as it has reacted during the
past two years. In an unprecedented manner, the world is linked in
a global struggle against a global problem.

There are reasons for hope, however, there is a great need to understand. We cannot yet speak as historians, with the lofty perspective that comes with the passage of time. We must try to understand, we must try to anticipate. We must use all the tools at our disposal to study what is happening, we can and should respond.

This meeting on "The Global Impact of AIDS" had historic importance. It was based on the effort to bring the researchers of many disciplines together to share what has thus far been learned. Let us draw strength from that common purpose.

GLOBAL IMPACT OF AIDS : OFFICIAL OPENING OF THE CONFERENCE

Anthony Newton, MP, HM Minister of Health

INTRODUCTION

I was very pleased to be invited to open this important international conference on the Global Impact of AIDS. I congratulate the London School of Hygiene and Tropical Medicine and the World Health Organization for jointly sponsoring the Conference, and I am pleased that my Department and the Overseas Development Administration have been able to make contributions towards its costs.

The timing of this Conference was particularly fortunate since it followed hard on the heels of the World Summit of Health Ministers on AIDS held here in London a few weeks ago.

The World Summit raised awareness of the problems posed by the disease throughout the world. 148 countries attended, over three-quarters being represented at Ministerial level. The Summit established a political consensus on the need for urgent national and international action on AIDS. This consensus was given concrete expression in the London Declaration, adopted at the Summit, which sets out a broad framework for AIDS prevention in which education and information are given the central emphasis.

The point I want to stress at this stage is that establishing a political consensus and setting a framework for prevention are of course only first steps. What is needed now is to build upon the increased awareness of the need for international cooperation and national action by turning statements of principle into specific policies and action throughout the world.

The theme of this Conference was the Global Impact of AIDS. A very great deal is encompassed in that short title and I would like to highlight two aspects. First, AIDS is indeed a global issue. The solution to it must be a global one involving a coordinated international effort. The World Health Organization has a central role to play in this. Its Global Programme on AIDS has done an impressive amount in a short space of time. The UK Government is giving its full support to this programme and we shall be providing £4.5 million to it in the coming year from the overseas aid programme.

Second, the enormous impact of AIDS. The Conference will be dealing with an impressive array of issues covering social, economic, legal and ethical aspects of the AIDS problem. In considering these subjects and in making proposals, I hope that the devastating impact of the spread of AIDS upon individuals will not be forgotten. When we contemplate the sobering figures of the numbers infected and the economic and social costs of the disease we may sometimes lose sight of the fact that each number in the column refers not just to a case or a point in a trend line, but to a person and a family; to the upheaval in their lives and the particular problems that they face.

AIDS provides a stern test not only of our science and technology but also of our compassion and of the fundamental value of our societies.

PUBLIC EDUCATION

The London Declaration acknowledged the vital role of information and education in the prevention of AIDS. In the UK we have adopted a step-by-step approach in our public education campaign. This has the aims first of raising levels of awareness and knowledge about the disease among the general population and then of persuading people, especially those most at risk, to take action to protect themselves and others.

Independent evaluation of the effectiveness of the first year of the campaign has shown that we have achieved considerable success in getting across to the general public basic facts about the disease and the ways of reducing the risks of infection. This progress is now being built on by the Health Education Authority which has taken over the running of the campaign. Last month the Authority launched the latest phase of the campaign, again aimed at the population as a whole, to sustain awareness of the continuing risks of HIV infection among the general public and to encourage them to adopt responsible attitudes to sexual behaviour.

Whether campaigns should be targetted at specific groups whose behaviour puts them at significant risk or whether they should be directed at the general population is, I am sure, a question that is being debated in many countries.

In the UK, although research has shown widespread public support for our campaign, the approach of targetting the general population has been criticised in some quarters for being both unnecessary and alarmist. It is certainly true that so far, unlike the position in some other countries, we are aware of relatively few cases of HIV infection acquired as a result of heterosexual activity. Nevertheless I believe it is right in the UK to warn the general public of the continuing risks.

The essence of prevention is to act before a disease reaches substantial proportions in a population. So far the spread of the infection in the general population in the UK is limited and we wish it to stay that way. But there is a real risk that this spread could increase, and given the lethal nature of the virus and the long incubation period of AIDS we cannot afford to wait and see what happens. Not to act now would be irresponsible. The only responsible course is to ensure that everyone is aware of the risks and knows how to avoid them.

I am not suggesting all countries should take precisely the same path as we have. Each country must decide what is the best way of informing its citizens about the risks of HIV infection taking into account its culture and traditions. But I am certain of one thing; in the UK we have no other choice than to explain the facts as we know them as frankly and as simply as possible, if we are to fight this terrible disease effectively.

I know some are concerned that by advocating the use of condoms to reduce the risk of HIV infection, we are encouraging promiscuity.

I do not believe this to be the case. What I do believe is that people in this country are now more aware of how AIDS is caused and of the measures needed to avoid or reduce the risk of contracting or transmitting it. This progress has only been possible through open discussion of facets of life which, for understandable reasons, are offensive to some. It means talking openly about matters such as the need to change sexual behaviour, about the dangers of injecting drugs, or about the importance of condoms in reducing the risk of spreading the AIDS virus.

MONITORING AND PREDICTIONS

It is axiomatic that if we are to plan the provision of services for all aspects of the care of people with HIV-related illness, we need reliable information on the numbers of people likely to need such services. It is also important to consider the longer-term impact of AIDS on societies and economies.

In order to ensure that we have the most effective systems for surveillance and monitoring the Government's Chief Medical Officer, Sir Donald Acheson set up an expert group under Dr Joe Smith, Director of our Public Health Laboratory Services, to advise on improvements to current arrangements. His group have now reported and have made a number of wide-ranging recommendations which we are considering carefully. We shall be publishing their report very shortly and seeking views on its proposals.

Turning to predictions of future numbers, the first question to ask is whether reliable predictions can be obtained? I am told that the mechanics of such forecasting at least in the short-term is not a problem. But predictions can be only as reliable as the information which is fed in. In the case of HIV infection, there are so many crucial pieces of biological and behavioural information which are missing or only partly understood that there will inevitably be major uncertainties surrounding any estimates which are produced.

This, however, is not an argument for not attempting to make estimates; it is merely an argument for producing and interpreting any predictions with caution, having regard to the precise assumptions that have been used in making them. Then as more facts accumulate, the predictions can be modified and planners can try to plan flexibly, knowing that they are planning within a given range of uncertainty.

Since predictions are so important, we asked Sir Donald Acheson to set up a second expert group to prepare the best possible predictions of the numbers of people with HIV infection and AIDS that we can expect in England and Wales. Obviously, the further ahead we seek to look into the future, the greater the uncertainty will be. For that reason the group will be looking at predictions only for the next two to five years.

I am very pleased to announce that Sir David Cox of Imperial College, one of the country's most eminent statisticians, has agreed to be the group's chairman. The group will begin its task within the next few weeks, and I am sure that the results of their work will be of immense value in helping us to ensure that service provision is as effective and efficient as possible.

Internationally, I know that much effort is being put into developing predictions of the demographic and economic implications of the spread of the infection. The UK Government, under the aid programme, has been pleased to be able to support Sir David's colleague, Professor Roy Anderson in taking forward elements of this work.

In my remarks I have touched on only a handful of questions out of the vast number to which AIDS gives rise. During this Conference you will be addressing many more. I doubt that you will achieve complete unanimity on how they should all be tackled, but, given both the complexity of the issues involved and the huge diversity of backgrounds and perspectives of those here, I am not certain that such unanimity would necessarily be desirable.

What I am sure of is that this Conference can do a great deal to clarify the issues and to crystallise the problems. By so doing it can play an influential part in ensuring that the crucial decisions that all countries face are based on considered advice and facts, not prejudice and assumption. In this way, to quote the closing words of the London Declaration, it will help to "begin now to slow the spread of HIV infection". It could not have a better purpose.

Part I: EPIDEMIOLOGY

The Global Impact of AIDS, pages 3-7
© 1988 Alan R. Liss, Inc.

1.   WORLDWIDE EPIDEMIOLOGY OF AIDS

J Mann

Director of the Global Programme on AIDS, World
Health Organization

This is the first meeting of its kind to address what we have
called the third epidemic. The third epidemic - that of response
and reaction, social, cultural, political and economic to the
pandemic of HIV infection and AIDS. Today, less than seven years
after AIDS was first recognised, fewer than five years after the
etiologic agent was discovered, we have an excellent grasp of the
modes of HIV transmission, a relatively good idea of the
worldwide epidemiology of HIV and we are beginning to develop
an integrated view of HIV dynamics as a function of individual,
social and biomedical determinants.

I will briefly review the principal elements of what we
know, starting with modes of HIV spread. Despite some things you
may have read recently, the modes of HIV spread have not
changed. Indeed, the modes of spread from the beginning of our
knowledge of this virus to now and all over the world have
remained the same. This virus is sexually transmitted, is
transmitted through direct contact with blood, and is transmitted
perinatally from mother to child. There is no evidence of spread
from toilet seats; there is no reason to think that those paper
covers that you can use to cover toilet seats will protect you
against AIDS. There is no evidence of spread through insects;
there is no evidence for casual contact spread; this message is a
message in which we should have confidence and which we should
repeat and repeat and repeat again.

As of the first of March 1988, there have been a total of
81,433 cases of AIDS officially reported to the World Health
Organization from 133 countries around the world. Forty-two of
these countries are in the Americas, 41 are in Africa, 27 are in

Europe, 23 are in Asia and Oceania. If we look at these reported cases, nearly three-quarters (74%) are from the Americas, 12% have been reported from Africa, 13% from Europe and the remaining 1% from Asia and Oceania. There are now 49 countries in the world that each report more than 50 cases of AIDS.

We all know that the number of AIDS cases reported is only part, in some cases a large proportion and in some cases a small proportion of the actual number of AIDS cases. The reasons for this are clear, as it is sometimes not possible to make a clinical or laboratory-confirmed diagnosis; in some countries the reporting infra-structure is weak; and in some countries, including industrialised countries, there may be reluctance on the part of certain health providers to report, or fatigue at reporting all AIDS cases. There is also at times political reluctance to report on the full scope of this disease because there remains in minds of some a stigma attached to having AIDS in the country. If we look at the worldwide picture of AIDS today, we can distinguish three basic patterns of HIV infection and AIDS; I would like to briefly describe them. The first pattern involves North America, Western Europe, Australia and New Zealand. In these areas, the sexual transmission of the virus is predominantly homosexual although heterosexual transmission has been, and is continuing to occur. In these areas, HIV transmission by blood transfusion is prevented because blood transfusions are screened, but bloodborne spread is still occurring through sharing of needles and syringes among persons with self-injecting behaviours. Finally in these areas of the world there is transmission from mother to child but fortunately, relatively few women are infected and therefore there are relatively fewer instances of transmission to children.

The second pattern includes a good deal of Africa, and parts of the Caribbean. In these areas the sexual transmission is heterosexual, although there is some homosexual transmission. In these areas, transmission by blood does not involve intravenous drug use but involves blood transfusions still not yet screened everywhere for HIV. Transmission by blood also involves the re-use of needles and syringes, for medical and other purposes, which have not been properly sterilized between each use. Finally, a relatively larger proportion of the infected people are women of child-bearing age and therefore there is a large and growing tragedy of HIV infection in newborns and children in these parts of the world.

In the third part of the world - Asia, the Middle East and North Africa - the virus appears to have arrived more recently, yet HIV infections are occurring and have occurred. Many of the early infections were associated with direct contact with other parts of the world, but there is increasing evidence of transmission within these countries. The virus is certainly present in Asia yet it has not yet taken full hold even in the major risk behaviour groups. In summary, the world is not, strictly speaking, uniform in terms of the current extent of AIDS and HIV infection yet the modes of spread are the same and the strategy is fundamentally the same throughout the world.

I would now like to raise some issues for your consideration at the beginning if this important Conference, the first conference that is addressing the Third epidemic - the social and cultural and political dimensions of this problem - which is as integral and great a part of the AIDS problems as the virus itself.

First I would like to reflect on a curious situation. The political, social and cultural dimensions of disease have always been with us. Think of the influenza pandemic of 1918-1919, of malaria today, of smallpox, of plague. Yet where are the studies of economic, social and political impact from these diseases? What was learned during those diseases, what knowledge became institutionalised from experiences like the Black Death or malaria? Where is the literature and art of malaria or diarrhoeal disease? It took a political philosopher, Albert Camus, to make of the disease plague a social and cultural metaphor accessible to us all and to write a book that has a tremendous amount of meaning for those working against AIDS.

I believe that we are actually now witnessing the birth of a new paradigm of health. I think that we are in the process of experiencing a change, a fundamental change, in the way we look at health, at illness, at life, at society. Like any paradigm that is emerging there is no clear break between the past and future but we are in the midst of this process and I would like to indicate to you some of the pieces that I feel we can recognize in this paradigm.

First, there is an unprecedented political commitment, as was expressed at the recent London Summit of Health Ministers. There has never before been the kind of political discussion and political commitment and political sensitivity to a disease globally as we are seeing with AIDS today. Actually, this is the first disease to meet four criteria for what might be called a new kind of global disease. The first criterion is that it is a global problem. Secondly, it is also thought of and understood and spoken

of as a global problem. Thirdly, it is known about worldwide. Last
week I was in China and we did a little survey in the streets of
Beijing. Ninety percent of the people who were interviewed had
heard of AIDS and about 90% of these correctly stated that sexual
transmission is the major mode of spread. This is a remarkable
phenomenon: you cannot go anywhere in the world and find people
who have not heard about, spoken about or seen something about
AIDS. Fourth and finally, AIDS is being combatted at a truly
global level. This is different from smallpox eradication. Smallpox
eradication was a programme to eradicate smallpox from the
developing world on behalf of the whole world. In contrast, AIDS
prevention and control is a struggle in which the industrialised
countries are as deeply engaged, as deeply committed and
threatened as the rest of the world. Thus, AIDS is a global
problem, it is thought of as global, it is known about to an
unprecedented extent around the world and it is being combatted
on a global level.

   Media and communications have played a fundamental,
perhaps **the** fundamental role. Indeed our world is different in that
regard from the world of the past. We are living in a world which
is dramatically different in terms of communication from the
world in which smallpox was eradicated. I think that we
underestimate this too frequently or perhaps we trivialise it.
People's consciousness and awareness, their understanding and
their information are absolutely vital to the world view they hold
and which they project in their societies. I think we must return
to the time of Europe when the Americas were first discovered,
when John Donne referred to that "new found land" to capture the
excitement that a change in worldview can bring. Our view is
irrevocably global and we are linked in a global network, an
increasingly global society.

   Another component of this new paradigm is that we
recognise that walls don't work. I had the privilege the other day
of being at the Great Wall of China and asked my Chinese
colleagues : "Did it work - that Wall?" The answer was that walls
do not protect and our world is finally coming to terms with that
fact. Thus, the Chinese Ministry of Health stated that AIDS
cannot be stopped at the borders of China or any country. The
costs of isolation that are implied by a wall are too high.
Geography cannot protect; we are all in a world in which walls
represent a danger of isolation, not a source of protection.

   There is also in this paradigm a unique linkage between
human rights and health. Isolation and exclusion of the individual,

the group, the national or international level creates a danger both for the person or group that is excluded and for the rest of us. We know that in AIDS, we must not divide the world into "them" and "us"; we must include those who are infected with us. Again, in China, the Government explicitly stated that Chinese who are infected will be kept within society, kept at their job, at their work and that their identity will be protected and kept confidential.

I think we need an international human rights network to monitor discrimination and human rights issues related to this health issue - AIDS.

This is needed because discrimination in any part of the world threatens us all. It threatens those who live in an area where discrimination is allowed to occur and it threatens others living in other parts of the world because it opens the door to that kind of discrimination there as well. We have to be linked not just in fighting a disease but in protecting the human rights that are important, not only in themselves, but because the violation of human rights in the fight against AIDS would be itself a danger to public health. We must protect human rights because we want to effectively control AIDS as well as protecting rights for their own sake; thus as a world community we need to know when and where and how discrimination occurs - we need to be alerted to it and we need to fight it collectively.

Ladies and Gentlemen, we are participants and we are also witnesses. We have the duty of witnesses during this AIDS epidemic to report, to testify, to be present and to record. We are also the participants and the creators. You are going to hear during this Conference about the data many have collected, the studies underway, and the contribution being made to our deepening knowledge of AIDS. In this epidemic, as never before, we must study, we must learn, we must explore the meaning of health.

And therefore, although we live in a world that is threatened by unlimited destructive forces, we have become, unwittingly perhaps, architects through our engagement in AIDS, in the building of a new vision, a personal vision, a national vision, a global vision. I believe you know and I hope you feel, that in the way that we fight against AIDS, we fight for health and for life itself, together on this planet - a new view, a new paradigm - the discovery of what we can do in our "new found land".

The Global Impact of AIDS, pages 9-15
© 1988 Alan R. Liss, Inc.

2.   DYNAMICS OF HUMAN IMMUNE DEFICIENCY VIRUS
      (HIV) EPIDEMIC - THE GHANAIAN EXPERIENCE

A R Neequaye[1], L Osei[2], J AA Mingle[1,2], G Ankra-
Badu[1], C Bentsi[3], A Asamoah-Adu[3], J E
Neequaye[4,1].

University of Ghana Medical School, Accra.[1]
Noguchi Memorial Institute for Medical Research,
Legon, Accra.[2] Ministry of Health, Public Health
Laboratories, Accra.[3] Burkitt's Tumor Project,
University of Ghana Medical School, Accra[4]

INTRODUCTION

      Acquired Immune Deficiency Syndrome (AIDS) was
described for the first time in Africans not long after its
description in the United States of America in 1981 (Clumeck et
al, 1984). Since then the disease has been described in Central
Africa, East Africa (Piot et al, 1984) and other African countries
(Neequaye et al, 1987, Denis et al, 1987). Many of these countries
have identified people at high risk of infection with the HIV.
Homosexuality and intravenous drug abuse are important risk
factors in America and other developed countries, whereas
heterosexual spread and spread by prostitution are more
important risk factors in many African countries. Needless to say,
effective control measures in any community must take
cognisance of factors which place people in that community at
high risk of HIV infection.

      This study takes a look at the causal factors that have
characterised HIV infection since its first discovery in Ghana in
March 1986.

MATERIALS AND METHODS

      In October 1985, the Government of Ghana in response to
global concern for this disease established a National Technical
Committee on AIDS (NTCA) to advise it on all matters relating to
the spread and control of AIDS in Ghana. In November 1985, the

Noguchi Memorial Institute for Medical Research in collaboration with Tokyo University, established a retroviral serological testing centre at Legon. Other testing centres have since been established in the four regional hospitals, namely Korle-Bu, Kumasi, Tamale and Sekondi-Takoradi to minimise spread of infection through blood transfusion. Laboratory technicians have also been trained to man 15 of the 48 transfusion centres in the country for visual reading of the Wellcozyme ELISA testing of donated blood.

Soon after its foundation, the NTCA produced and circulated educational materials including the World Health Organization (WHO) clinical case definition on AIDS to all doctors in Ghana, who were requested to send serum samples and relevant data on all patients who satisfied the WHO case definition for AIDS. In addition serum samples were obtained from a section of the general population including blood donors, prostitutes, patients attending a clinic for sexually transmitted diseases (STD). Sexual contacts of HIV sero-positive individuals were also screened. Since the first few positive cases we saw gave a history of stay in neighbouring countries, particularly Côte d'Ivoire, hospitalised patients with such history were screened automatically.

HIV antibody testing was by ELISA (Wellcozyme) and confirmation by Indirect Immunofluorescent Antibody Testing and Western Blot.

RESULTS

As at 31st December 1987, there were 276 sero-positive cases in Ghana. These were made up of 242 females and 32 males. They were identified from various groups as indicated by Table 1.

Regional Distribution of HIV Infection

Sero-positive people had been recorded from eight of the ten regions in Ghana by 31st December 1987. The regions with none recorded were the Northern and Upper West Regions.

52% of the cases came from the Eastern region alone, followed by Greater Accra Region and the Ashanti Region. These three Regions contributed more than 80% of the total cases. It is of interest to note that the cases from the Eastern Region came from a small area at the south eastern corner. Females greatly outnumbered the males, except for the Western Region where equal numbers were recorded for both sexes. The Western Region is adjacent to the Côte d'Ivoire border.

TABLE 1.   Groups that were Screened

Groups of People	No. Screened	No. Positive	% Positive
1. Blood donors	5480	6	0.11
2. Local prostitutes	236	5	2.12
3. Female prostitutes returning from Côte d'Ivoire with disease	335	199	59.40
4. Patients with sexually transmitted diseases	107	5	4.67
5. Infants from HIV positive mothers	7	7	100.0
6. Healthy people seeking certificate for travel	300	2	0.67
7. Other Ghanaians with history of stay in neighbouring countries including Senegal, Nigeria, Togo and Burkina Faso	215	33	15.35
8. Patients reporting at the hospitals	214	20	9.35

**TABLE 2.   Regional Distribution of HIV Infection in Ghana
March 1986 - December 1987**

Region	Male	Female	Total	%
Western	4	4	8	2.9
Central	-	6	6	2.2
Greater Accra	16	46	62	22.5
Eastern	6	139	145	52.5
Volta	1	7	8	2.9
Ashanti	1	22	23	8.3
Brong Ahafo	4	11	15	5.4
Northern	-	-	-	-
Upper East	-	1	1	0.4
Upper West	-	-	-	-
Not stated	-	8	8	2.9
Total	32	244	276	100.0

Age and Sex Distribution of HIV Infection

70% of our cases were found in the sexually active age
group of 20 - 40 years, with the peak incidence being in the 25 to
29 age group. Seven cases were found in the under 1 year age
group, having contracted the infection from their HIV positive
mothers.

No cases have been recorded in the 60 years and above age
group.

TABLE 3.   Age and Sex Distribution of HIV Infection in Ghana
March 1986 - December 1987

Age Group	Male	Female	Total	%
Under 1	3	4	7	2.5
1 - 4	-	-	-	-
5 - 9	1	-	1	0.4
10 - 14	1	-	1	0.4
15 - 19	-	15	15	5.4
20 - 24	-	57	57	20.7
25 - 29	8	54	62	22.5
30 - 34	6	44	50	18.1
35 - 39	1	23	24	8.7
40 - 44	3	9	12	4.3
45 - 49	2	7	9	3.3
50 - 54	-	3	3	1.1
55 - 59	-	2	2	0.7
60+	-	-	-	-
Not stated	7	26	33	12.0
Total	32	244	276	100.0

DISCUSSION

During the economic crisis of Ghana in the late seventies and early eighties, many Ghanaians both professional and unskilled left the country to make a living elsewhere. Most of the professionals went to places like Saudi Arabia, the United States of America and Europe. The unskilled, however, were more likely to go to the neighbouring West African countries such as Côte d'Ivoire, Burkina Faso and Togo. Some travelled as far as Senegal, Liberia and Nigeria. To give an idea of the numbers involved in this migration, over a million Ghanaians living in Nigeria were repatriated in 1984. During this period of exodus to neighbouring countries a lot of young Ghanaian women found their way to Côte d'Ivoire. Some went by their own efforts but others were actively recruited by older Ghanaian women who had been resident for some time in Côte d'Ivoire. Many went without knowing what work they would do, and finding no other means of support resorted to prostitution. This earned them valuable foreign exchange. When they visited Ghana on festive occasions such as Easter and Christmas, they were usually well dressed and their apparent wellbeing persuaded their friends to join them in their "good life" in Côte d'Ivoire. Most of them were from the Eastern Region of Ghana, a region which has traditional trade links with Côte d'Ivoire. The local women call it "going to French". In one small Eastern Region Hospital alone, by December 1987, 50 HIV positives, mostly AIDS cases, had been identified. Forty-five of these had a history of travel to Côte d'Ivoire and the rest to other neighbouring countries. The reasons they gave for travelling were diverse. Some went to trade, others were lured into working in "Chop bars" and some admitted going to earn money through prostitution. In the course of time, some of these young girls became sick. They could no longer work to support themselves. They are returning home in search of treatment which is expensive in Côte d'Ivoire. It is these young women who are returning with the disease. This explains why most of the cases are females from the Eastern Region.

The majority of patients returning from Côte d'Ivoire have AIDS or AIDS Related Complex. In 1986, female/male ratio was high, 11 : 1. By December 1987, however, the ratio had fallen to 7.6 : 1. The reason for the fall, we believe, is due to Ghanaians in Ghana becoming infected and beginning to spread the disease locally. These are mostly asymptomatic. Thus, we expect in time that the sex ratio will approximate unity and we anticipate a second wave of local AIDS cases in 2 - 3 years.

Some of the asymptomatic sero-positives who have no personal history of travel have had sexual links with prostitutes in neighbouring countries who returned home on festive occasions and a few with prostitutes working locally. In Accra, a total of 5,480 blood donors have been screened between June 1986 and

December 1987 and six were HIV positive. These were not pre-selected for risk behaviour. Out of 300 healthy Ghanaians wishing to travel abroad to countries needing AIDS clearance certificate, such as the United States of America, Saudi Arabia, Egypt, Germany, etc, 2 were positive, giving a seroprevalence rate of 0.67 per cent.

CONCLUSION

In Ghana the first wave of HIV sero-positives has been in female prostitutes who had worked in neighbouring West African countries, in particular Côte d'Ivoire. Initially, the female/male ratio was 11 : 1. However, a trend towards a lower ratio is being observed as the infection spreads from these women into the local population. As in the East African countries, prostitution is likely to be a major factor in the transmission of the disease.

REFERENCES

Clumeck N, Mascart-Lemone F, De Maubeuge J et al (1984). Acquired immune deficiency syndrome in black Africans. Lancet 1: 642

Denis F, Barin F, Gershy-Damet T et al (1987). Human T-lymphotrophic virus type III (HIV) and type IV in Ivory Coast. Lancet 1: 408-411

Neequaye A R, Ankra-Badu G A, Affram RK (1987). Clinical Features of HIV infection in Accra Ghana. Ghana Medical Journal 23: 3-6

Piot P, Quinn T C, Tachman H et al (1984). Acquired immunedeficiency syndrome in a heterosexual population in Zaire. Lancet 2: 65-69.

The Global Impact of AIDS, pages 17–20
© 1988 Alan R. Liss, Inc.

3.   HIV INFECTION IN DEVELOPING COUNTRIES :
EMERGING CLINICAL PICTURES IN AFRICA

Tebebe Yemane-Berhan

All Africa Leprosy and Rehabilitation Training
Centre (ALERT), affiliated with the Armauer Hansen
Research Institute (AHRI), WHO Collaborating
Centre for Training in Leprosy, PO Box 165, Addis
Ababa, Ethiopia.

It is indeed a difficult task to speak and discuss about this
important subject: the emerging clinical spectrum associated with
HIV infection in Africa. This difficulty is partly explained by the
complex relationship between the existing endemic infectious
diseases in Africa and the newly recognized HIV infection. Many
endemic diseases in Africa are known to activate HIV replication
and/or to immunosuppress infected individuals. As an indirect
effect of this, there may be an increased susceptibility to HIV
infection in exposed individuals.

The microbial infections may serve as co-factors of HIV
infection by increasing HIV viral replication and expression or by
modulation of the host immune system. On the other hand the
immune deficiency caused by HIV infection may contribute to a
particular pattern for the clinical manifestations of the existing
endemic infectious diseases. So when discussing the clinical
manifestations associated with HIV infection in Africa one may be
tempted to summarize it as something like a magnification of the
prevalent infectious diseases with violent and fatal progression.

The difficulty in making clinical diagnosis to HIV infection
is one of the major problems in determining the prevalence of
AIDS in Africa. The revised WHO case definition of AIDS at
Bangui, Central Africa, has been shown to be specific (89-93%)
and quite sensitive (55-60%) in adults (Colebunders et al., 1987;
Berkley, 1988). Hence one has to look carefully into the pattern
of clinical pictures observed on African AIDS patients.

My presentation will be limited to a few clinical

manifestations that I think are showing the emerging spectrum of HIV infection in Africa, particularly in adults.

STDs constitute a major medical and social problem in African countries. The rate of gonorrhoea per 100,000 population in Kampala is 10,000, in Nairobi 7,000 and in Addis Ababa 8,000 (Attili et al., 1983; Tebebe et al., 1987).

In Africa where heterosexual transmission of HIV infection is predominant, 40-60% of the population is in the most sexually active age group.

Cumulative cases of AIDS and ARC are attributed to the heterosexual transmission of HIV. This heterosexual transmission is further amplified by the high prevalence of sexually transmitted diseases. Several observations indicate that males having STDs are significantly associated with HIV infection particularly if it is acquired from a prostitute.

The clinician having a role to play in the prevention and control of any disease has to be aware more than ever of the different consequences resulting from a diagnosis of STD, especially when open genital lesions are present. Here the golden rule of STD, contact tracing, becomes highly important. In cases where repeated gonorrhoea and chancroid have been contracted from prostitutes, 18% of the male clients are seropositive for HIV (Harmann, 1988).

Now, I would like to mention one general symptom which may be called generalized body weakness. This well known syndrome was considered among the minor symptoms, but it is constantly observed in AIDS patients that it can be qualified as a clinical spectrum emerging to the front line. This constantly observed clinical manifestation has even been proposed as one of the major symptoms in the clinical case definitions of AIDS in Africa (Pallaugy et al., 1987).

This clinical spectrum may be defined as an extreme lassitude disabling the patients to perform routine acts of the daily life.

This syndrome of weakness is not explained by any of the different associated clinical manifestations, not even explained by weight loss observed in these patients. What is also surprising is that this weakness may be associated with our other minor symptoms (dermatological manifestations, oral candidiasis etc...).

One minor sign which has drawn our attention is the symptom of dry unproductive and persistent cough without any correlation with the chest x-ray findings. This has been observed in more than 80 percent of the cases from Ethiopia and Uganda.

We have also observed dementia as a primary manifestation of HIV infection. It is well known that neuropsychiatric manifestations have been commonly reported in AIDS patients.

The particularity I would like to stress is more relevant to patients presenting with psychiatric disorders as a first manifestation resulting from infections with HIV. These are patients treated primarily in psychiatric institutions and then manifesting disseminated tuberculosis. Based on this manifestation, the clinician may suspect the possibility of tuberculosis meningitis in a background of disseminated tuberculosis retrospectively. In spite of anti-tuberculous treatment death follows. With autopsy the diagnosis of disseminated tuberculosis is confirmed, but no sign of tuberculous meningitis is found. Histological examination of the brain tissue revealed lesions of viral encephalitis (Negesse, 1987).

Diffuse aggressive form of Kaposi's sarcoma is a well known manifestations associated with HIV infection. The only remark I would like to make is the appearance of Kaposi's sarcoma in children in a few parts of Africa, especially in Zambia (Rolfe & Wels, 1987).

Another new picture we are observing in Africa is acne. Patients at the age of 35 and over who never had acne before, come to clinics with full blown acne and no other signs or symptoms. These patients have been shown to develop AIDS 6-8 months after the acne (Masawe, 1988).

Previously, there have been rare incidences of psoriasis in West Africa. However, recent experiences showed that psoriasis cases which are related to HIV infection are growing steadily (Obasi, 1987).

Among the emerging dermatological manifestations related to HIV infections, exanthemata with macular and maculopapular exanthemata and vesicular or vesiculopapular exanthemata are more frequently seen in some parts of Africa.

One of the major diseases that had shown a tremendous come back with the AIDS epidemic both in the developing and the developed world is TB. Of the first few reported cases of AIDS from Ethiopia, more than 30 per cent had pulmonary TB. Serosurveys among TB patients in Kinshasa, Zaire and Uganda showed 30-40 per cent seropositivity to HIV (Mann et al., 1986; Berkely, 1988). Glandular TB, scrofuloderma, which is commonly seen in children is now being observed in adults. There is an increased trend in the frequency of TB meningitis as well.

Finally, in relation to the various clinical pictures that are emerging in Africa, and the role of important factors such as tropical diseases, malnutrition and lack of resources, we are left without an answer for what we see in Africa today as far as HIV infection is concerned. This, therefore, is as good a time as any to look back, and analyze the existing situation in order to come up with a better clinical case definition for HIV infection in Africa.

REFERENCES

Attili V R et al (1983). Med J Zambia. 19-21.

Berkley S. Report on Ugandan AIDS cases. Salzburg seminar (Austria) Feb. 1988.

Colebunders R, Francis H, Izaley N et al (1987). Evaluation of a clinical case definition of acquired immuno deficiency syndrome in Africa. Lancet i: 492-494.

Harmann O R M. Paper presented at the 4th Pan-African Congress of Dermatology (PAFCODERMA) Accra, Feb. 1988.

Mann J M et al (1986). JAMA 256: 346.

Masawe A E J. Personal Communication, Feb.1988.

Negesse Y. Personal Communication, 1987.

Obasi O E. Personal Communication, 1987.

Pallangyo K L, Mbanga U M, Mugusi F et al (1987). Clinical case definition of AIDS in African adults. Lancet ii: 972.

Rolfe M, Wels H G (1987). Kaposi's sarcoma in Zambian children. AIDS 1: 259-260.

Tebebe Y B, Yalem A, Abera G et al. A study in the treatment of male acute uncomplicated gonorrhoea Norfloxacin 800mg. and Trimethoprim 160mg. + Sulphamethoxazole 800mg. , 5th African Regional Conference on Sexually Transmitted Diseases, Harare, Zimbabwe, June 1987, Abstracts, p. 46.

The Global Impact of AIDS, pages 21-25
© 1988 Alan R. Liss, Inc.

4. THE EFFECTS OF THE AIDS EPIDEMIC ON THE
    TUBERCULOSIS PROBLEM AND TUBERCULOSIS
    PROGRAMMES

Gary Slutkin, J Leowski, J Mann

Global Programme on AIDS, and Tuberculosis Unit,
World Health Organization.

Immunosuppression has been long known to worsen the
course of tuberculous infection. Persons with malignancy or who
use immunosuppressive drugs have an increased rate of
tuberculosis. Now there is evidence for an increased rate of
progression from asymptomatic to overt tuberculosis for persons
co-infected with HIV. The result may be an increased number of
cases of tuberculosis in the coming years in some regions of the
world.

This report discusses the effects of the HIV/AIDS epidemic
on the tuberculosis problem and will also point to other effects of
the AIDS epidemic on tuberculosis control programmes. Sources
of data for this report include information contributed by the
International Union Against Tuberculosis (IUAT), the Tuberculosis
Surveillance Research Unit, the U.S. Centers for Disease Control,
the New York City Health Department, and other national and
international sources.

THE CURRENT TUBERCULOSIS SITUATION

The most recent estimates of the World Health Organization
and the IUATLD are that 8 to 10 million new cases of tuberculosis
occur annually and that there are approximately 3 million deaths.
Several countries have case rates of 100 to 300 per 100,000. In
several countries five to 15% of all deaths are reported as due to
tuberculosis. In many developing countries, rates of tuberculosis
infection seem to be declining, but by only 1 to 3% per year, and
in some, rates may not be declining. In several countries, rates of
population increase outweigh the tuberculosis rate declines and
the patient-load remains constant.

Persons and Groups with M. tuberculosis Infection - with Co-infection of HIV

For the purpose of this discussion, it should be useful to view tuberculosis as rising from a pool of persons previously infected with the organism M. tuberculosis, some of whom are also co-infected with HIV. It then becomes relevant to consider first the prevalence of infection with M. tuberculosis.

Most data today on tuberculosis infection are derived from skin test surveys in children. Most of the studies done in sub-Saharan Africa and Southeast Asia show annual rates of infection of 1 to 3% a year, a prevalence of infection of 10-30% for 10 year olds, leading to estimates of at least 30 to 60%, for adults. Recent skin test results for Latin America born adults tested in San Francisco have found 50 to 90% of adults with tuberculosis infection. The same range has been found for Southeast Asian adults tested in the same situation.

Evidence for an Increased Risk of Tuberculosis among Persons Co-infected with HIV

Some evidence for an increased risk of tuberculosis among persons co-infected with HIV comes from a study performed by the New York City Health Department. In this study, the HIV antibody status of 519 intravenous drug users had been known from testing performed at a methadone clinic. The names of the HIV infected and non-infected persons were matched to the tuberculosis registry of New York.

Twelve of 279 intravenous drug users who were HIV-infected developed tuberculosis, as compared to 0/240 in the HIV non-infected group (p less than .001; lower bound 95% confidence intervals of odds ratio 3.1). It is not possible to calculate the risk of tuberculosis from this study method and longitudinal studies are needed.

Further evidence for an increased risk of tuberculosis for dually infected persons comes from the finding of high rates of HIV infection among tuberculosis patients in several countries. As should be expected, this has been found in those areas of the world where infection with both organisms are prevalent. Rates of HIV seropositivity in tuberculosis patients are 3 to more than 20 times the rates found in the general population in these countries. In Zaire, tuberculosis patients had 7 times the prevalence of a control group matched for age, sex and residence. These findings are best explained by an increased rate of tuberculosis among persons co-infected with HIV, in other words, with over-representation of this group. Alternative explanations, i.e. of enhanced transmission by sexual practices or needles among those patient groups, are not tenable, in particular in all of the locations where this has been found.

Possible Effects on Populations

If immunosuppression from HIV were to have an effect on populations, we would expect to see this effect also in those regions of the world or in those population sub-groups where both infections are common, including the inner cities of the U.S. and Central and Eastern Africa.

The numbers of reported tuberculosis cases in the United States from 1953 to 1986 show that until 1984, there had been a relatively constant rate of decline of about 5% a year. Flattening of the curve is seen in 1985 and then an increase in 1986. From 1984 to 1985 there was a decrease of only 0.2% (or 54 cases) nationwide. 1986 was the first year in which there was a substantial increase in indigenous tuberculosis morbidity since uniform national reporting had begun. It is worth noting that the excess in cases was greatest in the 25-44 year age group, and that there was no increase in young children, suggesting increased endogenous reactivation rather than increased transmission.

The largest increase in the U.S. occurred in New York City, although increased numbers were reported in 25 states and Washington D.C. (New York has approximately 1/6th of the world's currently reported AIDS cases and a middle range tuberculosis problem among American cities. The HIV prevalence rate of infection in IV drug users in New York City is 40-60% in some groups.) The number of reported cases of tuberculosis in New York increased from 1981 to 1986 by just over 50% in this time period. Matching of tuberculosis and methadone registries showed that an increasing number of tuberculosis cases as IV drug users, the group with the majority of HIV related disease in New York.

For Africa we were able to find two tuberculosis surveillance systems which had sufficient information, from Tanzania and Burundi; however, caution is necessary in the interpretation of these data. The Tanzanian reporting system became national in 1979, and complete by 1982. This was followed by a flattening of the curve suggesting a new relatively constant rate of reporting. Although we see an increase since 1983, it is still too early to blame HIV, because improved treatment with short course chemotherapy was introduced at the same time. This has a known effect of attracting cases. An improved utilization of the health services is also believed to be an important factor accounting for some of the increase in case numbers seen in Burundi.

Although there are complicating factors, these trends require our attention. The effect of tuberculosis in Africa could be large because many persons also have asymptomatic tuberculous infection.

The Effect of HIV/AIDS on Tuberculosis Programmes

Besides the **possible effect** of increasing the number of tuberculosis patients to which a programme must provide service, there are important qualitative changes for tuberculosis control in the HIV/AIDS era. New problems include concern about this new population of HIV co-infected persons, and reports about possible altered safety or efficacy of the basic tuberculosis control practices.

Concerns of Tuberculosis Programs and Workers for TB Patients who are or may be Co-infected with HIV include that of Health Worker Safety

Tuberculosis workers must now face the challenge of additional concern for their own safety, a concern for all health workers in HIV infected areas; however, tuberculosis workers in many locations will be caring for more HIV infected persons than most clinics. Needles are used in this setting for tuberculin skin testing and for streptomycin treatment injections and we have seen that there are many HIV infected TB patients.

Questions arise as to if and when TB programmes should do HIV testing. The value of such programmes is not yet clear. Heightened concerns are seen for confidentiality and counselling. And tuberculosis programmes have new questions as to the need for follow-up, referral, and contact tracing for one or both diseases.

Concern About Possible Altered Safety or Efficacy of Current Anti-TB Practices

The available anti-tuberculosis strategies and tools, although limited, have become firmly established. Now there are occasional reports that question whether HIV infected persons respond differently, or require modifications of existing guidelines in use. For example, HIV positive persons are frequently anergic on tuberculin skin testing. More importantly, the clinical and radiographic picture of tuberculosis is different, with more persons having non-pulmonary and serious presentations. There are reports of relapses using conventional anti-TB therapy and the U.S. CDC has different recommendations for treatment of HIV co-infected persons.

There have also been a few case reports of local and possible disseminated reactions to BCG which have led to a modification in the WHO/EPI recommendation to exclude its use in symptomatic HIV infected children. Lastly, but most importantly, regarding the use of these tools, it is now **absolutely necessary** that equipment used for streptomycin injections be properly sterilized if streptomycin is to be included in the regimen.

SUMMARY

There is now evidence for an increased rate of progression from asymptomatic to overt tuberculosis for persons co-infected with HIV. There are early trends suggesting an increased number of cases in some regions where both infections are common. Tuberculosis programmes at all levels have other new challenges as well as numbers. **Research, guidelines, advocacy and support are needed.** Our immediate needs are for **improved surveillance** and focused research to **better define the magnitude of the problem** and to forecast future impact. Improved surveillance is needed, in particular for infection by both HIV and *M. tuberculosis.* A serologic marker for tuberculous infection would help this work greatly.

This is an extremely fertile area for research as dozens of new research questions are raised. The key will be to perform studies which are sufficiently focused to provide the most needed answers as soon as possible. One key need is properly designed and coordinated longitudinal studies to determine the true rate of tuberculosis (and AIDS) among dually infected persons, and to serve as a background for possible intervention studies. Studies on infectivity, clinical patterns, results of treatment, adverse drug reactions and the value of chemoprophylaxis are also needed.

The World Health Organization is actively developing a plan for prioritizing, coordinating and facilitating control and research in this area.

The Global Impact of AIDS, pages 27-33

5.   THE EPIDEMIOLOGY OF AIDS IN THE CARIBBEAN AND
     ACTION TO DATE

C J Hospedales, S Mahabir

Caribbean Epidemiology Centre (CAREC), P O Box
164, Port of Spain, Trinidad

INTRODUCTION

     The Caribbean Epidemiology Centre (CAREC) has been the
surveillance centre for communicable diseases in the Caribbean
since 1975. It has 19 member countries* which vary in population
from 7.5 thousand to 2.4 million, with a total population of 6.4
million. In addition, regular reports are received on the
occurrence of communicable disease from most other countries in
the region.

     This report is based on cases of AIDS meeting the
WHO/CDC definition reported to CAREC by the national
epidemiologists of the 19 member countries. Early cases were
reported to CAREC in a non-standardised fashion but late in 1985,
a special system of quarterly surveillance was introduced by the
Pan American Health Organisation, which all the countries now
use and which permits better analyses of the situation. To
complement this, more timely surveillance of cumulative cases
and deaths is maintained by telephone, telex and whenever
CAREC's staff visit countries or vice versa.

AIDS STATUS

     The first case of AIDS was reported from Trinidad and

---

*   Anguilla, Turks & Caicos Islands, Virgin Islands (UK),
     Monserrat, Cayman Islands, St. Christopher/Nevis, Bermuda,
     Dominica, Antigua, St. Vincent, Grenada, Saint Lucia,
     Belize, Bahamas, Barbados, Suriname, Guyana, Trinidad &
     Tobago and Jamaica.

Tobago in 1983. By 31st December 1987, 652 cases of AIDS were reported to CAREC with a 63% mortality rate. Seventeen of the 19 member countries have reported at least one case, though five countries (Bermuda, Bahamas, Jamaica, Barbados and Trinidad and Tobago) account for the vast majority of reported cases (Table 1). The cumulative prevalence rate for all the countries was 10.2 per 100,000 population. Six countries have similar or greater rates than the United States, while most countries had a rate greater than the United Kingdom.

TABLE 1. Cumulative AIDS Cases for 19 CAREC Member Countries Ranked by Rate Order

Country	Mid 1987 Population (000s)	Cumulative Cases (31.12.87)	Rate per 100,000 Population
Bermuda	59.4	71	120
Bahamas	235	176	75
Turks & Caicos Is.	8.5	5	59
Anguilla	7.5	2	27
Barbados	256	52	20
Trinidad & Tobago	1230	231	19
Cayman Islands	20.1	3	15
St Vincent	109	9	8
Grenada	117	8	7
Saint Lucia	140	10	7
Dominica	80.2	5	6
Antigua	82.4	3	4
St Christopher/Nevis	52.1	1	2
Belize	166	4	2
Surinam	385	9	2
Jamaica	2400	49	2
Guyana	988	14	1
Virgin Islands (UK)	13.6	0	0
Montserrat	13.6	0	0
All Countries	6363.4	652	10.2

UK Rate/100,000 = 2.2
US Rate/100,000 = 20.7

Beginning in 1983, there has been an exponential increase in the number of cases reported, with a doubling time in one year (Fig. 1). If this continues, there are likely to be some 5,000 cumulative reported cases by the end of the decade. Table 2 shows the distribution of cumulative cases by age and sex for the 375 (56%) of cases that can be classified. 72% of cases were 15-44 years old. Nine percent of cases were under 5 years old, reflecting increasing mother-to-child transmission. The male/female ratio was 3 : 1.

TABLE 2.   Cumulative AIDS Cases by Age and Sex

Age	Male	Female	Total	(%)
-1	13	8	21	(5.6)
1-4	7	5	12	(3.2)
5-14	2	1	3	(0.8)
15-24	35	16	51	(13.6)
25-34	110	41	151	(40.3)
35-44	58	11	69	(18.4)
45-54	42	9	51	(13.6)
55+	13	4	17	(4.5)
TOTAL	280	95	375	(100)

Male : Female Ratio = 3 : 1

39% occurred among homosexual/bisexual men. 51% occurred among heterosexuals (Table 3). This is in contrast to North America and Europe, where the majority of cases have been among homosexual or bisexual males. Several reasons exist for the low proportion of cases which can be classified. These include late presentation in a moribund state with death soon after admission, lack of personnel to do the interviewing necessary and the reporting of cases and deaths before reporting age, sex and risk factor data.

TABLE 3.   Cumulative Adult AIDS Cases by Risk Factor and Sex

Risk Factor	Male	Female	Total	(%)
Bisexual Male	36	-	36	(12.5)
Homosexual Male	77	-	77	(26.7)
IV Drug Abuser	18	1	19	(6.6)
Haemophiliac	1	-	1	(0.4)
Heterosexual Contact	78	70	148	(51.3)
Blood Transfusion	1	2	3	(1.0)
No Risk Factor	3	1	4	(1.4)
TOTAL	214	74	288	(99.9)

Note: Information is given for only those cases that can be classified.

CHANGES IN AGE, SEX AND RISK FACTOR DISTRIBUTION

An increasing proportion of new cases is aged 15-29 years, perhaps reflecting an increased manifestation of AIDS in this younger, more sexually active population. An increasing proportion of new cases is female. A rapidly increasing proportion of new cases is attributable to heterosexual transmission. This is in between the North American and African experience, but appears to be shifting towards the latter.

DISCUSSION

Outside of North America, the Caribbean has generated more than 10% of the cases in the Americas from 2% of the population. (There are problems with this statement, however, as many of the early cases acquired their infection abroad e.g. homosexual men and migrant farmworkers travelling to North America.) Indeed, some Caribbean countries (Bermuda, Bahamas, Barbados and Trinidad and Tobago) have some of the highest per capita rates of reported cases in the world. This, perhaps, together with the high rate of occurrence in Haiti, led to the description of the Caribbean as an area of "high risk" in some of the early reports. However, the Caribbean is not homogeneous. Trinidad and Tobago and the Bahamas have large numbers of cases compared with Jamaica and Guyana, where the epidemic is now taking off (Fig. 1).

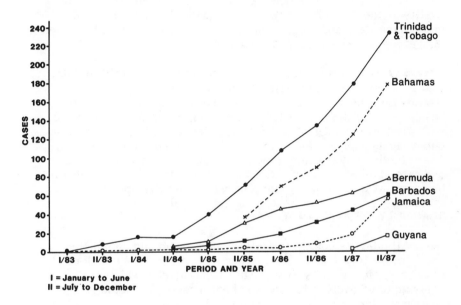

Figure 1. Cumulative Cases of AIDS in Six Caribbean Countries by Six Month Periods, 1983-1987.

Having said that, however, certain common patterns exist with respect to risk factors. In most of the territories, the early cases tend to be among homosexual/bisexual men, but as the epidemic progresses, the pattern of transmission becomes increasingly heterosexual. This is also true of Haiti, the Dominican Republic and the French Departments (Martinique, Guadeloupe and French Guiana). One exception is Bermuda, where the majority of cases are associated with intravenous drug abuse.

The rapid increase in heterosexual transmission among reported cases may be exaggerated by the reluctance of homosexual and bisexual men to admit their sexual orientation. That heterosexual transmission is increasing however, is suggested by the decreasing male:female ratio. This is in keeping with the observation that most Caribbean homosexuals tend not to be exclusively homosexual: most are bisexual. A corollary of increasing numbers of women with HIV infection is an increasing number of children with AIDS: to date, some 9% of AIDS cases reported to CAREC have been less than 5 years old.

There is a pressing need to improve the completeness and quality of the information so as to describe the AIDS epidemic more accurately and confirm or refute the apparent rapid changes in age, sex and risk factor distribution.

Since HIV has a long incubation period, the pattern of AIDS that is being seen today reflects what was happening with transmission several years ago. It is highly likely that the virus has penetrated the population to a much greater degree than the AIDS data would suggest and the male:female ratio, among those currently acquiring their infection, has declined even further. Given the long incubation period, information on the prevalence and rate at which new infections occur over time (incidence) will be essential to monitoring the progress of the HIV epidemic.

SUMMARY OF ACTION SO FAR

All member countries are very concerned and committed to the fight against AIDS, but have been hampered by the lack of resources. Most have National AIDS Committees, which are evolving/have evolved beyond the health sector to include representatives of other sectors e.g. education.

Plans and programs are variable in completeness and state of implementation. They were refined and further developed during an AIDS Programming and Funding Workshop in November 1987, organised by CAREC/PAHO and funded by WHO. Areas of need, common to all countries, were identified during the workshop and the elements of a sub-regional project were agreed (laboratory services, education, counselling). This has been submitted for funding to donor agencies and will be executed by CAREC, which has a coordinating role in the Caribbean for AIDS prevention and control.

With funding from WHO's Global Program on AIDS (WHO GPA), CAREC has established a team led by a Medical Epidemiologist to support member countries' efforts against AIDS. Additionally, CAREC will house a GPA Caribbean Education and Information Centre.

Activities in countries, to date, have included HIV seroprevalence studies and knowledge - attitude - behaviour surveys; national AIDS conferences; public education utilising leaflets and newspapers; radio, television and local art forms such as reggae; education of health care workers; community-based distribution of condoms. CAREC has supported several of these activities. At the time of writing, 15 countries are screening donor blood for HIV antibody with confirmatory testing at CAREC. The other four are in the process of acquiring the technology.

The Global Impact of AIDS, pages 35–41
© 1988 Alan R. Liss, Inc.

6.   EPIDEMIOLOGY OF AIDS AND HIV INFECTION IN THE
UNITED STATES

Richard M Selik, Gary R Noble, W Meade Morgan,
Timothy J Dondero, James W Curran

The Centers for Disease Control, Public Health
Service, U.S. Department of Health and Human
Services, Atlanta, Georgia 30333.

Between June 1, 1981 and March 7, 1988, 55,167 patients
with AIDS were reported in the United States and U.S.
territories. The ratio of males to females was 11.2 to 1. AIDS
patients are classified in exposure categories according to their
presumed means of acquiring human immunodeficiency virus
(HIV) infection. Sixty-four percent were homosexual or bisexual
men, 18% were intravenous-drug abusers (IVDAers), and 7% were
both. Heterosexual transmission of HIV was presumed responsible
for AIDS in 2,189 (4%) patients. Of these, 918 (1.7%) were born
in countries where heterosexual transmission is believed to
account for most AIDS cases, and 1,271 (2.3%) others had
heterosexual partners either with AIDS or at increased risk of
AIDS. The male-to-female ratio in the latter group was 1 to 3.5.

RACIAL/ETHNIC DIFFERENCES

The numbers of AIDS patients in Hispanic and black (non-
Hispanic) populations were disproportionately high: 26% of AIDS
patients were black and 14% Hispanic, whereas these groups
composed only 12% and 7% of the population, respectively. The
disproportion was even greater for AIDS cases directly or
indirectly related to intravenous-drug abuse (IVDA): 45% were in
blacks and 24% in Hispanics. Forty-five percent of blacks and
45% of Hispanics with AIDS were IVDAers or had heterosexual
contact with IVDAers, compared with 14% of whites (non-
Hispanic) with AIDS (Table 1). Of black and Hispanic children
(age less than 13 years) with AIDS, 60% and 73%, respectively,
had mothers who were IVDAers or whose sex partners were
IVDAers, compared with 31% of white children with AIDS.

TABLE 1. Distribution of AIDS Patients[1] by Exposure Category for Different Racial/Ethnic Groups in the United States and U.S. Territories (Reported as of 7 March 1988)

Exposure Category	White	(%)	Black	(%)	Hispanic	(%)	Other	(%)	Total	(%)
Homosexual/bisexual men without IVDA[2]	25861	(78.4)	5269	(37.4)	3457	(45.6)	266	(71.5)	34853	(63.3)
Homosexual/bisexual men with IVDA	2553	(7.7)	971	(6.9)	498	(6.6)	14	(3.8)	4036	(7.3)
Heterosexuals with IVDA	1908	(5.8)	4933	(35.0)	2673	(35.3)	20	(5.4)	9534	(17.3)
Heterosexuals whose sex partners had IVDA	181	(0.6)	453	(3.2)	226	(3.0)	2	(0.5)	862	(1.6)
Heterosexuals whose sex partners had other risks[3]	198	(0.6)	1067	(7.8)	55	(0.7)	6	(1.6)	1326	(2.4)
Children whose mothers had IVDA or had sex partners with IVDA	61	(0.2)	287	(2.0)	145	(1.9)	3	(0.8)	496	(0.9)
Children whose mothers had other risk factors[4]	30	(0.1)	137	(1.0)	15	(0.2)	2	(0.5)	184	(0.3)
Transfusion of blood or clotting factors	1563	(4.7)	272	(1.9)	162	(2.1)	38	(10.2)	2035	(3.7)
Undetermined means of acquiring HIV infection[5]	644	(2.0)	700	(5.0)	344	(4.5)	21	(5.6)	1709	(3.1)
Totals	32999	(100.0)	14089	(100.0)	7575	(100.0)	372	(100.0)	55035	(100.0)

1. Excluding 132 patients of unknown race/ethnicity.
2. History of intravenous-drug abuse.
3. Includes 918 adults without other identified risk factors who were born in countries where heterosexual transmission of HIV is believed to account for most AIDS cases.
4. Includes 88 children whose mothers or mothers' sex partners were born in countries where heterosexual transmission of HIV is believed to account for most AIDS cases.
5. Includes patients on whom risk information is incomplete (due to death, refusal to be interviewed, or loss to follow-up), patients still under investigation, and completely investigated patients for whom no specific risk factor was identified.

TABLE 2. Distribution of AIDS Patients by Geographic Region[1] for Different Exposure Categories in the United States and U.S. Territories[2] (Reported as of 7 March 1988)

Exposure Category	New York City	(%)	Other NE Region	(%)	Midwest	(%)	South	(%)	West	(%)	US Territories	(%)	Total	(%)
Homosexual/bisexual men without IVDA[3]	6345	(18.2)	4043	(11.6)	3105	(8.9)	9390	(26.9)	11864	(34.0)	178	(0.5)	34925	(100.0)
Homosexual/bisexual men with IVDA	564	(13.9)	547	(13.5)	280	(6.9)	1093	(27.0)	1476	(36.5)	85	(2.1)	4045	(100.0)
Heterosexuals with IVDA	3748	(39.2)	3342	(34.9)	367	(3.8)	1375	(14.4)	467	(4.9)	265	(2.8)	9564	(100.0)
Heterosexuals whose sex partners had IVDA	262	(30.4)	284	(33.0)	30	(3.5)	202	(23.4)	60	(7.0)	24	(2.8)	862	(100.0)
Heterosexuals whose sex partners had other risks[4]	315	(23.7)	234	(17.6)	65	(4.9)	601	(45.3)	109	(8.2)	3	(0.2)	1327	(100.0)
Children whose mothers had IVDA or had sex partners with IVDA	193	(38.9)	155	(31.2)	19	(3.8)	78	(15.7)	25	(5.0)	26	(5.2)	496	(100.0)
Children whose mothers had other risk factors[5]	32	(17.2)	31	(16.7)	16	(8.6)	96	(51.6)	11	(5.9)	0	(0.0)	186	(100.0)
Transfusion of blood or clotting factors	134	(6.6)	369	(18.1)	286	(14.0)	688	(33.7)	543	(26.6)	22	(1.1)	2042	(100.0)
Undetermined means of acquiring HIV infection[6]	414	(24.1)	275	(16.0)	127	(7.4)	573	(33.3)	313	(18.2)	18	(1.0)	1720	(100.0)
Totals	12007	(21.8)	9280	(16.8)	4295	(7.8)	14096	(25.6)	14868	(27.0)	621	(1.1)	55167	(100.0)
Corresponding population in millions (1980 census)	7	(3.1)	42	(18.3)	59	(25.8)	75	(32.8)	43	(18.8)	3	(1.3)	229	(100.0)

1. The regions consist of the following states:– Northeast: Connecticut, Maine, Massachusetts, New Hampshire, New Jersey, New York, Pennsylvania, Rhode Island, Vermont; Midwest: Illinois, Indiana, Iowa, Kansas, Michigan, Minnesota, Missouri, Nebraska, North Dakota, Ohio, South Dakota, Wisconsin; South: Alabama, Arkansas, Delaware, District of Columbia, Florida, Georgia, Kentucky, Louisiana, Maryland, Mississippi, Oklahoma, North Carolina, South Carolina, Tennessee, Texas, Virginia, West Virginia; West: Alaska, Arizona, California, Colorado, Hawaii, Idaho, Montana, New Mexico, Nevada, Oregon, Utah, Washington, Wyoming.

2. Includes 608 patients in Puerto Rico and 13 in other U.S. territories.

3. History of intravenous-drug abuse.

4. Includes 918 adults without other identified risk factors who were born in countries where heterosexual transmission of HIV is believed to account for most AIDS cases.

5. Includes 88 children whose mothers or mothers' sex partners were born in countries where heterosexual transmission of HIV is believed to account for most AIDS cases.

6. Includes patients on whom risk information is incomplete (due to death, refusal to be interviewed, or loss to follow-up), patients still under investigation, and completely investigated patients for whom no specific risk factor was identified.

GEOGRAPHIC DIFFERENCES

The numbers of AIDS patients in New York City and in the western region of the United States were disproportionately high: 22% of AIDS patients resided in New York City and 27% in the West, whereas these areas contained only 3% and 19% of the population respectively. Of AIDS cases in heterosexual IVDAers, however, 39% were in New York City, but only 5% were in the West (Table 2). The proportion of cases directly or indirectly related to IVDA was 40% in New York City, 47% in the remainder of the North East, and constituted the majority of cases in New Jersey (62%) and Puerto Rico (64%) but under 20% in other regions.

TRENDS

The annual number of AIDS patients reported in each exposure category has increased every year from 1981 through 1987. Mathematical modelling of AIDS trends has led to projections that 73,000 cases will be diagnosed in 1991 alone, with a cumulative total of 270,000. As the numbers of cases in some exposure categories have increased faster than those in others, the proportion in some categories has increased, while the proportion in others has decreased (Table 3). The proportion of cases presumed due to heterosexual contact with persons in high-risk groups (homosexual men, IVDAers, hemophiliacs) or with persons known to have HIV infection has increased from 1.1% of cases reported in 1982 to 2.8% in 1987. Associated with this increase was an increase in the proportion of cases in women from 7.1% to 7.9%. The proportion of cases in persons who were not in high-risk groups, but were born in countries where heterosexual transmission is believed to account for most cases, decreased from 6.4% in 1982 to 1.2% in 1987.

HIV-ANTIBODY SEROPREVALENCE

HIV-antibody surveys (Centers for Disease Control, 18 December 1987) have shown that the prevalence of HIV infection parallels the distribution of AIDS cases by sex, race/ethnicity, geographic area, and exposure category. The HIV-antibody prevalence in homosexual men was generally between 20% and 50%, and in IVDAers ranged from below 5% in most of the country to 50%-60% in the New York City area, northern New Jersey, and Puerto Rico (Table 4). The prevalence was about 70% in persons with haemophilia A and 35% in those with hemophilia B and did not vary geographically. Based on HIV prevalence

TABLE 3. Percentage Distribution of AIDS Patients by Exposure Category for Different Years of Report, 1982 - 1987, in the United States and U.S. Territories

	1982	1983	1984	1985	1986	1987
AIDS patients reported :	706	2103	4589	8358	13252	21184
Exposure Category						
Homosexual/bisexual men without IVDA*	60.5	61.0	64.5	65.8	64.5	63.1
Homosexual/bisexual men with IVDA	8.6	9.6	9.2	7.2	7.4	7.0**
Heterosexuals with IVDA	16.7	17.8	17.4	17.0	17.0	16.8
Heterosexuals whose sex partners had IVDA	0.8	0.7	1.0	1.2	1.7	1.8**
Heterosexuals whose sex partners had other risks	0.3	0.4	0.3	0.4	0.8	1.0**
Heterosexuals born in certain countries @	6.4	4.1	2.4	1.7	1.6	1.2**
Children whose mothers had IVDA or had sex partners with IVDA	0.8	0.8	0.7	0.9	1.0	0.8
Children whose mothers were born in certain countries @	0.3	0.5	0.2	0.2	0.1	0.1**
Children whose mothers had other risk factors	0.0	0.0	0.0	0.1	0.2	0.2**
Transfusion of blood or clotting factors	2.3	2.0	2.1	3.2	3.4	4.3**
Undetermined means of acquiring HIV infection @@	3.3	3.1	2.3	2.2	2.4	3.6**
Totals	100.0	100.0	100.0	100.0	100.0	100.0

*   History of intravenous-drug abuse.

**   Significant change (p is less than 0.05, Armitage's chi-square test for linear trend).

@   Countries where heterosexual transmission of HIV is believed to account for most AIDS cases.

@@   Includes patients on whom risk information is incomplete (due to death, refusal to be interviewed, or loss to follow-up), patients still under investigation, and completely investigated patients for whom no specific risk factor was identified.

TABLE 4. HIV-Antibody Prevalence in Selected Populations in the United States, 1985 - 1987*

Population	Prevalence Range %
Homosexual/bisexual men	10-70
Intravenous drug abusers	0-61
Hemophiliacs	
Type A	26-92
Type B	15-52
Heterosexual partners of HIV infected persons	10-60
Pregnant or parturient women	0-2
Prisoners **	0-17
Female prostitutes **	0-45
Military recruit applicants	
Men	0.24
Women	0.04
First-time volunteer blood-donors	
Men	0.07
Women	0.02

*   Source : Centers for Disease Control. Human immunodeficiency virus infection in the United States: a review of current knowledge. MMWR 1987; 36 (suppl no. S-6): 22-35

**   A substantial proportion of persons in these groups may be intravenous-drug abusers.

estimates for persons in the various HIV exposure categories and estimates of the populations of these groups, the number of persons with HIV infection in the United States has been estimated to be 1.0 - 1.5 million in 1986-1987. The prevalence of HIV infection in heterosexual partners of persons with HIV infection or at recognized risk ranged from less than 10% to 60%. The prevalence in 1,253,768 applicants for military service tested between October 1985 and September 1987 was 0.15%. The prevalence was higher in black and Hispanic applicants (0.51% and 0.22% respectively) than in white applicants (0.07%). The prevalence in women attending pre-natal clinics ranged from 0.0% at 2 private clinics in the midwest to 1.7% in a public hospital in Puerto Rico. In women delivering babies in Massachusetts, HIV-antibody prevalence was 0.2%, and in 3 New York City municipal hospitals, it was 2.0%-2.4%.

In the United States, most cases of AIDS and HIV infection occur in homosexual/bisexual men, IVDAers, hemophiliacs, and the sex partners and children of persons in these groups. Recommendations for preventing infection in these high-risk groups have been published (Centers for Disease Control, 14 August 1987). The general heterosexual, non-drug-abusing population has been much less involved, although the proportion of cases in this category may be increasing slowly. The epidemic is most likely to spread into this group by heterosexual contact with persons who have multiple sex partners, some of whom are IVDAers or bisexual men.

REFERENCES

Centers for Disease Control. Human immunodeficiency virus infection in the United States: a review of current knowledge. MMWR 18 December 1987: 36 (Suppl no. S-6): 1-48.

Centers for Disease Control. Public Health Service guidelines for counselling and antibody testing to prevent HIV infection and AIDS. MMWR 14 August 1987; 36: 509-515.

Morgan W M, Curran J W (1986). Acquired immunodeficiency syndrome: current and future trends. Public Health Rep 101: 459-465.

The Global Impact of AIDS, pages 43–52
© 1988 Alan R. Liss, Inc.

7. GEOGRAPHIC FACTORS AND HUMAN
IMMUNODEFICIENCY VIRUS INFECTION AMONG
HOMOSEXUAL MEN AND INTRAVENOUS DRUG
ABUSERS FROM THE NORTHEASTERN PART OF ITALY

D Serraino[1], S Franceschi[1], E Vaccher[2], S
Saracchini[2], U Tirelli[2]

Epidemiology Unit[1] and Medical Oncology[2], Centro
di Riferimento Oncologico, Aviano (PN), Italy

The acquired immunodeficiency syndrome (AIDS) epidemic
has already spread worldwide. The population groups affected by
AIDS, or infected with the human immunodeficiency virus (HIV),
differ widely from one country to another, in relation to the
different modes of virus transmission. For example, the major
source of AIDS cases have been homosexual and bisexual men in
the U.S., the U.K. and northern Europe, heterosexuals in Africa
and intravenous drug addicts (IVDAs) in Spain and Italy (Curran
et al., 1988; Instituto Superiore di Sanitã, 1988).

AIDS cases have increased rapidly in Italy in the last years,
in particular among IVDAs (Fig. 1), who are at present by far the
group at highest risk (62% of reported cases). Italian homosexual
and bisexual men, on the contrary, have been involved so far to a
lower extent than in other countries (21% of AIDS cases)
(Instituto Superiore di Sanitã, 1988).

A similar picture emerges from seroprevalence data on HIV
infection. Italian IVDAs show prevalence of HIV positivity among
the highest in Europe, up to 76% (Angarano et al., 1985), whereas
the few seroepidemiological studies conducted among Italian
homosexuals reported a frequency of HIV infection lower than
20% (Vitale et al., 1987).

STUDY DESIGN

In order to assess prevalence and patterns of spread of HIV
infection in high-risk groups in the northeastern part of Italy, a
physical examination was performed and a blood sample taken
from 313 parenteral drug addicts (229 men and 84 women,

median age: 25 years) self-referred to five Centers for Drug-Addicts Assistance, and 112 homosexuals and bisexual men (median age : 34 years), who voluntarily attended the AIDS Outpatient Clinic at the Centro di Riferimento Oncologico of Aviano.

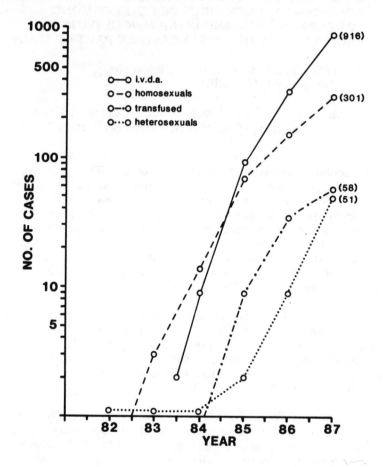

Figure 1. Cumulative Number of AIDS Cases in Adults by Risk Group, Italy 1982 - 1987.

Information was elicited by means of a questionnaire on sociodemographic factors, long-distance travels in the last three years and sexual habits (number of partners per year, anal and oral sexual practices, use of condoms) etc. Antibodies against HIV were determined in a single laboratory by a commercial

enzyme linked immunoabsorbent assay (ELISA), with
confirmation by western blot.

In order to measure the influence of various characteristics
on the risk of acquiring HIV infection, the relative risks (RRs)
and their 95% confidence interval (CI) were computed from data
stratified by age and, when appropriate, sex by the Mantel-
Haenszel procedure (Mantel and Haenszel, 1959). For drug
addicts, a multiple logistic regression (MLR) equation, including
terms of age, sex, residence, year when drug addiction began,
long-distance travels, sexual behaviour and place of examination,
was fitted by the method of maximum likelihood (Breslow and
Day, 1980). Further details on risk factors for HIV infection in
IVDAs have been provided elsewhere (Franceschi et al., 1988).
Owing to the few HIV seropositive homosexuals it was not
possible, apart from age, to control for the effect of other
potential confounding factors.

**TABLE 1.   HIV Antibodies in 313 Drug Addicts by Age and Sex.
Italy, 1984 - 1987**

	HIV POS N	(%)	HIV NEG N	(%)	MH–RR * (95% CI)
Age (years)					
0-24	48	(35)	88	(65)	1**
25-29	39	(32)	83	(68)	0.86
					(0.51-1.45)
30 +	7	(13)	48	(87)	0.28
					(0.12-0.64)
Sex :					
Men	68	(30)	61	(70)	1**
Women	26	(31)	58	(69)	0.98
					(0.56-1.70)

*   Relative risk (RR) estimates, adjusted for age and sex by
     the Mantel-Haenszel (MH) procedure and 95% confidence
     intervals (CI).

** Reference category

RESULTS

Intravenous Drug Addicts

Ninety-four IVDAs (30%, 95% CI: 24-36%) were seropositive to HIV antibodies. Drug addicts younger than 30 were seropositive nearly three times more frequently than older ones, whereas seropositivity rates were similar between the two sexes.

TABLE 2. HIV Antibodies in 313 Drug Addicts by Geographical Factors and Prostitution. Italy, 1984 - 1987

	HIV POS N (%)		HIV NEG N (%)		MH-RR** (95% CI)	MLR-RR@ (95% CI)
Province of Residence :						
Udine, Gorizia	14	(9)	134	(91)	1*	1*
Pordenone	58	(48)	63	(52)	8.55	13.40
					(4.66-15.68)	(6.10-29.41)
Other	22	(50)	22	(50)	10.67	9.42
					(4.80-23.33)	(3.66-24.23)
Travels in the last 3 years :						
Within region	15	(20)	59	(80)	1*	1*
Within Italy	34	(35)	62	(65)	2.09	2.96
					(1.02-4.27)	(1.24-7.08)
Out of Italy	39	(31)	95	(69)	1.76	2.61
					(0.88-3.51)	(1.16-5.86)
Prostitution						
No	82	(28)	210	(72)	1*	1*
Yes	11	(55)	9	(45)	4.68	2.09
					(1.55-14.10)	(0.78-9.23)

* Reference category
** Relative risk (RR) estimates, adjusted for age and sex by the Mantel-Haenszel (MH) procedure and 95% confidence intervals (CI).
@ Multiple logistic regression (MLR) relative risk (RR) estimates, including terms for age, sex, province of residence, year at starting of drug addiction, travels in the last three years, prostitution and place of examination.

Apart from needle sharing, by far the most important means of HIV spread among IVDAs and admitted by all the interviewed subjects, the strongest determinants of the risk were province of residence and long-distance travels. IVDAs living in Pordenone province showed a prevalence of HIV seropositivity of 48%, but those living in Udine and Gorizia provinces had an overall prevalence of less than 10%. Such large difference was not affected by allowance for various potential confounding factors (MLR-RR of Pordenone vs Udine and Gorizia provinces : 13.4, 95% CI : 6.1-29.4) (Table 2).

Long-distance travels exerted a similar, though smaller, influence. Drug addicts who had travelled out of their region of residence in Italian cities or out of Italy (mainly in northern Europe) in the last three years showed, after allowance for several potential confounding factors, an almost three-fold greater risk of being HIV seropositive than those who had not left Friuli-Venezia Giulia region (MLR-RR of travelling out of Italy vs region only: 2.6, 95% CI: 1.2-5.9) (Table 2).

Also, being a prostitute, admitted only by female IVDAs, substantially increased the probability of HIV infection. However, the relative risk was not significant after allowance for possible confounding factors (MLR-RR of being prostitute : 2.1, 95% CI: 0.8-9.2) (Table 2).

Homosexual and Bisexual Men

Twenty-two of the present group of homosexual and bisexual men were seropositive to HIV antibodies (20%, 95% CI: 12-27%). The prevalence of seropositivity increased with age; in homosexuals over 39 it was twice that of those younger than 30 (Table 3).

Geographical factors seemed to play a role on the risk of HIV infection although to a lesser extent than among IVDAs. Homosexuals who had travelled in northern Europe and in the U.S. showed respectively a two-fold and a four-fold higher risk of HIV seropositivity than those who had not travelled abroad (RR for travelling in Europe: 2.1, 95% CI: 0.8-5.7; for travelling in the U.S.: 4.2, 95% CI: 0.8-23.2). At variance with what was found among IVDAs, homosexuals living in Udine and Gorizia provinces and in Pordenone province had similar HIV seropositivity rates (16% and 17% respectively), whereas those living in other cities of the northeastern part of Italy (25% of seropositivity) showed no significantly increased risk of HIV infection (Table 3).

No elevation of risk was seen among the homosexuals who admitted to being prostitutes. Only two of them (8%) were seropositive (Table 3).

TABLE 3. **HIV Antibodies in 112 Homosexual and Bisexual Men by Various Characteristics. Italy 1984 - 1987**

	HIV POS N	(%)	HIV NEG N	(%)	MH-RR * (95% CI)
Age (years)					
0-29	6	(14)	37	(86)	1**
30-39	9	(20)	35	(80)	1.59
					(0.51-4.92)
40 +	7	(28)	18	(72)	2.40
					(0.71-8.09)
Province of residence:					
Udine, Gorizia	7	(16)	37	(84)	1**
Pordenone	4	(17)	20	(83)	1.11
					(0.29-4.25)
Other	11	(25)	33	(75)	1.72
					(0.59-5.00)
Travels in the last 3 years:					
Italy	10	(14)	60	(86)	1**
Europe	9	(26)	26	(74)	2.06
					(0.75-5.67)
U.S.	3	(43)	4	(57)	4.24@
					(0.76-23.24)
Prostitution :					
No	20	(23)	67	(77)	1**
Yes	2	(8)	23	(92)	0.33
					(0.07-1.58)

* Relative risk (RR) estimates, adjusted for age by Mantel-Haenszel (MH) procedure and 95% confidence intervals (CI).
** Reference category
@ Exact confidence interval

HIV seropositivity was three times more frequent among homosexuals who reported thirty-five or more sexual partners per year, in comparison to those who admitted fewer than ten (RR :3.3, 95% CI: 0.9-12.0). The frequency of receptive sex, both anal and oral, did not seem to influence substantially the probability of being infected (Table 4).

TABLE 4. Sexual Habits and HIV Infection in 112 Homosexual and Bisexual Men. Italy, 1984 - 1987

	HIV POS N	(%)	HIV NEG N	(%)	MH-RR * (95% CI)
Number of partners**per year :**					
Less than 9	4	(12)	28	(88)	1@
10 - 34	9	(25)	27	(75)	2.09 (0.60-7.29)
More than 35	7	(37)	12	(63)	3.30 (0.91-12.02)
Anal receptivesex :					
Some partners	12	(18)	55	(82)	1@
Most partners	10	(23)	34	(77)	1.32 (0.51-3.42)
Oral receptivesex :					
Some partners	6	(21)	23	(79)	1@
Most partners	15	(19)	66	(81)	0.94 (0.31-2.82)

* Relative risk (RR) estimates, adjusted for age by the Mantel-Haenszel (MH) procedure and 95% confidence interval (CI).

** It does not include homosexuals who admitted to be prostitutes.

@ Reference category.

Long-distance travel and number of sexual partners seemed to exert an independent effect on the probability of acquiring HIV infection (Table 5).

TABLE 5. Risk of HIV Infection by Travels and Number of Sexual Partners in 112 Homosexual and Bisexual Men. Italy 1984 - 1987

	Number of sexual partners per year:		
	Less than 10	10-34	More than 34
Travels in the last 3 years:			
No	1*	2.22	4.00
Yes	2.50	5.55	7.14

* Reference category

DISCUSSION

The present survey had obvious limitations, not only because it was restricted to two high-risk groups, not representative of the general population, but also because no rigorous sampling framework was applied to the IVDAs and homosexual communities. Collected information came from self-referred subjects, who may have differed substantially from those who did not attend either the Centers for Drug Addicts Assistance or the AIDS Outpatient Clinic. This lack of information on source population was especially important in a group as the present one, largely constituted by asymptomatic individuals. Furthermore, such selection mechanisms were likely to be different in IVDAs as compared to homosexuals.

Comparison of risk factors for HIV infection in such two groups, little overlapping in Italy, can be useful to cast light on the spread of HIV in Italy. The age distribution of IVDAs and homosexuals was substantially different; the risk of infection among homosexuals seemed positively correlated with age, while for IVDAs the opposite was true, addicts younger than 25 being three-fold more often HIV positive as compared to those older than thirty.

The important role played by geographical factors in the transmission of HIV infection is well documented. On account of the divergent life-styles of the population studied, however, main risk factors are different in such two groups (Biggar et al., 1984; Weiss et al., 1986). The data from the present study, conducted in an area of Italy amongst those at lowest risk for AIDS, were consistent with the hypothesis that HIV may have spread among homosexuals through sexual contacts in high-risk areas. The risk of acquiring the infection was particularly high for those homosexuals who had sexual contacts in the U.S. in the last three years. It is likely that over time, as the prevalence of seropositivity increases in the northeastern part of Italy, a greater role for number of sexual partners and anal receptive intercourse will emerge.

IVDAs, on the average, travelled less often than homosexuals. It is not surprising, therefore, that, within geographical factors, place of residence seemed to affect IVDAs' risk of being infected much more strongly than their long-distance travels. For IVDAs the study area can be divided into two parts: one high-risk area (Pordenone province), with a prevalence of HIV infection as high as in the largest Italian cities, and one low-risk area (Udine and Gorizia province). Such a marked difference had no obvious explanation, since these provinces are, geographically and economically, very similar. However, one of the biggest U.S. military bases (Aviano) in Western Europe is located in the Pordenone province. The presence of this base could offer a possible explanation for the difference in seropositivity rates, taking into account that one third of the female drug addicted prostitutes in Pordenone province reported U.S. soldiers among their clients (Tirelli et al., 1986).

In conclusion, whereas the greatest effort must be done in Italy in order to discourage needle-sharing among IVDAs, an effective counselling strategy towards Italian homosexuals may still be effective to prevent the AIDS epidemic reaching, in this group of individuals, the size documented in other countries.

REFERENCES

Angarano G, Pastore G, Monno L, Santantonio T, Luchena N, Schiraldi O (1985). Rapid spread of HTLV-III infection among drug addicts in Italy. Lancet ii: 1302.

Biggar R J, Melbye M, Ebbesen P et al (1984). Low T-lymphocyte ratios in homosexual men. Epidemiologic evidence for a transmissible agent. JAMA 254: 1441-1446.

Breslow N E, Day N E (1980). "Statistical methods in cancer research". Lyon: IARC scientific publication No. 32.

Curran J W, Jaffe H W, Hardy A M, Morgan W M, Selik R M, Dondero T S (1988). Epidemiology of HIV infection and AIDS in the United States. Science 239: 610-616.

Franceschi S, Tirelli U, Vaccher E et al (1988). Risk factors for HIV infection in drug addicts from the northeast of Italy. Int J Epidemiol 17: 162-167.

Instituto Superiore di Sanitã. Centro Operativo AIDS. Roma. Bulletino Epidemiologico Nazionale, 11 February 1988.

Mantel N, Haenszel W (1959). Statistical aspects of the analysis of data from retrospective studies of disease. J Natl Cancer Inst 22: 718-748.

Tirelli U, Vaccher E, Sorio R, Carbone A, Monfardini S (1986). HTLV-III antibodies in drug-addicted prostitutes used by US soldiers in Italy. JAMA 256: 711-712.

Vitale F, Portera M, De Crescenzo L et al (1987). AIDS in Sicily: prevalence of antibodies to human immunodeficiency virus (HIV) in low and high risk groups. Eur J Epidemiol 3: 278-283.

Weiss S H, Ginzburg H M, Goedert J J et al (1986). Risk factors for HTLV-III infection among parenteral drug users. Proc Am Soc Clin Oncol 5: 3.

The Global Impact of AIDS, pages 53–60
© 1988 Alan R. Liss, Inc.

8. PREVALENCE OF RISK-PRONE SEXUAL BEHAVIOUR IN THE GENERAL POPULATION OF NORWAY

J M Sundet, I L Kvalem, P Magnus, L S Bakketeig

Department of Epidemiology, National Institute of
Public Health, Oslo, Norway.

INTRODUCTION

It is well known that sexual intercourse is one of the main
channels of HIV transmission. Seen in this perspective, there is a
conspicuous lack of knowledge about the prevalence of risk-
prone sexual behaviour in the general population.

MATERIALS AND METHODS

These data are based on the responses to an anonymous
postal questionnaire. The respondents were asked to answer
questions about number of partners during lifetime and more
recently, both same-sex and opposite-sex. Also they were asked
about type of intercourse. This questionnaire was sent to a
random sample of the Norwegian population aged 18 through 60
years late autumn 1987. The sample size was 10,000 which is
about 0.5% of the total Norwegian population in this age
interval. The sample was drawn from the population registry by
the Central Bureau of Statistics of Norway. About 63% of the
sample responded to the questionnaire. The age and sex
distribution of the responding group is shown in Table 1.

TABLE 1. Response Percentages

Age	Males	Females
18-31	60	72
32-45	56	62
46-60	48	55

Two main trends may be noted. Females were more willing to answer than males; and young persons more than old persons. Except for a certain over-representation of high education groups and urban areas, the respondent group was fairly representative of the population. A further argument for representativity is the fact that the percentage reporting having been HIV tested is very near to the actual population percentage (approximately 10%).

RESULTS

Homosexual and bisexual practice among the males in the respondent group, a total of 3.5% reported that they had at least one same-sex partner up to the present. The corresponding numbers among females were 3.0%. The age and sex distribution of persons reporting at least one same-sex partner up to the present is displayed in Table 2.

TABLE 2. Percentages with Homosexual Experience Lifespan

Age	Males (%)	Females (%)
18-31	4.7	4.8
32-45	3.1	2.1
46-60	1.8	0.6
TOTAL	3.5	3.0

The percentages are generally slightly lower among females than among males. Also, they are lower among older persons. This last trend may both be due to repression because of guilt and shame, and a real difference between young and old persons with respect to same-sex practice.

The percentages reporting at least one same-sex partner during the last three years are displayed in Table 3.

TABLE 3. Percentages with Homosexual Experience Last Three Years

Age	Males (%)	Females (%)
18-31	1.3	2.2
32-45	0.6	0.4
46-60	0.3	0.1
TOTAL	0.9	0.9

These numbers may be a more reliable indication of actual behaviour among persons with same-sex practice.

We have further sub-grouped persons with same-sex practice into those who have reported only same-sex partners, and those who have reported partners of both sexes, and the resulting percentages are displayed in Table 4.

TABLE 4. Percentages of Persons Reporting Same-Sex Practice

	Males (%)	Females (%)
Only same-sex	17	25
Both sexes	83	75

The relatively low numbers of those who reported only same-sex partners, both for males and females, are noteworthy. Thus, between 75 and 83% of those who reported at least one same-sex partner up to the present, also reported partners of the opposite sex. It may be added that about 60% reported more opposite-sex than same-sex partners.

Partner turnover among those with the same-sex partners.

It may be of interest to study intensity of partner turnover among persons with same-sex partners relative to those with only opposite-sex partners. Table 5 indicates that those with same-sex partners tend to report more partners than those with only opposite-sex partners. It is seen that persons reporting same-sex partners tend to have a larger partner turnover than those reporting only opposite-sex partners.

TABLE 5. Lifespan Number of Partners by Sex and Homosexual Experience

Total No. of Partners	With Homosexual Experience		Without Homosexual Experience	
	Males (%)	Females (%)	Males (%)	Females (%)
1-5	28	31	51	70
6-10	20	29	22	19
11-50	45	32	23	11
50 +	7	8	4	0

In Table 6 the number of sexual partners of those reporting only same-sex partners and those who reported partners of both sexes is shown. The main tendency is that persons reporting partners of both sexes tend to report a larger number of partners than those who have had only same-sex partners.

TABLE 6. Number of Partners Among Homosexuals and Bisexuals Lifespan

Total No. of Partners	Homosexual		Bisexual	
	Males (%)	Females (%)	Males (%)	Females (%)
1-5	56	65	20	18
6-10	0	26	25	30
11-50	25	9	51	41
50 +	19	0	4	11

The frequency distribution of the number of sexual partners during the last three years among those reporting at least one same-sex partner up to the present is displayed in Table 7.

TABLE 7. Frequency Distribution in (%) of Number of Same-Sex Partners Last Three Years

Number of Partners	Males (%)	Females (%)
0	78	75
1-10	16	23
11-50	4	2
50 +	2	0

Only about 25% reported same-sex partners in this period. Could this relatively low percentage indicate a behavioural change?

Partner turnover among heterosexuals.

There are two groups to be discussed here: married and cohabitees, which was 70% of the respondents, on the one hand, and singles on the other. Table 8 displays the percentages by sex and age of presently married or cohabitees who reported at least one adulterous sexual relationship up to the present. Again there are two main trends: except for the youngest group, males tend to be more adulterous than females, and young persons more than old.

TABLE 8. Out of Marriage/Cohabitation Sexual Activity Lifespan

Age	Males (%)	Females (%)
18-31	15	14
32-45	27	13
46-60	20	8
TOTAL	22	12

Table 9 displays the number of partners during the last three years among those reporting at least one adulterous relationship during their present marriage/cohabitation.

TABLE 9. Sex Outside Marriage/Cohabitation Last Three Years

Total No. of Partners	Males (%)	Females (%)
0	29	27
1-10	68	71
11-50	3	2
50 +	0	0

It is of some interest to note that over 70% reporting at least one adulterous relationship at all, also report out of wedlock partners also during the last three years. The frequency distribution of number of partners during the last 3 years among heterosexual males and females who are at present single is displayed in Table 10. 65% of all the single males and 68% of the females reported at least one partner in this period. It may be noted that the number of partners tend to be quite low for both sexes; but somewhat larger among males than among females.

TABLE 10. Sexual Activity Among Singles Last Three Years

Total No. of Partners	Males (%)	Females (%)
0	35	32
1-10	59	65
11-50	5	3
50 +	1	0

Anal Intercourse

Table 11 shows the percentages of those with only same-sex partners and those partners of both sexes who reported at least one anal sex partner. The corresponding percentages for heterosexual males and females are also included.

TABLE 11. Percentage of Anal Intercourse Partners Lifespan

	Males	Females
Only same-sex partner	25	–
Both sexes	51	48
Heterosexual	10	14

The low percentage among those with only same-sex partners is noteworthy. Actually, the prevalence of anal intercourse is considerably higher among those with partners of both sexes, which in turn is higher than those among heterosexuals. To the extent that anal intercourse is particularly riskfull with regard to HIV infection, these numbers may indicate that there is a spread potential from the male bisexuals to the heterosexual group. Owing to the much larger number of heterosexuals, there is a quite substantial spread potential among heterosexuals.

SUMMARY

The results from this study may enable us to estimate the number of practising homosexuals and bisexuals in any population comparable to the Norwegian one in this respect. The data on partner turnover and the prevalence of anal sex in the heterosexual part of the population may indicate a considerable spread potential of the HIV virus.

The Global Impact of AIDS, pages 61–65
© 1988 Alan R. Liss, Inc.

9. HIV AND INTERNATIONAL TRAVEL *

James Chin

**Global Programme on AIDS, World Health
Organization, Geneva.**

It is very clear that whatever its origin, AIDS is now a
pandemic problem. Its etiologic agent, the human
immunodeficiency virus (HIV) is now present in virtually every
major city in the world as a result of international travel of
infected persons and infected blood products. My presentation
will address two of the current major issues regarding HIV and
international travel. The first is what the current risk of
acquiring an HIV infection during international travel may be and
the second is how effective would HIV antibody screening of
international travellers be to prevent the further spread of AIDS.

I refer you to the three major global patterns of AIDS/HIV
which Dr Mann described (pp. 3-7). The explanation for the
existence of these three patterns includes the apparent date of
HIV entry and/or period when HIV began to spread extensively in
the population, the relative importance of the three modes of
HIV transmission, and details of sexual and other social risk
behaviour in the population. It needs to be emphasized that these
three patterns represent generalizations which cannot be broadly
applied to any specific country or area. The specific prevalence
and pattern of HIV infections can and do vary widely within
areas of a given pattern.

The global patterns and prevalence of HIV infections varies
widely from country to country and within countries, but the

---

* Adapted from a manuscript authored by C Fordam von Rey,
Jonathan M Mann and James Chin, submitted to the Journal of
the American Medical Association (JAMA).

routes of HIV transmission have been documented to be the same throughout the world. HIV is predominantly transmitted from an infected person to an uninfected person by homosexual or heterosexual intercourse. HIV is also effectively spread by contaminated blood – in transfusions, or by use of unsterile needles and syringes. The other major mode of HIV transmission –from an infected mother to her infant before, during or shortly after birth is not relevant to a review of the risk of HIV infection and international travel. Therefore, we can conclude that the social/sexual behaviours that put a traveller at risk of acquiring HIV infection are similar worldwide.

It follows then that preventative measures against sexual transmission of HIV are identical worldwide, regardless of whether the individual is a traveller or a resident of a given area. The risk of sexual acquisition of an HIV infection can be eliminated by avoiding penetrative sexual intercourse (vaginal or anal) or reduced by avoiding such contact with persons who have multiple sexual partners, such as prostitutes, and by the use of condoms.

The risk of acquiring HIV infection from infected needles or blood while travelling is increased in areas where HIV is prevalent and routine screening of blood for HIV antibodies has not been fully established. International travellers are at a very low risk of exposure to contaminated needles or blood (unless they are IV drug users). This low risk of blood exposure to HIV can be further minimized by avoiding injury prone behaviour (with its attendant risk of transfusion) and by seeking health care, when required, at medical facilities with adequate blood donor testing and instrument sterilization capabilities. Such medical facilities can usually be identified by resident consulates or embassies.

All travellers need to be informed that HIV is not transmitted by casual contact. Use of any public conveyance by persons infected with HIV does not result in any risk of infection for others sharing the same conveyance. HIV is also **not** transmitted by coughing or sneezing, by eating food which may have been prepared by an HIV infected person. One expert group which evaluated the theoretical risk of acquiring an HIV infection from mosquitoes essentially concluded that it would take the equivalent of several thousand bites from mosquitoes whose individual feeding on an HIV infected person had just been interrupted, in order for them to transmit an HIV infection.

It can be concluded that international travel is as safe today as it ever has been, and it can also be safe from HIV infections if travellers adhere to simple precautions regarding sexual behaviour and receipt of injections or blood.

Now to turn to the second major issue. The emergence of the AIDS epidemic on a global scale has prompted some countries, primarily pattern III countries, where the current prevalence of AIDS/HIV is very low, to consider HIV screening of international travellers in an attempt to exclude HIV infected persons and thus retard HIV spread within the country.

According to the International Health Regulations of the World Health Organization, the only health document that can be required from international travellers is a valid vaccination certificate against yellow fever. Nevertheless, some countries have considered requiring proof of HIV negative status or screening entering travellers for HIV infection. Most countries have rejected such proposals after more careful consideration of the costs and benefits of such measures.

Since HIV infection is now present in every region of the world and in virtually every major city, even total exclusion of foreign travellers would be unlikely to prevent the introduction and spread of HIV infection within a country. This would be especially true for those countries where large numbers of international travellers are returning citizens. In addition, since some individuals with early HIV infection cannot be identified with existing serologic tests (i.e. during their "window" period), no screening programme, even if applied to all entering or returning travellers could completely prevent HIV introduction into any country. Furthermore, screening travellers, who in general are at a low risk of HIV infections would also be likely to identify more false positive than true positive persons. (Most countries would have to exclude diplomats from any mandatory testing of entering or returning travellers and it has not been documented that diplomats are a non-risk group for HIV infection.)

Logistical issues posed by screening travellers would be enormous. These include decisions about whether to screen before, at entry, or several months later, what to do with the traveller while awaiting test results, and a whole series of complex data management, laboratory control, legal and ethical issues.

Travellers with "AIDS free" certificates might engender a false sense of security. No internationally recognized certification of test results exists and besides, how long would such a certificate be valid for - a week, a month, a year? The costs of HIV testing of all international travellers would be enormous. In 1986, close to 100 million travellers crossed international borders legally by air travel alone. Land border crossings would add hundreds of millions if not billions of international border crossings per year. At a cost of at least a few dollars per test, the expense of screening all international travellers would be staggering. Thus, in addition to being relatively ineffectual, screening programmes for international travellers would divert scarce health resources from more effective control/prevention efforts. For these reasons, a panel of experts convened by the World Health Organization a year ago in March 1987 concluded that HIV screening programmes for international travellers would "at best and at great cost, retard only briefly the dissemination of HIV both globally and with respect to any particular country".

The non-effectiveness and total impracticability of screening all international travellers aside, some governments have or are considering imposing HIV testing on all non-nationals who intend to stay a few months to a few years. If this policy is critically and objectively evaluated, it can be shown that the risk of introduction and the risk of spread of HIV within any country is as great, if not greater from returning nationals who have been abroad for months to years. Excluding returning nationals clearly undermines the public health justification for such HIV screening programmes and makes the screening appear particularly discriminatory. Ultimately, the prevention of HIV transmission will be dependent upon the behaviour of both the entering or returning traveller, and resources would be better allocated to changing these behaviours.

Up to now, I have been talking about international travellers in general, non-specific terms and my conclusions regarding HIV risks apply to the vast majority of international travellers. There is, however, one specific group of international travellers who comprise a very high risk group for acquiring and, if infected, spreading HIV - I'm talking about the international sex tourist. Sexual tourism is a difficult problem to address. That it exists cannot be denied, but specific documentation of the extent of such tourism is hard to come by. If we can somehow divorce this complex and sensitive problem from all of the moral, legal, social and economic issues, and focus on how this public health problem can be addressed, we come back to the main theme of my talk -that HIV infection is primarily transmitted as a result of an individual's behaviour whether he or she is an international traveller or not. Passing laws to prohibit international sex or trying to screen all tourists who may be on a sex tour will clearly not be effective.

Public efforts at controlling the spread of HIV, whether it be national or international, are more likely to succeed if they focus on education for behaviour change rather than on offical actions which may be considered the "right" things to do, but which are both not feasible nor effective.

REFERENCES

1.   Piot P, Plummer F A, Mhalu F S et al (1988). AIDS: an international perspective . Science 239: 573-579.

2.   World Health Organization (1987). Report on International Travel and HIV Infection. WHO/SPA/GLO/87.1.

3.   Office of Technology Assessment (OTA), United States Congress. Do Insects Transmit AIDS? A staff paper in OTA's series on **AIDS-related Issues,** September 1987. For sale by the Superintendent of Documents, US Government Printing Office, Washington, D.C. 20402.

The Global Impact of AIDS, pages 67–77
© 1988 Alan R. Liss, Inc.

10. INTERNATIONAL POPULATION MOVEMENTS AND AIDS: Patterns, Consequences, and Policy Implications

Michael Micklin and David F Sly

Center for the Study of Population, Florida State University, Tallahassee, Florida, USA.

Rational policies designed to sever the link between international population movements and the spread of AIDS should be based on evidence appropriate to the complexity of the issues involved.

To our knowledge, only one study published to date has examined the empirical relationship between international population movements and AIDS. Darrow and his collaborators (1986) reported correlations between the number of cases of AIDS and two other STDs (syphilis and hepatitis B) in the United States in the early 1980s and several measures of international movement, including the number of immigrants from Haiti and African nations, the number of U.S. citizens travelling overseas, the number of foreign citizens visiting the United States, and the number of intercity and total passenger miles of air travel. Results show that the prevalence of syphilis and hepatitis B were highly associated with immigration from Africa (but not Haiti), U.S. travel abroad, foreign visitors to the United States, and airline miles, with correlations ranging from 0.65 to 0.93. The number of AIDS cases was associated only with immigration from Africa, airline miles, and travel to the U.S. by foreigners, though the correlations were somewhat lower than those for the other STDs. Although these data suggest a relationship between population movements and sexually transmitted disease, they permit, as the authors recognize, only limited inference.

In the interest of expanding our knowledge of the relationship between international population movements and the prevalence of AIDS, we have constructed a data set containing multiple indicators of both classes of variables. The AIDS data are based on the number of cases reported to the WHO Global Program on AIDS as of 31 January 1988. Information is available for 133 countries (i.e., those reporting at least one case) and is analyzed in terms of the total number of cases, the number of cases per 100,000 population, and the number of cases per 100,000 population between the ages of 25 and 39.

There are three principal types of international population movement, each containing at least two sub-categories. **Permanent Movers** include both documented and undocumented immigrants/emigrants and refugees. **Temporary Residents** consist of guest workers, diplomatic and military personnel, and students. **Travellers** include persons visiting another country for business purposes and tourists. For a variety of reasons, data on international population movements are of dubious quality. Definitions differ among countries, reporting is incomplete, and, with some exceptions (e.g., immigrants and students), data on the characteristics of the movers are not available. Obviously, research based on these data must be interpreted cautiously.

We looked for data on international population movements for two periods: the mid 1970s, prior to the onset of the AIDS epidemic, and the mid 1980s, after the disease had spread widely. Because this study is exploratory, we wanted to obtain as wide a range of data for as many countries as possible, reflecting both movements into and out of countries. From the 1977 and 1985 United Nations **Demographic Yearbook** we collected information on the number of long- and short-term immigrants, tourists, holiday visitors, business travel arrivals, cruise passenger arrivals, student arrivals, returning residents, long- and short-term emigrants, tourist departures, holiday departures, business departures, cruise passenger departures, and student departures. The United Nations **Statistical Yearbook** for 1975 and 1985 yielded data on student entries and departures. Finally, data on the number of refugees in various nations as of 1987 was obtained from the United Nations High Commissioner for Refugees. The number of countries for which this information was available varied considerably, ranging from 131 countries for student departures in the 1980s to 15 countries for cruise passenger departures in that same period. Of the 55 measures of international population movement used in this study, only 12 are based on data for less than 25 nations.

Table 1 presents some basic indicators of AIDS prevalence, population structure, and the volume of international population movements for the world and its major geographic regions.

TABLE 1. Indicators of AIDS Prevalence, Total Population, Population Aged 25-39, and Total Departures and Arrivals for the World and its Major Geographic Regions

	AIDS Cases Reported to WHO by 1-31-88	Mid 1980s Population (thousands)	Mid 1980s Persons 25 - 39 (thousands)	Total AIDS Rate per 100,000	AIDS Rate Per 100,000 25 - 39	Mid 1970s Total Arrivals (thousands)	Mid 1980s Total Arrivals (thousands)	Mid 1970s Total Departures (thousands)	Mid 1980s Total Departures (thousands)
WORLD	77353 (157)*	4557060 (148)	961906 (148)	1.69	8.01 (147)	441485 (105)	792679 (86)	111928 (96)	186788 (71)
AMERICAS	58609 (44)	664315 (43)	148842 (43)	8.88	39.64 (42)	110055 (35)	402622 (29)	24910 (31)	87339 (21)
EUROPE	8939 (28)	770075 (28)	171108 (28)	1.17	5.26 (28)	298154 (23)	325671 (22)	62907 (24)	75311 (22)
ASIA	221 (26)	2586515 (24)	543046 (24)	0.01	0.04 (24)	23768 (15)	52830 (16)	18194 (14)	23557 (14)
AFRICA	8839 (46)	512437 (44)	93142 (44)	1.76	9.66 (44)	6248 (24)	5556 (13)	5776 (20)	4445 (7)
OCEANIA	745 (13)	23718 (9)	5768 (9)	3.37	13.87 (9)	3260 (8)	5999 (6)	141 (7)	136 (7)

* Number of countries for which data are available.

Sources : World Health Organization Global Program on AIDS, United Nations
Demographic Yearbook, United Nations Statistical Yearbook.

Of the 77,353 cases of AIDS reported to the World Health Organization as of 31 January 1988, 75 per cent are in the Americas (66 per cent in the United States) and another 23 per cent are divided almost evenly between Europe and Africa. Obviously, the Americas, with only 15 per cent of the world's population and the United States, with only about five per cent, have highly disproportionate shares of the total number of AIDS cases. When crude and age-specific AIDS rates are considered, the Americas again rank highest, but are followed by Oceania, Africa and Europe respectively. Rates for the Americas are roughly three times those for Oceania, four times those for Africa, and eight times those evident for Europe. The pattern of international population movement also varies by region, and appears to have shifted somewhat between the mid 1970s and the mid 1980s. For the earlier period, European countries accounted for over half of the total number of arrivals and departures (68 per cent and 56 per cent respectively), followed by the Americas (25 and 22 percent) and Asia (5 and 16 percent). By the mid 1980s the Americas accounted for about half of both departures and arrivals (51 and 47 percent, respectively), followed by Europe (41 and 40 percent) and Asia (16 and 12 percent). In short, although the total number of international arrivals and departures increased (with minor exceptions) over this period in all regions, the concentration of movement shifted from Europe to the Americas, particularly the United States. Taken together, the nations of the Americas and Europe, which account for about 87 percent of the current AIDS caseload, are either the origin or destination of around 90 percent of international population movements. The other high prevalence region, Africa, is neither a major sender nor a major recipient of international movers.

Examination of the relationships among the AIDS prevalence indicators shows that the crude rate and the age-specific (25-39) rate are highly correlated (r = .978 to .999) at the global level and within geographic regions (Asia, Africa, Europe and the Americas). The total number of cases is not significantly related to the crude and age-specific rates when all countries are considered, or within the Asian and American regions; it is, however, moderately related to both the crude and age-specific rate for countries in Europe and Africa (r = .60 to .70). Total population size is related to AIDS prevalence only for the Americas (r = .848), which probably reflects the relatively large number of cases in a few populous countries (e.g. The United States, Brazil, Canada and Mexico).

TABLE 2. Zero-order Correlations Between Indicators of AIDS Prevalence (Number of Cases, Crude Rate, Age-specific Rate) and Indicators of International Arrivals for Selected Countries.

	Period[1]	Number of Cases		Crude Rate[2]		Age Specific Rate[3]		Number of Countries
		Total Movers	Movers per Capita	Total Movers	Movers per Capita	Total Movers	Movers per Capita	
Students (In Country)	E	.867	.091	.863	.313	.830	.297	41
Students (In Country)	L	.919	.069	.099	.003	.100	-.002	72
Refugees (In Country)	L	.654	-.017	.420	.216	.334	.224	72
Total Arrivals	E	.141	-.039	-.003	.608	-.009	.589	105
Total Arrivals	L	.853	-.016	.078	.554	.007	.546	85
Long Term Immigrants	E	.318	-.016	.146	.196	.107	.165	72
Long Term Immigrants	L	.553	-.032	.318	.304	.295	.302	44
Short Term Immigrants	E	.294	-.064	.158	-.131	.122	-.141	31
Short Term Immigrants	L	.108	-.107	.017	-.207	-.105	-.225	21
Tourist Arrivals	E	.089	-.043	.002	.425	.005	.420	76
Tourist Arrivals	L	.148	-.059	-.044	.574	-.051	.576	66
Holiday Arrivals	E	.769	-.046	.081	.752	-.077	.732	48
Holiday Arrivals	L	.267	-.056	-.031	.542	-.039	.532	50
Business Arrivals	E	.644	-.047	.342	-.072	.257	-.088	44
Business Arrivals	L	.380	-.046	.014	.908	.007	.894	45
Transient Arrivals	E	.052	-.067	-.063	.713	-.073	.653	52
Transient Arrivals	L	-.007	-.083	-.095	.676	-.104	.608	39
Cruiseship Arrivals	E	.971	-.083	.108	.795	.139	.829	39
Cruiseship Arrivals	L	.054	-.090	.209	.163	.292	.204	23
Students Arrivals	E	.990	.008	.728	.076	.687	.075	20
Students Arrivals	L	.996	.086	.966	.053	.944	.034	19
Residents Returning	E	.071	-.036	-.013	.051	-.014	.044	59
Residents Returning	L	-.0456	-.052	-.027	.297	-.031	.291	33
Other Arrivals	E	.006	-.052	.078	-.024	.060	-.018	53
Other Arrivals	L	.996	.272	.091	.669	.084	.654	36

1 Early = mid 1970s; Late = mid 1980s.

2 Per 100,000 Population.

3 Per 100,000 Population between 25 and 29 years of age.

International population movements can be differentiated according to whether they represent arrivals to, or departures from, a given country. This distinction is important because of its implications for efforts to control the spread of AIDS. Countries with high prevalence of AIDS may be less concerned about the HIV status of arriving persons than countries with moderate to low prevalence levels if the volume of arrivals is low; on the other hand, if many people are entering the country, officials may be concerned over the HIV status of incoming persons regardless of the current level of AIDS prevalence in the resident population. Perhaps the more critical question is whether international departures are coming disproportionately from high prevalence countries. If so, the question of whether HIV testing should be conducted at the country of origin may be debated more seriously.

Following this line of reasoning, we have separated our analysis according to whether the data represent arrivals or departures. Tables 2 and 3 relate three AIDS prevalence measures to indicators of international arrivals at the global and regional levels, respectively. The number of countries on which the correlations are based differs because of the unavailability of certain arrival indicators for some countries. At the regional level, we exclude Asia and Oceania due to the low number of AIDS cases reported in these regions to date.

Table 2 shows that the number of AIDS cases is positively related to all but two of the 23 arrival indicators, and 10 of these correlations are at least moderate in size (.50 or larger), including those for the number of foreign students and refugees in the country, the number of long- and short-term immigrants, and the number of holiday, business, cruise passenger and student arrivals. Pre-AIDS (early) indicators are just as likely to show a moderate to strong relationship with the number of cases as are the post-AIDS (late) indicators. Moreover, when population size of the receiving country is controlled (column 2), all the relationships considered become so weak they are insignificant.

Relationships between the crude AIDS rate and the arrival indicators are at least moderate in only three cases: the number of foreign students in the country and student arrivals (both early and late). However, when population size is controlled, the coefficients shift dramatically. Nine arrival indicators now show at least a moderate relationship with the crude AIDS rate, none of which were that large when population size was uncontrolled. These per capita arrival indicators include the total number

TABLE 3. Zero-order Correlations Between Indicators of AIDS Prevalence (Number of Cases, Crude Rate, Age-specific Rate) and Indicators of International Arrivals for Selected Countries By Region.

	Period[1]	Number of Cases		Crude Rate[2]		Age Specific Rate[3]		Number of Countries
		Total Movers	Movers per Capita	Total Movers	Movers per Capita	Total Movers	Movers per Capita	
Americas								
Refugees (In Country)	L	.936	-.059	.941	.050	.936	.020	16
Total Arrivals	E	.323	-.085	-.003	.700	-.016	.684	34
Total Arrivals	L	.976	-.065	.059	.528	.048	.520	28
Long Term immigrants	E	.762	-.063	.331	.187	.262	.167	20
Long Term Immigrants	L	.922	-.092	.554	.256	.522	.265	13
Tourist Arrivals	E	.700	-.090	.128	.487	.081	.490	27
Tourist Arrivals	L	.001	-.108	.001	.559	-.009	.554	25
Holiday Arrivals	E	.794	-.100	.035	.751	.035	.740	19
Holiday Arrivals	L	.608	-.124	-.005	.499	-.012	.490	20
Business Arrivals	E	.674	-.157	.406	-.296	.343	-.306	14
Business Arrivals	L	.675	-.108	.020	.921	.013	.916	15
Transient Arrivals	E	.880	-.097	.284	.876	.272	.811	21
Transient Arrivals	L	.879	-.109	.258	.858	.219	.777	14
Residents Returning	E	.259	-.090	-.021	.028	-.029	.016	22
Other	E	-.021	-.092	.055	-.001	-.035	.026	18
Other	L	.998	.329	.035	.875	.023	.863	18
Europe								
Tourist Arrivals	E	.359	-.158	.145	.332	.177	.343	26
Tourist Arrivals	L	.793	-.099	.527	.385	.555	.382	20
Students	E	.889	.403	.441	.659	.444	.665	22
Students	L	.960	.530	.515	.665	.526	.681	21
Refugees	L	.808	-.021	.517	.365	.528	.372	17
Total Arrivals	E	.436	-.031	.241	.325	.281	.331	23
Long Term Immigrants	E	.856	.250	.517	.496	.536	.475	21
Long Term Immigrants	L	.496	-.255	.351	.312	.377	.291	19
Africa								
Tourist Arrivals	E	.113	-.210	-.132	-.171	-.118	-.171	25
Tourist Arrivals	L	-.178	-.219	-.262	-.214	-.258	-.215	16
Students	L	-.123	-.289	-.167	-.254	-.167	-.266	22
Refugees (In Country)	L	.089	.076	-.031	.208	-.029	.205	25
Total Arrivals	E	-.086	-.196	-.215	-.185	-.210	-.187	23
Total Arrivals	L	.164	-.317	-.032	-.269	-.034	-.271	13

1. Early = mid 1970s; Late = mid 1980s.

2. Per 100,000 Population.

3. Per 100,000 Population between 25 and 29 years of age.

(early and late), and tourist (early), holiday (early and late), business (late), transient (early and late), and cruise passenger (early) arrivals. The pattern of relationships is thus erratic and does not permit any obvious substantive interpretation.

We also calculated an age-specific AIDS prevalence rate based on the population 25-39 years of age and related it to the gross and per capita arrival indicators (columns 5 and 6). The unsystematic pattern of relationships evident for the number of cases and the crude AIDS rate is repeated. Only three indicators of total movers are of at least moderate strength (number of students in country and both early and late student arrivals), while nine indicators of per capita arrivals show a sizeable association with the age-specific AIDS rate (early and late total arrivals, late tourist arrivals, early and late holiday arrivals, late business arrivals, early and late transient arrivals, and early cruise passenger arrivals).

Table 3 considers selected relationships (those for which we had data for at least 10 countries) at the regional level. The pattern of relationships between AIDS prevalence measures and indicators of international arrivals for the Americas and Europe is similar to that observed at the global level. Considering the number of cases reported, the majority of indicators of total movers show moderate to strong associations, but when population size of the receiving country is controlled, all but a few of the relationships are eliminated. As at the global level, both the crude and age-specific AIDS rates for the Americas and for Europe are related to a number of arrival indicators, but the size of the coefficient is often considerably different for total and per capita mover measures (though more consistent for the European countries). For Africa, the observed relationships are uniformly weak and frequently negative.

Data for departures are presented in Table 4. Because of insufficient data for regional level only the global pattern will be examined. While a number of indicators of the total number of departures are at least moderately related to the total number of AIDS cases, these associations disappear when the size of the sending population is controlled. Indicators of total departures do not appear to be even moderately related to either the crude (column 3) or the age-specific (column 5) AIDS rates. However, a number of moderate to strong relationships are evident for departures per capita (columns 4 and 6). Both the crude and age-specific AIDS rates are correlated with per capita indicators of total departures (early and late), long-term emigrants (late), the

Table 4. Zero-Order Correlations Between Indicators of AIDS Prevalence (Number of Cases, Crude Rate, Age-Specific Rate) and Indicators of International Departures for Selected Countries

	PERIOD[1]	Number of Cases		Crude Rate[2]		Age-Specific Rate[3]		
		Total Movers	Movers per Capita	Total Movers	Movers per Capita	Total Movers	Movers per Capita	Number of Countries
Total Departures	E	.456	-.048	.205	.543	.014	.529	93
Total Departures	L	.826	-.039	.088	.747	.092	.745	69
Long-term Emmigrants	E	.605	-.088	.048	.310	.027	.247	59
Long-term Emmigrants	L	.796	-.095	.302	.735	.298	.714	37
Short-term Emmigrants	E	-.027	-.100	-.015	-.107	-.009	-.111	23
Short-term Emmigrants	L	-.118	-.120	-.188	-.128	-.207	-.141	17
Tourists	E	.273	-.060	-.019	-.616	-.026	.599	59
Tourists	L	.664	-.056	.038	.938	.041	.931	43
Holiday	E	.258	-.122	-.062	-.105	-.071	-.108	31
Holiday	L	.757	-.075	-.075	.988	-.072	.987	20
Business	E	.258	-.196	-.071	-.158	-.078	-.173	28
Business	L	.799	-.057	-.100	.828	-.099	.827	18
Transient	E	.058	-.075	-.044	.719	-.052	.703	35
Transient	L	.011	-.114	-.067	.836	-.074	.826	21
Education	E	.811	-.058	.013	-.074	.018	-.076	20
Residents Leaving	E	.706	-.050	.382	-.067	.304	-.073	46
Residents Leaving	L	.389	-.125	-.046	.642	-.047	.641	26
Other	E	.216	-.105	-.039	.041	-.038	.036	34
Other	L	.993	.102	.960	.059	.952	.054	29

[1] Early = mid 1970's; Late = mid 1980's

[2] Per 100,000 population

[3] Per 100,000 population between 25 and 39 years of age

number of tourists leaving (early and late), holiday departures (late), business departures (late), transient departures (early and late), and the number of residents leaving the country (late). Of the various relationships considered in this study, this latter set offers the most consistent, if not obviously interpretable results. The higher the crude and age-specific AIDS rates in a country, the higher the volume of departures per capita. However, because these relationships are seen for both the early (pre-AIDS) and late (post-AIDS) periods, this finding does not suggest that people are leaving their countries to escape the threat of contracting AIDS. Rather, it implies only that countries with a high rate of AIDS cases are more likely to be origins for international population movements than are low prevalence countries. Whether the population of movers contains a high or low proportion of HIV infected persons is an open question that cannot be answered on the basis of available data.

POLICY RESPONSES AND IMPLICATIONS

Whether real or imagined, the threat of an increased risk of spreading HIV infection and AIDS through international population movements has resulted in restrictive reactions by some governments (World Health Organization, 1987; Panos Institute, 1988). Several types of international movers are being affected. Foreign students are now required to submit to HIV screening by the governments of Belgium, Costa Rica, Czechoslovakia, the Federal Republic of Germany, India and the Soviet Union. Foreign workers have reportedly been singled out for screening by Kuwait, South Africa and the United Arab Emirates. Nationals returning from abroad must undergo HIV testing in Bulgaria, Cuba, Iraq, South Africa, and the Soviet Union. The Soviet government has indicated that foreign diplomats may be screened, depending on the judgement of "competent ministries" and the nature of existing treaties. Finally, a number of countries - Bulgaria, China, Costa Rica, Cuba, the Federal Republic of Germany (though apparently only the State of Bavaria), Iraq, the Philippines, Thailand, and the United States - have implemented HIV testing for all or most foreign immigrants and persons desiring long-term residence.

Clearly, all sovereign states "........ claim the exclusive authority to decide who shall enter and who shall become a citizen" (Weiner, 1985). However, states vary considerably in terms of what Weiner (1985) calls "rules of entry and exit", i.e., the conditions under which aliens are allowed to enter or are barred from entering a country and the conditions under which citizens, residents, or visitors are allowed or forced to leave a country. While little research has been conducted on the determinants or consequences of variations in these access rules, it appears that in at least some countries health status is a significant consideration (Druhot, 1986). Thus there is some legal precedent for national governments to require that persons seeking entry prove they are not infected with the AIDS virus.

Nonetheless, a World Health Organization consultant group (1987) has concluded that mandatory screening of international travellers is unlikely to reduce the rate of spread of HIV to and within countries. This would be true even for a country that has no HIV infection, assuming that nationals travelling abroad would have to be re-admitted even if they tested positive.

The dilemma of how to protect simultaneously the public health and the rights of individuals and social groups believed to threaten public health is not easily resolved. However, those who would promote policies that restrict commonly recognized rights of selected classes of persons have the responsibility of demonstrating that the threat is real and that the restrictive action will be effective. With regard to the contribution of international population movements to the spread of AIDS, the available evidence does not justify assumption of a causal connection. Policies that would restrict international movement or discriminate against travellers are therefore premature, at best.

REFERENCES

Darrow W W, Gorman E M, Glick B P (1986). The social origins of AIDS: social change, sexual behaviour and disease trends. In Feldman D A., Johnson T M (eds): "The Social Dimensions of AIDS: Method and Theory", New York: Praeger, pp 95-107.

Druhot D M (1986). Immigration laws excluding aliens on the basis of health: a reassessment after AIDS. J Leg Med 7: 85-112.

Panos Institute (1988). Travel Restrictions, AIDS Watch 1.

Weiner M (1985). International migration and international relations. Pop Dev Rev 11: 441-55.

World Health Organization (1987). Report of the Consultation on International Travel and Aids. WHO/SPA/GLO/87.1 Geneva: Special Program on AIDS.

Part II: THE IMPACT

The Global Impact of AIDS, pages 81-93
© 1988 Alan R. Liss, Inc.

11.   IMPACT OF AIDS ON SOCIAL ORGANIZATION

M Carballo and M Carael

Global Programme on AIDS, World Health
Organization, Geneva, Switzerland.

Three main points deserve mention in regard to the impact
of AIDS on social organization. The first is the remarkable
attention AIDS has already generated among policy makers,
health scientists and the public. Against a backdrop of other
chronic health problems, many of which still continue to provoke
a far greater morbidity and mortality, AIDS has assumed a
visibility and predominance rarely seen in respect of a health
issue. The second is how little is known about the social and
behavioural aspects of HIV transmission and, hence, about what
might be the ultimate implications for society. The third is that
although concern has mounted with regard to its increasing
spread, with respect to the absence of a vaccine or therapy, with
respect to the democratic character of its transmission, few
major changes have been made in the design of national health
and social services to accommodate and deal with the potential -
or indeed already being experienced - impact of AIDS.

In questioning what AIDS will mean for patterns of social
organization, however, we must also acknowledge that given the
paucity of data currently available, few of those questions can
be answered with any definitiveness. By raising them the need
for contingency planning may be highlighted, and the possible
role of health and social services emphasized.

We have heard that three relatively distinct patterns of
AIDS epidemiology have emerged. Each has its own implications
for social organization. In North America, Western Europe and
Australia, HIV infection has tended to focus around homosexual
acts and drug injecting with shared needles and syringes. A
second pattern, more specific to East, Southern and Central

Africa, parts of the Caribbean and Latin America, involves heterosexual transmission and affects equal numbers of men and women. The implications of this pattern for perinatal transmission of AIDS are obvious with between 30-60% of all infants born to infected mothers themselves being infected. In the Pacific and Asian regions, the prevalence of AIDS is low and is primarily linked to sexual contact with infected individuals from countries in North America, Northern Europe and Africa.

Population maintenance is a cornerstone of social organization and how AIDS might affect this has been addressed already. AIDS is unique in that unlike previous epidemics which have typically affected the very young and the very old, it primarily attacks those in the 20-40 year old bracket, at the peak of their reproductive careers. In a typical Pattern I country, the national mortality rate among 25-34 year old men will increase by two-thirds due to AIDS over the next three years. By 1991 the number of deaths among men in this age group will be greater than the total number of deaths from the four current major causes of death - traffic accidents, suicides, heart disease and cancer (Curran, 1985). This mortality will occur primarily among homosexual men and men using drugs by injection with needle sharing. Few reliable data are available on the extent of bisexuality, making it difficult to predict how AIDS related to homosexual acts will eventually impact on female mortality or reproductive health.

In the case of drug injecting behaviour, however, it is increasingly clear that drug injectors - male or female - constitute a direct link to the heterosexual, and not necessarily drug using, community. Their impact on the pediatric community has also become apparent in many cities in North America and Europe where the majority of cases of perinatally acquired HIV infection is related to drug injecting among one or both parents.

Given the covert nature of drug injection and the lego-political and social proscriptions against drug use, it may be difficult to reach drug injectors in many societies with the education, counselling and treatment that are necessary for effecting changes in needle-sharing behaviour, if not drug use. A continued spread of HIV infection among drug injectors, with continued implications for infant and young child mortality, can therefore be anticipated for some time, especially where innovative outreach programmes are not developed or effective (WHO, 1988).

It is in Pattern II countries, where AIDS is heterosexually transmitted and where ratio of infected men to women is 1 : 1, that the implications of the epidemic could have the greatest impact on population and reproduction. In a city of 1 million inhabitants where 40% of the population i.e., 400,000 can be expected to fall in the 20-50 year old age range, then over 2,000 AIDS-related deaths can be anticipated in 1991, raising the adult mortality rate in that city by over 100%. In areas where 10% of pregnant women are HIV-infected (and current estimates for some cities range between 5% - 30%), the increase in infant mortality due to HIV may be in the order of 40 per 1,000, rising accordingly with increasing levels of maternal infection. What the longevity for perinatally infected infants is remains unclear. Other intercurrent infections and poor socio-economic and environmental conditions are likely to influence adversely the well-being of these infants. Irrespective of exacerbating or attenuating factors, however, infant and young child mortality will inevitably increase.

Children who are not necessarily infected but who are dependent for care and nutrition on adults or older siblings, who themselves become ill or die, will also be placed at greater risk of malnutrition and other infectious diseases as a result of inadequate care and nurturing. This may be especially so in subsistence economy situations, or any situation where infant and young child health is already and has traditionally been seriously challenged.

In societies where formal social welfare systems are poorly developed, older people are also often dependent on younger, economically active family members for sustenance and support. There is a strong possibility that AIDS will impact, albeit indirectly, on their quality of life and ultimately on their health, although it is perhaps too early to assess how mortality rates in these older populations will be affected.

In considering these epidemiologic patterns we must, nevertheless, bear in mind that HIV seroprevalence rates are far from geographically uniform. Within Pattern II countries, for example, they vary from 0% to 28% according to the urban area in question, and between cities and rural areas (Piot and Carael, 1988).

In those cities where the current prevalence of HIV infection is estimated to be around 25-30% of the adult population (ibid), the long-term impact of HIV infection will be considerable, in terms of morbidity and mortality, particularly if effective control and prevention measures are not quickly introduced, accepted and followed by the populations concerned.

In many Central and Eastern African countries, however, rural populations still account for 90% of the total population; with current prevalence rates that range between 1 and 2%, these populations are for now at a much lower risk of significant increases in mortality and related change in demographic structures as a result of HIV infection. The exceptions may be certain rural areas of Tanzania and Uganda where there has been sizeable population movement in recent years (due to civil strike and military campaigns), and where up to 10% of selected rural adult populations are currently HIV infected (Mhalu et al, 1987; Carswell, 1987). But no matter what individual national variations obtain, the mortality differentials that have emerged in recent years between rural and urban settings (10-20% lower in urban than rural) (Akoto and Tabutin, 1987) and which are the product of higher educational levels, better environmental sanitation and access to medical care in urban areas, may nevertheless be diminished. This may go on to alter the way in which urban centres are perceived by rural people and may, in turn, influence existing patterns of rural-urban migration.

Urbanization and Social Networks

Urbanization and the social networks of rapidly growing cities throughout much of the Third World has become an important issue for health planners for many reasons in addition to AIDS. Most urban areas of developing countries have received large influxes of permanent and seasonal rural migrants who have been typically characterized by their age and sex selectivity. Young, single migrants have predominated. The areas they move to are typically ill-served by both social and health services; in many countries they remain only marginally employed and employable.

Where, in addition, these new migrants cannot draw upon well established community affiliations, social support for those individuals and families with HIV-related problems may be less spontaneous and more difficult to mobilize.

Anecdotal information from some countries suggests that resultant "out" migrations of people seeking care and support from families still living in rural areas can be anticipated. How extensive such migrations may go on to be is difficult to assess and could change with time, especially as alternative socially adaptive mechanisms emerge. But where it does occur, the opportunities for onward transmission and spread of the disease to rural areas need to be considered.

Overall urbanization patterns in Central and Eastern Africa are unlikely to be affected, however. The growth of cities in this region is in the order of 6-8% per year; a half of this is now due to in-migration (United Nations, 1985). Unless cities become identified as foci of AIDS infection in the eyes of rural people, migration to cities will probably continue at the same rate as it has until now. On the other hand, where cities do become associated in the mind of the rural populations with risk of HIV infection and AIDS, those who traditionally move to and from urban areas, such as traders and seasonal migrants, may go on to be viewed with suspicion and this, in some degree, could begin to affect economic and cultural communication between rural and urban communities.

In many parts of Africa, where it has become normative for young people to go to urban centres for higher education, fears about exposure to AIDS may also begin to undermine this practice and temporarily influence existing processes of educational development.

On the other hand, in countries where the prevalence of HIV infection in rural areas is high and where urban centres are seen, rightly or not, as centres of specialized AIDS-related health care and treatment, the converse of this pattern of migration could emerge.

Health and Social Welfare Services

How health and social services will cope is of paramount importance. Traditionally a problem in resource poor countries, industrialized societies are also beginning to be concerned about the ability of their health and welfare systems to deal with AIDS.

In low income areas or developing countries coverage by the health and social welfare systems is at best limited and the possibility of comprehensive care being made available is questionable. Other long-standing health problems have themselves not been, to date, well responded to outside of major urban areas - be this at a tertiary, secondary or primary level - and it is unlikely that the added burden of AIDS can be met through existing systems with the type of broad medical and psychosocial support that is required in the context of AIDS.

That in some cities, 40% of all hospital beds are taken up with AIDS patients, suggests that already scarce resources are being seriously threatened and other health problems may be receiving less attention. How long the additional load can be managed will depend on local policy, the magnitude of the AIDS problem locally, the way in which the community perceives AIDS, the response of health care workers themselves, and the resources that can be mobilized to support the formal system.

Even in economically advantaged countries, the economic costs and manpower resources required to provide the medical care follow-up needed may go beyond the current capacity and design of many existing health and social welfare systems.

In parts of North America and Europe, alternative systems such as the Shanti Project of California, the Terrence Higgins Trust in the United Kingdom, or the Noah's Ark project in Sweden, have emerged. Often initiated, staffed and in many cases financed by high-risk persons and groups, these systems seem to be able to provide a quality of constant and appropriate psychosocial care including counselling that may ultimately be able to improve the possibility of those with AIDS remaining non-hospitalized for longer and with a better quality of life than would be the case in many hospital settings.

Where AIDS becomes more prevalent, it may be that alternative systems such as these will increase in number and coverage. In complementing the role and responsibilities of the formal health care system they may eventually create a model for other chronic disease care. Certainly, there are already instances of these programmes providing education, counselling and screening services to non high-risk groups and advice and training to health personnel from the formal system. In Sweden, the Noah's Ark programme has now become affiliated with the Swedish Red Cross which provides Noah's Ark with the benefit of a longer established infrastructure, while offering the Red Cross a source of knowledge and experience that is new and highly relevant to counselling needs in blood transfusion activities.

In rural areas where formal health care systems have traditionally been unable to provide the type and quality of coverage needed, reliance on traditional medicine and care is a well-established reality. These traditional services will probably be resorted to more than ever in the context of AIDS, particularly where allopathic medical care is associated with failure to cure AIDS (Carswell, 1988).

The Family

As a resource in health care, the family has traditionally proved important through previous epidemics, famine and wars. Especially in societies with extended kinship systems, the ability of the family to provide para-medical and psychological support has been well documented. The emergence of the nuclear family in some societies may have reduced this ability, particularly in countries that have experienced a rapid urbanization and accelerated disruption of traditional family systems. The nuclear units that have emerged in many recently urbanised situations are perhaps more fragile and less well supported than the nuclear families of established industrialized society, and certainly the extended family networks of traditional rural societies (Parkin and Nyamwaye, 1986).

There are again anecdotal reports from the United States and East Africa (Katabira E T, personal communication) that families may not be able to deal as spontaneously with AIDS as they have been with other health problems, and that the traditional reliance on extended kin systems may not be as warranted as it was in previous crisis situations. Any consideration of this dynamic needs to consider the possible impact which fear and misunderstanding about the transmission of AIDS, and the implications of AIDS for domestic life, have on the integration of the sick into everyday routines.

Patterns of divorce, separation and widowhood, may also change in some countries. In Africa, generally, rates of divorce and separation vary between 3 and 12% (Bongaarts et al, 1984), compared to other regions of the world such as the USA and UK where over 30% of marriages end in divorce. The numbers of divorced persons at any one time are low because of the tendency of divorced or separated men and women to remarry quickly. In areas where the prevalence of HIV infection is high, even low rates of divorce and separation followed by rapid remarriage or entry into new unions will increase the probability of exposure to infection. In some cities of Central Africa, married women who report having had more than one union, and women who are divorced, are already showing such an increased risk of HIV infection (Carael et al, 1988).

Whether knowledge or awareness about AIDS and its relationship to sexual behaviour and number of sexual partners will affect the stability of unions and monogamy remains to be seen. As the number of AIDS cases increases and as more information about AIDS becomes widely available, multiple partner promiscuity could become less common and unions more stable.

Alternatively, in areas where such indicators of AIDS as weight loss, frequent diarrhoea and lymphadenopathy are common and associated with other conditions as well as AIDS, misunderstanding about the symptoms of AIDS may give rise to stress in families where symptoms are wrongly associated with HIV infection.

Yet another scenario is that where the prevalence of heterosexual HIV infection is high, mortality differentials between men and women may lead to higher than usual numbers of men or women becoming widowed. As yet it is not clear whether the natural course of HIV infection varies by sex, although the potentially adverse impact of repeated pregnancies on maternal health has been raised (Weber et al, 1986). If this is the case, societies where frequent and unregulated pregnancies are the norm may see an increase in maternal mortality and hence larger numbers of widowed men. If in turn, the relationship between HIV infection and sexual behaviour becomes well established in the eyes of the community, the opportunities for remarriage by these men may be lessened.

Changes may emerge too in the perceived value of contraception and child-bearing. On the one hand, as HIV infection goes on to be associated with significantly heightened risks of pregnancy wastage and neonatal mortality, the pressure on women to reproduce may increase, further debilitating the mothers themselves and, in turn, increasing rates of infant and young child mortality. It is noteworthy that many areas where heterosexual HIV infection is common are the same areas where family planning has, to date, made few inroads, either in terms of acceptability or service delivery. Conversely, in societies where low fertility has become the norm, fear of sexually transmitted HIV infection may even further delay child bearing.

Over the last 20 years the age at first marriage has shown a tendency to increase, especially in urban settings. Changes in attitudes to sex outside stable unions, however, may ultimately strengthen the practice of early marriage where partners are sought because they are thought young enough to not have been sexually exposed to HIV. Certainly, in societies where female virginity at marriage or first union has traditionally been highly valued, the practice of marriage at puberty or near puberty could become more attractive. In sub-Saharan African societies, age at marriage varies between western Africa where the age of girls at first marriage ranges between 15 and 22 years, and East Africa where slightly later marriage is common (Bongaarts et al, 1984).

Changes in family structure are also likely to influence child-rearing and care practices. Death or persistent illness among child carers, regardless of cause, can place infants at risk of interrupted development. Where nuclear families are the dominant form, as in the United States and Europe, such adaptive mechanisms as temporary child fostering have become common and relatively well developed ways of dealing with the problem situations. These approaches are receiving renewed attention in the context of AIDS in the USA and parts of Western Europe, although adoption of HIV-orphaned or unwanted children remains problematic. In much of sub-Saharan Africa the need for adoption in the formal administrative sense has traditionally been pre-empted by extended family systems of taking in the offspring of kin who die. Grandparents, brothers or sisters, and others in the community have traditionally assumed the responsibility, for caring for orphaned children, according to local kinship systems and traditions (Bledsoe and Gage, 1987).

Indeed, child-rearing responsibilities, even when both parents are alive and well, have been shared among family members. Thus, in parts of urban East and West Africa it is not unusual for children to be sent back to rural areas to be brought up by elder family members or other relatives. Should the association of AIDS with urban life become more evident to young couples, the practice of sending younger children back to rural families may become more dominant.

What the long-term health and social impact of this practice might be is not clear. Ostensibly sound, it should however be noted that studies of malnutrition and growth retardation among young children have suggested that total care by non-biological mother can be a negative factor, especially where older people become the principal caretakers and are themselves either not aware of the needs of the child or are unable to provide the constant care and stimulation that young infants and children need (Carballo and Bankowski, 1981).

In general, urbanization has been associated with the liberalization of sexual taboos and controls (Page and Lesthaeghe, 1981). Where, till recently, it has been acceptable or normative for married men to have regular sexual partners outside of marriage, the AIDS epidemic could possibly make such relationships less acceptable. This, however, could lead to a higher emphasis and dependence on prostitutes.

Prostitutes, male or female, are increasingly at high-risk of infection with up to 80% of female prostitutes working in selected areas HIV-positive (Van de Perre et al, 1985; Plummer et al, 1987; Mann et al, 1986; CDC, 1987). It is perhaps too early to say whether prostitution as a widely practised occupation will change in response to AIDS. Legislation, as well as the personal preference of clients, may diminish the number and accessibility of prostitutes. Fear of infection may reduce recruitment into sex for money, and cause many who are already involved to seek other types of work. In Ethiopia, long before the AIDS epidemic, government policies sought to provide prostitutes with retraining in other types of work. Such initiatives may become more common.

CONCLUSIONS

At this point in the evolution of the AIDS epidemic, with its considerable geographic variability and its differential prevalence among men and women in different parts of the world, no easy conclusion can be reached with regard to its ultimate impact on social organization.

Population structures as such may not go on to be seriously altered if well designed and effective control and prevention measures are introduced. But there is, in the pattern of AIDS epidemiology typical of certain countries, the potential to elevate mortality among selected groups with subsequent effects on overall fertility behaviour and child survival rates. The question of the indirect impact of HIV infection and AIDS on the health of the very young and the very old merits close scrutiny.

The implications for primary health care, both from a preventive and a care point of view are equally obvious. Community based interventions will become increasingly necessary both in developed and developing societies. These interventions will need to relate to the characteristics of the groups or communities in need and may go on to benefit from a planning process that incorporates a more sensitive assessment of those characteristics than has traditionally been the case in the planning and formulation of health care programmes. It may be that the experience of responding to AIDS control and prevention needs will strengthen the concept and operation of primary health care approaches in general. Certainly, it is already highlighting the gaps that have existed in many formal health care systems, be this in terms of their ability to provide early and pre-emptive identification of health problems, surveillance, care or preventive education.

At the level of the family, the epidemic will probably bring about significant changes, especially in areas where the prevalence of AIDS is high. The day-to-day management of AIDS will place a load on family and friendship structures that goes beyond what has been called for previously. The psychological element of fear will need to be overcome, both with respect to caring for the ill as well as reproduction. Under the best of circumstances, support to families affected by AIDS may be required but what form this will take, or what is actually feasible, is not yet clear.

In the past, society has adjusted to a variety of problems because shared values and goals were easily generated. HIV infection and AIDS could provoke very varied attitudes, beliefs and levels of commitment among different individuals and groups, all of which could make the adjustment process more complex and laden with opportunities for conflict.

REFERENCES

Akoto E, Tabutin D. Inegalités Socio-économiques en Matière de Mortalité en Afrique au Sud du Sahara. Seminar on Mortality and Society in Sub-Saharan Africa, October 19-23, 1987, Yaoundé, Cameroon.

Bledsoe C H, Gage A. Child Fostering and Child Mortality in Sub-Saharan Africa. Seminar on Mortality and Society in Sub-Saharan Africa, October 19-23, 1987, Yaoundé, Cameroon.

Bongaarts J, Frank O, Lesthaeghe R (1984). The proximate determinants of fertility in Sub-Saharan Africa. Population and Development Review 10: 511-537.

Carael M, Van de Perre P, Lepage P et al (1988). Risk factors for HIV infection among heterosexual couples in Central Africa 1988. AIDS, in press.

Carballo M and Bankowski Z, (Editors) Child Abuse 1981, CIOMS.

Carballo M. The Critical Role of Counselling. World Summit of Ministers of Health on programmes for AIDS Prevention. London 26-28 January 1988.

Carswell J W (1988). Impact of AIDS in developing countries. Brit Med Bull 44: 183-202.

Carswell J W (1987). HIV infection in healthy persons in Uganda. AIDS 1: 217-221.

Curran J W, Morgan W M, Hardy A M, Jaffe N N, Darrow W W, Dowdle W R (1985). The epidemiology of AIDS: current status and future prospects. Science 229: 1352-1357.

Mahlu F, Bredberg-Råden U, Mbena E et al (1987). AIDS 1: 217-221.

Mann J. Global AIDS: Epidemiology, Impact, Projections and Global Strategy. World Summit of Ministers of Health on Programmes for AIDS Prevention. London 26-28 January 1988.

Mann J, Quinn T C, Francis H. Sexual Practices associated with LAV/HTLV-III Seropositivity among Female Prostitutes in Kinshasa, Zaire. International Conference on AIDS. Paris. June 23-25, 1986.

Morbidity and Mortality Weekly Report. CDC, 1987;36: 11

Parkin D, Nyanwaye D (eds) (1986). "Transformation in African Marriage". Manchester: Manchester University Press.

Page H J, Lesthaeghe R (eds) (1981). "Child-spacing in Tropical Africa. Traditions and Change". London: Academic Press.

Piot P, Plummer F A, Mahlu F S, Lamboray J L, Chin J, Mann J M. AIDS : an international perspective. Science, 1988; 1: 573-579.

Piot P, Carael M (1988). Epidemiological and sociological aspects of HIV infection in developing countries. Brit Med Bull 44: 68-88.

Plummer F A, Simonsen J N, Ngugi E N et al. Incidence of HIV and Related Diseases in a Cohort of Nairobi Prostitutes. 3rd International Conference on AIDS, Washington D.C. 105 June 1987.

Todaro M P. Internal Migration in Developing Countries. International Labour Office, 1976, Geneva.

United Nations, Estimates and Projection of Urban, Rural and City Populations 1950-2025: The 1982 assessment. United Nations, 1985, New York.

Van de Perre P H, Clumeck N, Carael M et al (1985). Female prostitutes: a risk group for infection with HTLV-III. Lancet 2: 524-526.

Weber D J, Redfield R R, Lemon S M (1986). AIDS : Epidemiology and significance for the obstetrician and gynecologist. Amer J Obstet Gynecol 2: 155-157.

World Health Organization (1988). Intravenous Drug Use and Risk of HIV Infection. Meeting Report, 23-25 November 1987. Geneva, WHO, in press.

The Global Impact of AIDS, pages 95–106
© 1988 Alan R. Liss, Inc.

12. THE IMPACT OF THE SPREAD OF HIV ON
POPULATION GROWTH AND AGE STRUCTURE IN
DEVELOPING COUNTRIES

R M Anderson

Parasite Epidemiology Research Group, Department
of Pure and Applied Biology, Imperial College,
London University, London SW7 2BB

INTRODUCTION

Prediction of the future course of the human
immunodeficiency virus (HIV) epidemic and its likely impact on
human population size and structure in developed and developing
countries presents many problems at present. There are a
number of possible approaches to making predictions. One
method is to fit simple empirical functions to available
longitudinal data on the incidence of either the disease AIDS, or
HIV infection, and extrapolate into the future. In developed
countries this approach has produced reliable short-term
projections over one to three years, but there is no a-priori
reason to assume that extrapolation is valid beyond a short time
span.

An alternative approach is to construct simple or complex
models of viral transmission within and between specified risk
groups, in a framework that captures the demographic process
that determines population size and structure. Models that
incorporate the underlying epidemiological and demographic
processes have the potential to give greater predictive power but
their value is restricted by the necessity for more and better
epidemiological data than are currently available (Anderson et
al, 1986; May and Anderson, 1987).

The need for a better understanding of the basic processes
that determine the typical course of infection in individuals, and
spread between people, is central to the problem of prediction.
Many uncertainties still surround key epidemiological factors.
These include the following: the fraction of those infected who

will proceed to develop AIDS and on what time scale; the
likelihood of vertical transmission from infected mother to child;
the pathogenicities of human retroviruses other than HIV-1 (e.g.,
HIV-2) that are currently spreading in certain countries; the
importance of co-factors such as genital ulcers in heterosexual
transmission; the probabilities of transmission from female to
male and vice versa; the degree to which the infectiousness of
infected patients varies throughout the long and variable
incubation period of the disease and patterns of sexual behaviour
in defined communitities. This is a depressing catalogue of
ignorance. Furthermore, the long and variable incubation period
of the disease, plus the many social, ethical and practical
difficulties that surround research in this field, imply that
epidemiological knowledge will only accumulate slowly via long-
term studies. However, the need to assess the magnitude of the
problem, even crudely, is urgent in order to facilitate the long-
term planning of public health authorities and international aid
agencies. This has stimulated a number of studies of the possible
demographic impact of AIDS in the developing world that employ
very simple mathematical models of the major demographic and
epidemiological processes (Anderson et al, 1988; May et al,
1988a; 1988b). The major conclusions of this recent research are
reviewed in this paper in the light of the available
epidemiological data.

EPIDEMIOLOGICAL DATA

We begin by considering the available quantitative data on a
series of key epidemiological processes that have been identified
via theoretical studies as central to an understanding of the
spread, persistence and impact of HIV infection. The degree to
which the virus will spread in a given community is largely
determined by the magnitude of the basic reproductive rate of
infection R_0. This quantity measures the number of secondary
cases of infection produced, on average, by one primary case in a
susceptible population. With respect to the horizontal component
of transmission (via sexual contact) in populations of adults, R_0
is defined as the probability of transmission, β, per partner
contact times the effective average rate of partner change, c,
times the average time period, D, during which an infected
person is infectious to others ($R_0 = \beta cD$) (Anderson et al, 1986).
The effective average rate of partner change is given
approximately by the mean rate of partner change, m, plus the
variance to mean ratio of partner change rates, σ^2/m
($c = m + \sigma^2/m$; see May and Anderson, 1987). The influence of the
variance on the magnitude of R_0 highlights the importance of

heterogeneity in sexual partner change rates to the spread of HIV. A small proportion of individuals with high rates of partner change (relative to the average) can make a disproportionately large contribution to the reproductive potential of the infection.

Data on the three components of R_0, namely, β , c and D is very limited at present. From studies of transfusion associated cases of AIDS in developed countries, the average incubation period is thought to be around 8-9 years (a lower bound on the estimate) (Medley et al., 1987). Whether individuals are infectious over the entire incubation period is uncertain at present. One hypothesis is that there are two periods of peak infectiousness, one soon after infection and one as a patient progresses via ARC to AIDS (Pedersen et al, 1987).

TABLE 1. Estimates of the rate of spread of HIV Infection from longitudinal serological data (data sources given in Anderson et al, 1988)

Location	Time period	Population surveyed	Doubling time	Parameter combination	Basic reproductive rate R_0 (D = 15 yrs)
Kenya, Nairobi	81-85	Prostitutes	1.0	0.75	11.2
Kenya, Nairobi	81-85	Men with STDs	1.7	0.48	7.2
Kenya, Nairobi	70-86	Pregnant women	2.9	0.31	4.6
Zaire, Kinshasa	70-86	Pregnant women	3.5	0.26	4.0
Uganda, Kampala	85-87	Pregnant women	1.1	0.69	10.3
Central African Republic	85-87	General population	1.1	0.66	9.9

In developing countries the incubation/infectious period may be somewhat less than in developed countries as a result of more frequent exposure to a larger range of opportunistic infectious agents (Piot et al, 1988; Quinn et al, 1986). Information on β and c is again very limited. However, an indirect estimate of the parameter combination βc can be obtained from longitudinal date recording the rate of spread of infection in a given population (Anderson et al, 1988). A series of estimates of βc, the doubling time in the prevalence of HIV infection, t_d, and the basic reproductive rate R_0 are recorded in Table 1 for various communities in developing countries.

Vertical transmission is an important component of any assessment of the impact of AIDS. Current estimates of the proportion of babies born to infected mothers who acquire infection range from 22 to 60% as recorded in Table 2. The disease AIDS appears to develop much more rapidly in infants than adults (Medley et al, 1987) and mortality amongst infected children in developing countries appears to be very high (Piot et al, 1988).

TABLE 2. **Percentage of babies born to HIV infected mothers who acquired infection via vertical transmission (data sources given in Anderson et al., 1988)**

Country	Sample size	Percentage infected
Europe	71	22
United States	88	33
United Kingdom	85	35
Central African Republic	25	44
Italy	24	58
France	56	59

The fraction of infected persons who will develop AIDS is uncertain at present. Current estimates from cohort studies in the United States and Europe suggest that 30-40% develop AIDS over an 8-9 year period although a higher proportion show some symptoms of immunodeficiency. It appears probable that a high fraction of infected people will develop full blown AIDS but the time scale of, and variability in, disease progression are unclear as yet. Once AIDS develops life expectancy is short in relation to the average incubation period, being of the order of 1 year.

DEMOGRAPHIC PARAMETERS

Much more is known about the basic demographic parameters in developing countries than about the key epidemiological processes. Birth and death rates tend to be much higher in developing countries than developed countries and, currently, net population growth rates in Sub-Saharan Africa for example range from 2 to 4%. In most developed countries net growth rates are close to 0%. Life expectancies from birth in Africa are approximately 50 to 55 years while crude live birth rates per 1000 head of population are typically in the range of 45 to 55 per annum (Anderson et al, 1988). Dependency ratios, defined as the number of children below age 15 years and elderly people over 64 years, divided by the number of adults between 15 to 64 years are typically around 1.0. In contrast the ratio at present in the United Kingdom is 0.5.

MODEL PREDICTIONS

The simple models developed in recent papers aim to provide a rough understanding of how AIDS deaths resulting from horizontal and vertical transmission might effect demographic patterns, of the time scales of such effects and of how the possibility of a decline in population size and change in population age structure depend on the demographic and epidemiological parameters. Study of these simplified models is a preliminary to future numerical work on much more complicated and realistic models when data quality, and general understanding of the epidemiology of infection and disease, improves. A major function of simple theoretical analysis is the identification of data needs in future research.

1. Population growth rates

The simplest of the models developed by Anderson et al, (1988) and May et al, (1988a,b) is based on the assumption of homogeneous mixing amongst sexually active adults. It therefore represents an extreme case since heterogeneity in rates of

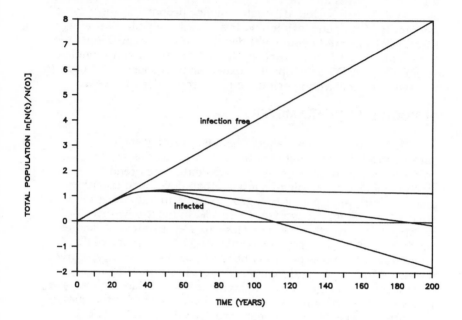

Figure 1. Population trajectories through time, recorded as the natural logarithm of population size at time t divided by population size at time t=0 when the infection was introduced, as predicted by a delayed recruitment model (Anderson et al, 1988) for various values of the fraction of healthy babies born to infected mothers. The top line denotes 4% growth in an uninfected population and the remaining trajectories from bottom to top denote predictions with the fraction of healthy babies set at 0.3, 0.5 and 0.7 respectively. Life expectancy of uninfecteds was set at 52 years, the incubation (=infectious) period was set at 8 years and the time delay to recruitment to the reproductively mature age class was fixed at 15 years. The rate of infection was set at 0.233 per capita per year. All infected were assumed to develop AIDS.

---

partner change, for example, where most heterosexuals have few sexual partners and a few have many, will act to reduce the demographic impact suggested in models based on homogeneity in mixing. With this caution in mind, the predictions of the simple models reveal that for a range of plausible parameter values AIDS is capable of changing population growth rates from positive to negative values over time scales of a few decades. An illustration of this prediction is displayed in Fig. 1 where population trajectories through time from the point of introduction of HIV infection are depicted for various combinations of parameter values.

The net growth rate of the population in the absence of infection was set at 4% and the top lines denote temporal change in an uninfected population in which the fraction of babies born to infected mothers who acquire infection (all assumed to die soon after birth) was set at 0.3, 0.5 and 0.7 (from top to bottom). The life expectancy of uninfecteds was fixed at 52 years, the incubation (=infectious) period was set at 8 years (with all infecteds developing AIDS on an average time scale of 8 years), the time period to recruitment to the reproductively mature age class was fixed at 15 years, and the doubling time of the infection in the general population in the early stages of the epidemic was assumed to be 3 years (Table 1).

With the assumption that all infecteds develop AIDS on some characteristic time scale (with an exponential distribution), a wide range of values for the parameters that define the rate of spread of infection (i.e. the parameter combination βc), the average incubation period (D), the fraction of healthy babies born to infected mothers and the population growth rate prior to the invasion of HIV, result in population growth rates changing from positive to negative as the infection spreads (Anderson et al., 1988). If we relax the assumption that all infecteds develop AIDS, the range of parameter values that result asymptotically in negative growth rates is somewhat reduced but it is still predicted to encompass plausible combinations as judged by the available data (Table 1). This is illustrated in Fig. 2 where the basic reproductive rate of infection, R_0, required to reverse the sign of population growth is displayed as a function of the fraction of infecteds who develop AIDS, f, and the fraction of healthy babies born to infected mothers, ϵ . In this particular example the populations growth rate prior to the invasion of HIV was set at 2% per annum and the incubation/infectious period was fixed at 15 years. Note that e must be small and f large if HIV is to induce negative population growth rates (i.e. plausible values for R_0).

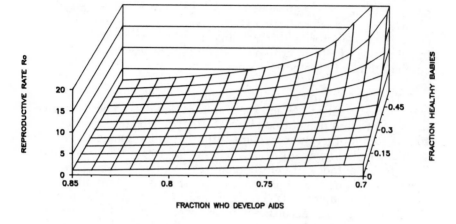

FRACTION WHO DEVELOP AIDS

Figure 2. The basic reproductive rate of infection required to reverse the sign of human population growth as predicted by simple delayed recruitment models of HIV transmission (see May et al., 1988a, b; Anderson et al., 1988). The critical reproductive rate is plotted as a function of the fraction of infecteds who develop AIDS and the fraction of healthy babies born to infected mothers. The incubation period of AIDS was fixed at 15 years and the life expectancy of uninfecteds was set at 52 years with a 2% population growth rate.

---

2. Time Scales

The period t_c, denoting the time taken before the population begins to decline after invasion by HIV (given that the prevailing demographic and epidemiological parameters permit this outcome), is given very approximately by :-

$$t_c \sim (\ln(1/\Delta))/(R_0-1)/\Delta-r)$$

where Δ is the fraction infected at time t=0, R_0 is the basic reproductive rate, D is the average infectious period and r is the pre-HIV infection population growth rate (May et al, 1988a,b). For low to moderate infection rates, like those observed in the general population in Zaire, Uganda, and Kenya, the time to the onset of population decline is predicted to be many decades (40-70 years).

3. Population age structure

Simple homogeneous mixing models of the transmission of HIV can be extended to encompass the full age structure of a population (May et al., 1988a,b; Anderson et al.,1988). This enables a rough assessment to be made of the impact of the spread of infection and deaths due to AIDS on the dependency ratio defined as the number of children below age 15 years and elderly people over 64 years, divided by the number of adults between 15 and 64 years. Recent studies of age structured models suggest that AIDS is unlikely to induce significant changes in the ratio (Anderson et al., 1988). On the one hand, the direct effects of mortality in the sexually active adult age classes due to AIDS tends to increase the ratio. On the other hand, the general depression of overall population growth rates due to the reductions in effective birth rates as a result of vertical transmission plus the death of reproductively mature adults, tends to increase the ratio. For some plausible ranges of values for the epidemiological and demographic parameters, age structured models predict a slight decrease in the dependency ratio (Fig. 3).

DISCUSSION

The three major predictions generated by the simple models that are outlined in the preceeding sections may be summarized as follows. AIDS may or may not reverse the sign of population growth rates depending on the magnitude of certain key epidemiological parameters. It is more likely to do so if a high fraction of those infected eventually develop AIDS and die and if the efficiency of vertical transmission is high (Fig. 2). Irrespective of the reversal of the sign of the growth rate, it appears probable that the disease will have a very significant impact on population abundance over the coming decades, in developing countries in which the infection is spreading rapidly in the general population. If the disease is able to reverse the trend of population growth, the time taken before the population begins to decline after the invasion of HIV is predicted to be long, of the order of a few to many decades. Whether or not AIDS will decrease or increase the dependency ratio within an infected population depends on the values of the major demographic and epidemiological parameters. For plausible values the disease is predicted to have little impact.

These conclusions are derived from deliberately simplified models and from limited data on key epidemiological processes.

As such, they must be accepted with great caution. As data

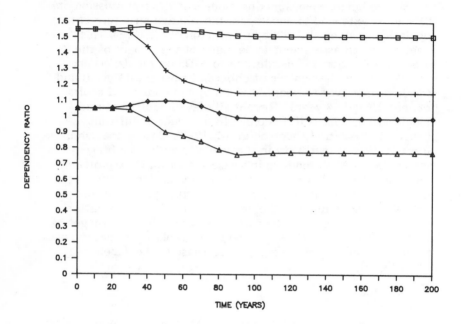

Figure 3. Temporal changes in the dependency ratio (ages less
than 15 and greater than 64/ages 15-64) as HIV spreads,
predicted by an age structured model that combines demographic
and epidemiological processes (Anderson et al., 1988). Four
different numerical simulations are recorded. In all the
maturation delay was set at 15 years and the life expectancy of
uninfecteds at 52 years with an incubation period of 15 years
where all infecteds develop AIDS. From top to bottom, 4%
growth rate and 0.7 healthy babies born to infected mothers, 4%
growth rate and 0.3 healthy babies, 2% growth rate and 0.7
healthy babies and 2% growth rate and 0.3 healthy babies.

─────────────

accumulates and biological understanding improves, more
complex and realistic models can be formulated. Of particular
importance is the need to incorporate heterogeneity in sexual
activity to mirror variability in sexual partner change rates and
age dependency in activity. Other issues that must be addressed
include the role of co-factors, such as other sexually transmitted

infections, in transmission and variability in infectiousness
throughout the long and variable incubation period. This latter
factor is probably of importance in both horizontal and vertical
transmission. In principal there is no great difficulty involved in
constructing simulation models to mirror these complications. In
practice, however, the major difficulty at present is obtaining
parameter estimates from empirical studies. There is an urgent
need for data on a series of key topics, namely; the distribution
of sexual partner change rates in defined communities; age
related changes in sexual activity; the incubation and infectious
periods of AIDS and HIV-1 in developing countries; the likelihood
of vertical and horizontal transmission throughout the long and
variable incubation period and the fraction of those infected who
will develop AIDS and on what time scale. Such information is
essential to improve the accuracy of predictive work.

ACKNOWLEDGEMENTS

I gratefully acknowledge financial support from the ODA,
PANOS and MRC. I have greatly benefited from discussions with
Robert May, Angela McLean, Graham Medley, Stephen Blythe
and Elke Konnings.

REFERENCES

Anderson R M, Medley G F, May R M and Johnson A M (1986). A
preliminary study of the transmission dynamics of the human
immunodeficiency virus (HIV), the causative agents of AIDS. IMA
J Math Appl Med Biol 3: 229-263.

Anderson R M, May R M, McLean A R (1988). Possible
demographic consequences of AIDS in developing countries.
Nature 332: 228-223.

May R M, and Anderson R M (1987) Transmission dynamics of
HIV infection. Nature 326: 137-142.

May R M, Anderson R M, McLean A R (1988a). Possible
demographic consequences of HIV/AIDS epidemics: I. Assuming
HIV infection always leads to AIDS. Math Biosc (in press).

May R M, Anderson R M, McLean A R (1988b). Possible
demographic consequences of HIV/AIDS epidemics: II. Assuming
HIV infection does not necessarily lead to AIDS. Lect Notes
Biomath (in press).

Medley G F, Anderson R M, Cox D R, Billard L (1987). Incubation period of AIDS in patients infected via blood transfusion. Nature 328: 719-721.

Pederson C, Nielsen C M, Vestergaard B F et al. (1987). Temporal relation of antigenaemia and loss of antibodies to core antigens to development of clinical disease in HIV infection. Brit Med J 295: 567-569.

Piot P, Plummer F A, Lamboray J, Chin J, Mann J M (1988). AIDS: the international perspective. Science 239: 573-579.

Quinn T C, Mann J M, Curran J W, Piot P (1986). AIDS in Africa: an epidemiological paradigm. Science 234: 955-963.

The Global Impact of AIDS, pages 107–110
© 1988 Alan R. Liss, Inc.

13. AIDS AND FAMILY PLANNING PROGRAMMES

Pramilla Senanayake and Anthony Klouda,

International Planned Parenthood Federation,
Regents College, Regents Park, London NW1 4NS

The International Planned Parenthood Federation (IPPF) is
the largest international Non-Governmental Organization (NGO)
working in the field of family planning. We work in over 120
countries. This paper in the main reflects the experience gained
from many of our member Family Planning Associations (FPAs)
who are currently working or plan to work in AIDS prevention
programmes.

The subject of AIDS and family planning will be discussed in
two broad areas. The first part will defuse some myths relating
to AIDS in family planning. Secondly, the positive linkages
between AIDS prevention and family planning programmes will
be discussed.

There are three myths about the way in which AIDS might
reduce population growth, and the role of FPAs in programmes
for population control (whether it is for increasing or decreasing
growth rates). Because some people believe FPAs generally to be
involved in a simple, or direct way in **reducing** population
growth, they think that FPA activities become irrelevant during
the AIDS crisis. This is to misunderstand totally the work of
FPAs. In fact, their work becomes **more** important during the
AIDS crisis, and this will become clearer as we defuse the myths
one by one.

The first is a myth that sexually active adults will die from
AIDS in sufficiently large numbers to reduce population by
lowering the number of births. In other words, it is believed that
there would be fewer adults capable of procreation and therefore
that no further efforts are needed in population control by FPAs.

This myth needs to be defused. Family planning programmes promote the health rationale for family planning. They do so by preventing pregnancies that are :-

- too early (births to girls under the age of 18)
- too late (births to women over 35)
- too many
- too close together (births spaced less than two years apart).

No family planning programme relies on increasing numbers of deaths for curbing uncontrolled population growth. On the contrary, family planning programmes strive to improve the quality and length of life and thus directly contribute to the decrease of population growth rates.

In most countries, the general mortality rates are very much higher than current AIDS mortality rates and will remain so for a long time. Family planning programmes attempt to reduce maternal and child mortality rates. Even maternal mortality rates - globally speaking - are far in excess of AIDS mortality rates. Worldwide, 500,000 women die each year from causes related to pregnancy, childbirth and puerperium. Most of these are preventable through family planning programmes. If mortality rates had been so simply linked to population, we would had had much more of an impact from other illnesses than from AIDS.

The second myth is that AIDS can give rise to higher infant mortality through infants themselves being infected, or because uninfected children may be more susceptible to higher mortality from being orphaned early in life and neglected due to social and economic factors. It is therefore postulated again that family planning programmes are irrelevant. Indeed, this myth should be defused. On the contrary, family planning programmes strive to :-

- save lives by reducing infant and child mortality
- ensure better health for children
- improve the quality of life

The third myth is that since a large number of AIDS deaths occur in the most economically productive age group, this, in turn, results in :-

- increased national poverty

- reduced socio-economic development
- increased mortality and morbidity.

This presumed cause of lowered population growth is again said to pre-empt the use of family planning programmes. No simplistic relationship exists between population growth, socio-economic development and productivity of particular groups. However, it is horrifying to suggest we do nothing about HIV control in order to curtail population growth, just as it is wrong to suggest we do nothing to curtail other deaths.

The next part of this paper will look at the positive linkages between AIDS prevention and family planning programmes.

What is the connection?

Because the mode of transmission is now predominantly sexual, FPAs are at the heart of its prevention. They are perhaps the only group that has the peculiar blend of qualities, experience and skills that are needed. They :-

- provide advice about reproductive health and sexual life to the age group most affected by HIV
- have skills in communication with defined groups
- have experience in counselling
- promote and teach the use of condoms
- give sexual education to young people
- develop programmes concerned with women's roles in development
- promote male involvement and reponsibility in family planning
- provide advice about contraception, which may be especially valuable for those who are infected by HIV.

Family planning programmes provide contraceptive choice for couples. Close links exist between the type of contraceptives couples may choose to use, and HIV transmission. For example, in family planning programmes, condoms are described as having a failure rate of up to 10%. When used regularly and properly, this failure rate can be brought down to as low as 1%. For couples who are currently using the so-called more reliable contraceptives such as injectables, oral contraceptives or voluntary sterilisation, would it be useful to recommend the additional use of a condom in order to prevent the transmission of HIV? These are the kinds of decisions that family planning programmes need to make in close consultation with those working in the AIDS field.

A further complication arises with regard to family planning clients who wish to become pregnant. They need to be advised with regard to the risks that they may run of infecting the infant if they are uncertain about their own, or their partner's HIV status.

In conclusion, it needs to be pointed out that, at the present time, there is no cure for AIDS. Therefore, there is a need for information that is practical and relevant for different groups to assist them in preventing themselves from being infected. This information needs to be relevant for different groups of people at risk. Family planning programmes have experience and expertise at reaching special groups - for example, young people. The family planning associations are a grass-roots network and are important for links with the hard-to-reach groups. However, the population implications of AIDS as identified earlier in this paper and defused as myths intensifies, rather than diminishes, the need for proper family planning services.

Finally, family planning programmes improve the quality of life by promoting optimum conditions for childbearing, for both mother and infant. To reiterate, these programmes endeavour to prevent those pregnancies which are :-

- too early
- too late
- too close
and - too many.

The Global Impact of AIDS, pages 111-117
© 1988 Alan R. Liss, Inc.

14.   IMPLICATIONS OF THE MEDICAL AND SCIENTIFIC
ASPECTS OF HIV AND AIDS FOR ECONOMIC
RESOURCING

A Griffiths

Director of Research, Health Management Institute,
5 Rue de Florisaat, Geneva 1206, Switzerland

INTRODUCTION

The purpose of this keynote paper is first, to explain the
basic inputs and problems in estimating the economic impact of
AIDS; second, to give an order of magnitude of the costs, and
finally to introduce some of the key economic issues.

The inputs for costing

So far, no global estimate of the economic impact of AIDS
has been attempted, and many national estimates have been
partial, covering only the cost (or price) of personal medical
care. (1) As the epidemic moves through its exponential growth
phase, the need for adequate estimates will become increasingly
urgent.

The basic inputs for assessing the economic impact of AIDS
are :-

1.   The numbers of AIDS cases by age and sex, now and in
     future years.
2.   Estimates of the morbidity and mortality associated with
     these cases - including their health and social care
     requirements, and working years lost.
3.   Cost estimates for the care required and for the working
     years lost.

1.   Expected numbers

Both present and future numbers of AIDS cases are

uncertain. The notification and recognition of cases are incomplete even in developed countries, for example by an estimated 20% in the USA, and by much more in developing countries. For example, it is most unlikely that only 5 of Nigeria's 100 million inhabitants have AIDS, as reported to WHO. Projections are still less certain. For example, the estimate of 74,000 new cases in the USA in 1991 is subject to a margin error from 46,000 to 92,000, (2) and the global estimate of 1.5 million cases by 1991 is even less certain.

The best immediate prospects for estimating expected numbers appear to be from simple models with limited but reliable data. The detailed data required for more sophisticated modelling are not likely to be available for some time. (3-4)

The main data requirements for estimating future numbers are :-

1)   The number of HIV positives.
2)   The rates of transmission between infected and uninfected groups.
3)   The incubation rates of the disease.

2.   Morbidity, mortality, health and social care and loss of work

Experience so far suggests that the best way to capture morbidity and mortality data is through patient records. The task would be considerably easier if hospital teams made an effort to maintain complete records, including care given by other services, and periods when patients' health prevents them from working. The main difficulties here are the logistics of data collection, incomplete recording, and two items that are hard to predict -therapy improvements, and changes in the strategies of care.

3.   Costing

The costs to consider may conveniently be classified in four groups, according to whether they are direct or indirect, visible or invisible. (5)

Direct costs are the costs of health and social care, including both personal care, and non-personal services such as blood screening and replacement, health education, staff training, and research.

Many cost estimates include only the **direct visible costs,** that is those included (visible) in health and social service accounts. However, there are also **direct invisible costs,** represented by services provided by family, friends and charities. Though unpaid, these services nevertheless represent a real consumption of resources, and hence a real cost.

These costs are often ignored, since they do not have to be covered in health agencies' budgets, and because there are usually few data from which to estimate them. However, their omission can lead to suboptimization in choosing care strategies. For example, a community care oriented strategy is almost certainly cheaper than a hospital based one. However, it may be considerably less economic than it at first seems if the costs of unpaid services are added, and may also place a heavy cost burden on families and other unpaid sources of care.

The main difficulty in estimating direct costs is that the unit costs of particular services are not known. Average costs or reimbursed prices have often been used instead. Experience suggests that both underestimate the real costs. (6)

Indirect visible costs are the costs of economic production lost through morbidity and mortality, including estimates for the value of unmarketed production, such as housekeeping tasks and subsistence agriculture. These costs have tended to be ignored by health authorities. However, as a fatal disease of young, mainly male adults, AIDS represents a substantial loss of working years. Studies in developed countries suggest that these costs are five to six times higher than the costs of health care and research. (7)

The fourth category of costs are **indirect invisible costs.** These are the costs of intangible reactions and lower quality of life through factors like pain, incapacity, fear, anxiety, isolation, stigma, depression etc. These costs are clearly important for AIDS, but are so difficult to evaluate that no study to date has attempted to estimate them.

4. Some orders of magnitude and financing issues

The most complete costing of AIDS so far done is that of Scitovsky and Rice for the USA. (7) It estimated the total cost of AIDS in current dollars in 1986 at $8.7 billion, of which $1.1 billion was for personal health care, over $0.5 billion was for research and other non-personal services, and the remaining $7.0 billion (80%) was the present value of the lifetime loss of economic production, almost all of it through premature death. In 1991, the estimated cost of the 144,000 cases expected to be alive is $66.5 billion: over $8.5 billion for personal health care, $2.3 billion for research and non-personal services, and $55.6 billion (84%) for the lifetime loss of production.

These numbers are large. They are still large when related to the number of AIDS cases and deaths. The estimated average cost of personal health care per case alive is $35,600 in 1986, and over $49,400 in 1991 (research and non-personal services excluded). The average value of the lifetime loss of production per AIDS death amounts to $600,000 for those dying in 1986, and over $800,000 for those dying in 1991.

However, these costs must be viewed against the perspective of total costs. The estimated cost of personal medical care for AIDS cases represents only 0.3% of all personal health care expenditure in 1986 and 1.4% in 1991. Annual growth in health care spending has often far exceeded this. The indirect cost of AIDS is more disturbing; it rises from 2.1% of all losses due to illness and death in 1986 to 12% in 1991.

Developed countries which have not done their own costings can probably obtain a reasonable order of magnitude estimate of the cost of AIDS by scaling the above costs per case and per death to GNP per capita and applying them to expected cases and deaths.

The overall conclusion is clear. For developed countries, the costs of AIDS are large but sustainable. The main economic issue is who will pay? How will the costs be shared? A widespread problem is that budgets and reimbursement rates are often below the real costs of care for AIDS patients. This problem takes on serious proportions when it is borne in mind that in most countries AIDS cases are concentrated in a few major urban areas and are more often cared for by the public hospitals and health services of these areas. (6,8) Thus, while only an estimated 0.06 beds per 1,000 population will be occupied by AIDS patients in the USA in 1991, these beds will be concentrated in a few areas like New York, Los Angeles, and San Francisco. However, this concentration is declining as the epidemic grows.

In a few developed countries, lack of health insurance or minimal cover are also problems. For example, in the USA 35 million people are estimated to be in this situation. Intravenous drug users frequently have little or no insurance, and AIDS sufferers who lose their jobs through their illness risk losing their job-related health insurance at the same time. In addition, insurers are increasingly refusing or restricting insurance cover for HIV positives and AIDS sufferers. Indeed, in Switzerland, one insurer is reported to have reduced reimbursement to AIDS patients considered to have knowingly risked infection. (9)

The situation for developing countries, with high levels of HIV infection and AIDS, notably in the African region, is much more serious. First they cannot hope to meet the very high costs of AIDS patients. For example how many developing countries spending as little as one or two dollars per capita or even less on drugs can afford $12,000 per year for the drug AZT for hundreds or thousands of patients? Nevertheless, resources will probably be transferred from primary care and rural areas to the large hospitals and other urban services pressed by large numbers of AIDS cases, and it will take some time before it is realized that without large increases in drug and other expenditures, the best policy is probably to allow patients to die as comfortably as possible at home.

Second, in African countries, and probably in many of the other developing countries not yet heavily infected, the principal mode of transmission is heterosexual. The population at risk is not relatively small groups of male homosexuals and intravenous drug users, but the whole sexually active population, so that very large numbers may be infected before transmission slows down. (10)

This problem is further compounded by the fact that effective prevention requires the use of the condom by a significant proportion of the population. Experience suggests that this is not likely to happen. First, health education explaining AIDS and promoting the use of condoms has not been easy in developed countries, it will be considerably harder in developing ones. Furthermore, experience from family planning programmes suggest that the condom has low cultural acceptibility, and is neither physically nor economically accessible to substantial proportions of the population.

In these circumstances the demographic effects of AIDS are likely to be considerable. In high prevalence populations the mortality rate in adults aged 20 to 50 years old could equal or exceed the death rate from all other causes. Child mortality rates, currently between 80 and 140 per 1000 live births could increase by 10-50% (half the babies born to HIV positive mothers are infected, and half of these die within the first two years). (10) Such an increase in mortality is also likely to decrease the birth rate. Overall, the demographic effects could well be analogous to those of a war.

Economically, since plentiful young labour is one of the few economic assets of developing countries, and the resources for capital substitution are very limited, the relative effects in terms of economic productivity are likely to be markedly greater than in developed countries.

CONCLUSION

In developed countries, despite the substantial costs of AIDS, the main requirements are institutional ones to ensure adequate and equitable funding. The loss of economic production, though considerable, would not appear to be large enough to have structural implications. In developing countries, however, both the direct and indirect costs of AIDS are likely to pose substantial problems, and the earlier they can be clarified the sooner appropriate action can be taken to limit and correct them.

REFERENCES

1. Sisk J E et al. The Costs of Aids and other HIV infections: Review of the Estimates. Staff paper Office of Technology Assessment, US Congress Washington DC, May 1987.

2. Morgan W M, Curran J W (1986) Acquired immunodeficiency syndrome: current and future trends. Public Health Rep. 101: 459-465.

3. Knox E G (1986). A transmission model for Aids. Euro J Epid 2: 165-177.

4. May R M, Anderson R M (1986). Transmission dynamics of HIV infection. Nature 326: 137-142.

5. Griffiths D A T (1981). Economic evaluation of health services. Concepts and methodology applied to screening programmes. Rev. Epidl. et sante publ. 29: 85-101.

6. Green J et al. Projecting the Impact of AIDS on hospitals. Health Affairs, Fall 1987, 19-31.

7. Scitovsky A A, Rice D P (1987). Estimates of the direct and indirect costs of acquired immunodeficiency syndrome in the United States 1985, 1986 and 1991. Public Health Rep 102: 5-17.

8. Andrulis D P et al (1987). The provision and financing of medical care for AIDS patients in US public and private teaching hospitals. JAMA 258: 1343-1346.

9. Coupables d'etre victimes, Hebdo, Lausanne, 1988, 25 Feb. 42-49.

10. Chin J. AIDS, the national response and the role of development organizations. Working paper, Surveillance, Forecasting and Impact Assessment Global Programme on AIDS, WHO Geneva, 1988.

The Global Impact of AIDS, pages 119-122
© 1988 Alan R. Liss, Inc.

15.   MEDICAL COSTS OF HIV AND AIDS IN BRAZIL

Hesio Cordeiro

President of the National Institute of Medical Care
and Social Welfare, Rua Mexico, 128-9 andar, Rio de
Janeiro, RJ CEP 20031, Brazil

Even prior to December 1982, when the cumulative
incidence of AIDS cases in the United States reached 879 cases,
absolute incidence was already being used as a measure of the
extreme seriousness of the syndrome. In 1984, with an
accumulated total of 7,025 cases, attempts were being made in
the United States to demonstrate the gravity and the
significance of the disease, not only through the measurement of
incidence but also through rates that would indicate, in relative
terms, the impact of the epidemic, as gauged by means of health
indicators. In this fashion, Curran and colleagues labelled as
"dramatic" the effect of AIDS on the "life expectancy" of the so-
called risk groups, among which there is a high incidence of the
disease. This statement may be made on the strength of a study
carried out in the United States for the determination of the
number of "lost potential years of life" due to AIDS and other
causes. According to this study, for single males between ages 25
and 44, in 1984 in the United States, the number of lost potential
years of life due to AIDS, was slightly lower than that attributed
to cancer. In Manhattan and San Francisco, 43% and 74%,
respectively, of the potential life expectancy lost were due to
AIDS.

In Rio de Janeiro, which in Brazil is the second in
importance from a political and economic standpoint and where
the number of AIDS cases is only exceeded by that for Sao Paulo,
69% of deaths between 1983 and 1986 were due to factors other
than disease, such as accidents, murders and suicides, whereas
AIDS accounted for only 5%.

Obviously, such reasoning, based on case frequency, would

lead to the conclusion that AIDS is not a significant health problem in Brazil. Nevertheless, we are certain that the relevance of the disease stems from the social factors involved.

AIDS, which started in economically hegemonic societies such as the United States and reached into such deeply ingrained areas of human concern as sex and death, stands out as a disease which may indiscriminately strike different sectors of society. Therefore, in a conservative society, something new like AIDS was inevitably bound to have the impact that we are presently witnessing.

We cannot, however, overlook the epidemiological context of AIDS in Brazil. In this connection, we must acknowledge the efforts made by the Brazilian Government, through the AIDS Prevention and Control Program, to use existing resources fully and effectively, despite structural and conjunctural hindrances and with due consideration given to our sanitary, social, political and economic situation.

HIV infection in Brazil is already affecting several sectors of society. Its impact is clearly seen in the economic, social, political, ethical and legal areas. One of the most serious consequences can be seen in the economic sector, where there has been a very sizeable increase in the cost of medical care services, which is the topic of our presentation. At this point, therefore, we should give you a general outline of the public health services which provide medical care in Brazil.

Brazil is politically organized as a federation of states which are in turn subdivided into municipalities. The federal, state, and municipal levels of health care are integrated, for the purpose of guaranteeing the right to health, to which the State believes every citizen is entitled. Two important ministries -the Ministry of Social Security and Welfare and the Ministry of Health - are responsible for preventive measures, medical care, and rehabilitation. The Ministry of Social Security and Welfare is in charge of assuring medical care to the population through the National Institute for Medical Care - INAMPS. At the present time, the Brazilian Public Health System is undergoing far reaching structural changes, as part of a nation-wide movement that aims at a thorough reform of the health sector. A unified and decentralized system is being set up for the purpose of concentrating both resource allocation and financial administration at the state and municipal levels. Resources come from mandatory social security withholdings from employees and employers. The resources allocated to INAMPS in 1987 and 1988 accounted for 36% and 31% respectively, of the total budget of the Ministry of Social Security and Welfare.

INAMPS provides medical care to the Brazilian population through hospitals and out-patient facilities of the public health care network and through the contracting of services from the private sector. At the present time 95% of AIDS patients are cared for at public hospitals.

To date, it has not been possible to figure out the direct cost of HIV infection in Brazil. A number of factors account for this, and special mention should be made of :-

* The shortage of health care facilities, particularly laboratory services, to meet the demand; and
* The fact that Brazil is dependent on the international markets for the purchasing of kits for HIV-diagnosis.

Actually, the only solution in which the serological confirmation of HIV infection is absolutely indispensible is for the control of transfusion blood and blood products. Nevertheless, the serological test is essential for the laboratory diagnosis of AIDS cases involving patients belonging to groups characterized by high risk behaviours, such as prostitutes, IV drug users, homosexuals, pregnant women, sexual partners of infected individuals.

The resources allocated for blood quality control, added to the resources required for in-hospital medical care, make the cost of care to AIDS patients quite high. The following data pertains to hospital costs and do not include costs related to outpatient care, home care, hospital-day and intangible costs, such as pain, misery, and the fact of becoming an outcast, all of which are essential and significant components of the social impact of AIDS.

The following indicators were used to calculate the cost of medical care for AIDS patients :

* average length of hospitalization;
* research and development;
* depreciation of fixed assets;
* bed occupancy indexes;
* medical, paramedical, and other personnel;
* drugs, with the exception of AZT;

* diagnosis procedures; and
* lethality rate.

A comprehensive analysis of these indicators led to the conclusion that the direct cost per patient-year in Brazil is equivalent to US $21,500.

In view of the fact that 95% of AIDS patients receive free medical health care, the annual cost of hospitalization alone is about US $ 25 million.

The following alternatives have been identified as an attempted solution for the problem of providing adequate health care to these patients in Brazil:-

*   Training of human resources in the field of health, since it is essential that health team personnel develop appropriate technical skills. This will make it possible for cases to be adequately diagnosed and to receive proper care, thus assuring the highest possible level of health support to patients.
*   Health care should be commensurate with the seriousness of the patient's condition. Alternate modalities of health care are being considered, such as out-patient, in-hospital, and home care.

We hold that the complexity of AIDS requires a multi-disciplinary approach to health care. It is indispensible to form multi-disciplinary teams, consisting not only of physicians, including infectious disease specialists and other specialists, but also other health professionals. Nurses, psychologists, laboratory personnel, and social workers are all key elements of such teams.

The participation of society, through organized volunteeer work, is also of special significance in the fight against this serious epidemic.

The obvious conclusion is, therefore, that there is an urgent need to join forces at all levels in order to stem the tide of this scourge of mankind. Only through solidarity and brotherhood among people will it be possible to meet this challenge and conquer such a formidable foe.

Brazil is fully aware that only through a great effort of international cooperation will mankind turn back the threat that the Acquired Immunodeficiency Syndrome represents in the Twentieth Century.

The Global Impact of AIDS, pages 123–135
© 1988 Alan R. Liss, Inc.

16. THE DIRECT AND INDIRECT COST OF HIV INFECTION
IN DEVELOPING COUNTRIES : THE CASES OF ZAIRE
AND TANZANIA

M Over[1], S Bertozzi[2], J Chin[2], B N'Galy[3],
K Nyamuryekung'e[4]

World Bank, Washington[1]; Global Programme on
AIDS, World Health Organization[2]; National AIDS
Control Programme, Zaire[3]; National AIDS Control
Programme, Tanzania[4].

INTRODUCTION

In this paper we present a summary of preliminary results of
studies of the direct and indirect cost of HIV infection in two
developing countries. If the presence of AIDS in a country
affects the demand for (as opposed to the supply of) its exports,
such effects would be additional to those considered in this
paper. Based on only a few weeks effort in each country, the
results are subject to revision as more thorough, definitive
studies are completed in these countries in the course of their
respective national AIDS control programs. But we expect even
these preliminary results to be of use to health care planners as
they begin to make resource allocations to the prevention and
treatment of HIV infection.

For the purposes of this paper, we define the direct cost of
a disease as the cost of treating those who suffer from it, and we
define the indirect cost as the value of the healthy years of life
it steals from society. Our goals are, first, to propose an
approach to estimating the direct and indirect cost of HIV
infection in a developing country and, second, to present
estimates of these quantities for each infected person. Since
reliable estimates do not yet exist for the total number of
infected persons in any single country in the world, it would be
inappropriate to use these estimates of infected person to
compute the total national cost at this stage of our knowledge.
However, one could compute hypothetical estimates based on a
variety of hypothetical rates of HIV infection. In a longer version
of this paper, we will present such hypothetical estimates.

DIRECT COSTS

A principal finding of the two case studies is that the direct cost per patient varies a great deal, even within a single country, depending not only on the particular clinical symptoms with which HIV infection manifests itself, but also on socioeconomic characteristics of the patient and medical and institutional characteristics of the health care options available to that patient. Therefore, rather than provide a single average figure for direct cost of HIV infection in any country, it is preferable to present a range of estimates together with an explanation of the causes of variation.

TABLE 1. Direct cost of HIV Infection per Symptomatic Adult (In 1985 US dollars)

Country	GNP per Capita	Direct Cost		
		Low	Mean	High
Zaire	170	132	-	1585
Tanzania	290	104	-	631
Caribbean Island	1000	-	2723	-
England	8460	-	10200	-
USA	16690	27571	-	50380

Sources :   Tanzania and Zaire: Joint WHO/World Bank estimates.
Caribbean Nation: Unpublished correspondence.
England: Johnson A M, M W Adler, J M Crown (1986). Acquired immune deficiency syndrome and epidemic of infection ...., Brit Med J 293: 491-492
United States, Low: Seage G R (1986). The economic impact of AIDS, JAMA 254: (22)
United States, High: Scitovsky A, M Cline, P Lee, (1986). Medical care costs of patients with AIDS in San Francisco, JAMA, 254: (22)

In Zaire the direct cost of health care per **symptomatic** HIV infected person ranges from a low of $ 132 to a figure twelve times as large of $ 1,585 (Table 1). In Tanzania estimated direct cost ranges from a low of $ 104 to a figure six times as large of $ 631. These estimates are expressed in 1987-88 US dollars converted at official exchange rates and attempt to include the financial costs of all resources used in the course of treatment, whether those costs are financed by the patient's family, by the government or by a charitable organization. However, they do not include an additional cost which health systems and their patients will be forced to bear if the epidemic continues to spread - the foregone health care that would have gone to patients crowded out of the system by AIDS patients. (In government and charitable health care systems which pay health care workers and other factors of production far less than their opportunity costs, there can be no presumption that the financial costs such as those computed here properly represent the cost of the foregone health care.) When more in-depth studies are performed, it will be important to examine the "crowding-out" issue more closely.

The estimates assume that every symptomatic HIV infected adult will seek at least some treatment from modern sector facilities. The low estimate is distinguished from the high estimate in each country by assumptions regarding the characteristics of the patient and the health care options faced by that patient. For example, in Zaire the low estimates assume that the patient restricts himself or herself to the relatively low cost care of the urban or rural "health zone" system, while the high estimates assume the patient ventures out into the higher-cost private health care market. In Tanzania the range of cost variation is smaller, but still important, as patients choose whether to seek the best available modern care or to remain in the village cared for by relatives.

How large are these costs? Although large compared to per capita health expenditures in these countries, these costs should instead be compared to per patient expenditures on other diseases. Studies to make these comparisons have not yet been performed, but we do not expect expenditures per patient for AIDS to greatly exceed those for other serious diseases of adults in the same countries.

Figure 1 presents the range of estimated cost for each of the two African countries together with estimates that are available for the United States, England and a Caribbean nation,

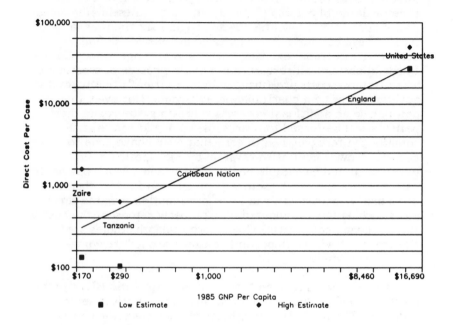

Figure 1. Direct cost vs GNP per Capita.

all plotted against gross national product (GNP) per capita on a
log-log scale. The figure demonstrates that there is a rough
correspondence between the direct cost of HIV infection in a
country and that country's economic situation. Countries in
which resources are limited are forced to spend less on each
patient; more prosperous countries permit themselves to spend
more. The pattern is quite similar to the one that relates overall
national health care spending to GNP per capita.

As countries turn to the preparation of treatment protocols
for AIDS patients, they will want to examine the range of
variation of actual costs within their own and neighbouring
countries. The World Bank and WHO are supporting the
development and refinement of cost estimates like those
reported here in order to contribute to this process. Countries
which are considering recommending treatment protocols which
are substantially more expensive than their physicians are
currently applying will want answers to a question not addressed

by this paper. How large are the additional health benefits currently obtained by the wealthier countries from their additional expenditures?

INDIRECT COSTS

The HIV virus, like other pathogenic organisms, deprives individuals of years of healthy, productive life and robs families of their loved ones. By applying a common method to the calculation of these indirect costs for each of the important diseases, one can compare the costs due to each individual disease and use these estimates as one input to decisions on allocating resources across diseases. We perform this computation in three steps.

First, we estimate the total number of future years of healthy life lost by an average HIV-infected person and by an individual who contracts each of a variety of other relevant diseases and we discount future lost years to the year of infection or contraction. In this paper we use a discount rate of 5%. We count years lost to disability from each disease as a portion of a year lost to death, although disability typically accounts for less than 10% of the years lost from the more important diseases. The first column of Table 2 presents the results for HIV infection and for 13 of the diseases thought to account for the most years of life lost in African countries. These figures show how many years of life could, in theory, be saved by the prevention or immediate cure of one case of each of these diseases. Note that preventing one case of HIV infection will save an estimated 8.8 discounted healthy life years. HIV infection ranks fifth on this measure, after sickle cell anemia, neonatal tetanus, birth injury and severe malnutrition, but ahead of childhood pneumonia, cerebrovascular disease, tuberculosis, measles, malaria and gastroenteritis. Figure 2 facilitates visual comparison among HIV infection and the other 13 diseases with respect to the number of life years which can be saved by averting a single case.

Second, we disaggregate the total future life-years lost from each disease into years lost in each of five age ranges which differ in their productivity implications. We assign a productivity weight to each age range relative to the productivity of a healthy adult aged fifteen to fifty. (Thus, age range zero to five is assigned a weight of zero, age range five to fifteen a weight of .20, age range fifty to sixty-five a weight of .85 and age range sixty-five plus a weight range of .25.) After

TABLE 2. Discounted Healthy Life Years Saved per Case
Prevented

No.	Disease Name	Discounted HLYs saved		Productivity Weighted Discounted HLYs saved	
		Value	Rank	Value	Rank
0	HIV Infection	8.8	5	6.2	5
1	Malaria	2.5	10	1.4	11
2	Measles	3.4	9	1.9	9
3	Pneumonia (Child's)	7.7	6	5.0	7
4	Sickle Cell	17.0	1	8.0	1
5	Severe Malnutrition	11.7	4	6.6	4
6	Prematurity	2.0	12	1.0	13
7	Birth Injury	14.7	3	7.7	3
8	Accidents	2.0	11	1.5	10
9	Gastroenteritis	1.0	14	0.5	14
10	Tuberculosis	5.5	8	3.9	8
11	Cerebrovascular	7.4	7	5.7	6
12	Pneumonia (Adult)	1.5	13	1.2	12
13	Tetanus (Neonatal)	15.3	2	8.0	2

Sources: Except for HIV infection, the diseases are ranked in
order of total number of healthy life days lost as
evaluated in Ghana Health Assessment Project Team,
International Journal of Epidemiology, 1981.

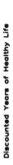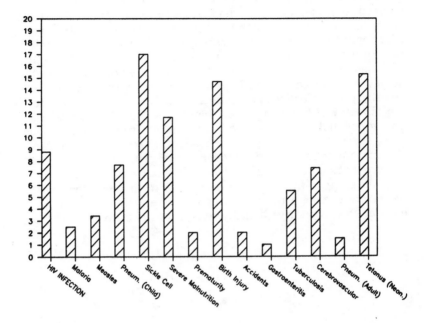

Figure 2. Healthy life years saved per case prevented.

weighting the future life-years lost by their productivity
weights, we again discount them to the year of infection or
contraction and use the totals to rank the relevant diseases as
shown in the third column of Table 2. Figure 3 contrasts the
number of productive healthy life-years lost per case with the
total number of life years lost. Because the productivity
weighting procedure discounts the less productive years, it
dramatically reduces the number of years of life lost per case
for childhood illnesses like sickle cell anemia and prematurity
and has a much smaller effect on adult diseases like
cerebrovascular disease and adult pneumonia. The effect of
productivity weighting on years lost from HIV infection is
intermediate between the childhood and the adult diseases,
because HIV infection strikes both adults and infants in Africa.
According to these calculations, every case of HIV infection
prevented saves about 6.6 discounted productive healthy life
years, more than preventing a case of all but four of the other
diseases.

If a decision-maker is interested only in reallocations of health care expenditures within the health care budget, there is no need to proceed further than we have to this point. By asking his or her staff to estimate the number of cases of each disease which will be prevented or cured by each of a variety of health care programs or mixes of programs within the available health care budget, the policy maker can choose the program mix which achieves the largest feasible gain of productivity weighted healthy years. However, suppose the decision-maker is located in the Ministry of Finance rather than in the Ministry of Health. This individual would want to know whether to reallocate money away from other, demonstrably productive sectors like transport and communication, to the prevention of diseases or perhaps to the prevention of a specific disease like AIDS. The computations we have done to this date are of no help to this decision. It is necessary to take a third step, attaching a monetary value to each of the productive healthy life years to be saved.

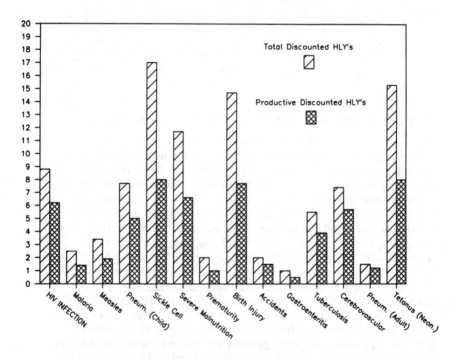

Figure 3. Productive healthy life years saved per case prevented.

There are two competing methods proposed in the health economics literature for valuing years of healthy life in monetary terms. One of these, called the "willingness-to-pay approach", has the advantage of capturing a portion of the psychic value that society attaches to saving a life, but the application of this method requires more in-depth study than has been possible to date. The other method, called the "human capital approach", is based solely on the economic return society receives for a year of the affected individual's labour, which is imperfectly measured by the individual's annual income. The "human capital approach" admittedly underestimates the value of the healthy life year of under- and unemployed individuals and perhaps overestimates the relative value of a life-year of an individual whose salary is based more on monopoly rents than on contribution to society. Nevertheless, weighting the productive years of healthy life lost to a disease by the average income per year can at least provide some provisional guidance to the decision-maker faced with the problem of inter-sectoral resource allocation. The problem is to know which average income to apply.

Each communicable disease affects a somewhat different socioeconomic cross-section of society. Diseases characterised by airborne transmission flourish in urban more than in rural residential patterns; those requiring insect vectors may affect both areas equally or be less prevalent in urban areas with partially effective vector control programs. However, because social and sexual intercourse are closely related, the incidence of sexually transmitted diseases like AIDS is likely to be more determined by socioeconomic strata within residential areas than by the geographic boundaries of those areas. As a working hypothesis we adopt the assumption that three general groups of the population must be distinguished, the rural, the urban with only a primary education and the urban with a secondary education or above.

Table 3 presents estimates for the average wage for each group in each country converted to 1987/1988 dollars and estimates the dollar value of discounted future years of healthy life lost in each of these three groups for each important disease. The ranking of HIV infection in the list of diseases remains unaffected by this procedure - it ranks fifth, with an indirect cost ranging from $ 890 to $ 2,663 in Zaire and from $ 2,425 to $ 5,093 in Tanzania.

TABLE 3. Dollar Value of Discounted Future Healthy Life Years (In 1985 Dollars)

	Zaire			Tanzania		
	Rural Adults	Urban Primary School	Urban Scndry School	Rural Adults	Urban Primary School	Urban Scndry School
Average Annual Income	144	287	431	391	626	821

No	DISEASE NAME						
0	HIV Infection	890	1780	2669	2425	3880	5093
1	Malaria	201	402	603	548	876	1150
2	Measles	273	545	818	743	1189	1561
3	Pneum. (Child's)	718	1435	2153	1956	3129	4107
4	Sickle Cell	1148	2296	3444	3129	5007	6572
5	Severe Malnutrition	947	1894	2842	2582	4131	5422
6	Prematurity	144	287	431	391	626	821
7	Birth Injury	1105	2210	3315	3012	4819	6325
8	Accidents	215	431	646	587	939	1232
9	Gastroenteritis	72	144	215	196	313	411
10	Tuberculosis	560	1119	1679	1526	2441	3204
11	Cerebrovascular	818	1636	2454	2230	3567	4682
12	Pneum. (Adult)	172	344	517	469	751	986
13	Tetanus (Neonatal)	1148	2296	3444	3129	5007	6572

TABLE 4. Total Cost per HIV Infected Individual (In 1985 US Dollars)

		Zaire		Tanzania	
Row No.	Cost Category	Low	High	Low	High
(1)	DIRECT COST Per Symptomatic HIV+	132	1585	104	631
(2)	Per HIV+ Individual	47	560	37	223
(3)	INDIRECT COST Per HIV+ Individual	890	2669	2425	5093
(4)	TOTAL COST Per HIV+ Individual	936	3230	2462	5316
(5)	RATIOS Indirect/Direct	19.1	4.8	65.9	22.8
(6)	Total/Per Capita GNP	5.5	19.0	14.5	31.3

NOTES:

Row (1): From table 1, various entries.
Row (2): A percentage of the Row (1) figure is allocated to year 1 according to the assumed percentage of people infected in year zero who would convert to AIDS in that year. The assumed percentages are 0.1% in each of the first two years and 6% in each subsequent year through the tenth. It is assumed that no conversion occurs after the tenth year so that a total of only 48.2% of HIV positives ever convert.
Row (3): From Row (0) of Table 3.
Row (4): Sum of Rows (2) and (3) above.
Row (5): Ratio of Row (3) to Row (2).
Row (6): Ratio of Row (4) to 1985 Per Capita Income.

TOTAL ECONOMIC IMPACT OF HIV INFECTION PER INFECTED PERSON

Table 4 collects in one place the low and high estimates of direct and indirect costs per case for HIV infection and other important diseases and computes their total. The estimates of direct cost per case of HIV infection are calculated from Table 1 by assuming the conversion rates to AIDS characteristic of the San Franciso cohort, and then discounting those costs to the year of infection, again at a discount rate of 5%. As stated above, the direct cost estimates are not yet available for other diseases.

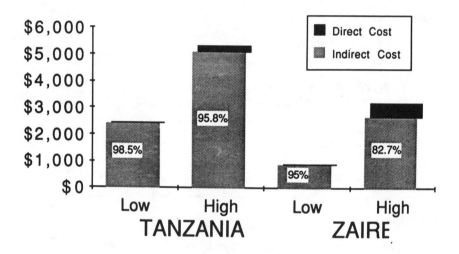

Figure 4. Relative sizes of direct and indirect cost estimates (in 1985 US dollars)

However, as in the case of HIV infection, we expect the indirect costs to dominate the direct costs for all important diseases. (Fig. 4)

Now suppose that the Ministry of Finance decision-maker knows that a certain quantity of financial resources could alternatively be allocated either to producing a known monetary benefit in the transport sector or to a health care program which would prevent a certain number of cases of a disease such as HIV infection. The figure in Table 4 will then permit that decision-maker to place a **minimum** monetary value on those prevented cases. In cases where this minimum produces a monetary return from the health sector investment which equals or exceeds that of the equal cost transport sector alternative, the decision-maker would be guided toward the health sector investment.

Of course the missing piece in this calculation is the cost of the various possible health care programs per case prevented. **In the case of communicable diseases, and especially of epidemics like that of HIV infection , calculation of this cost must take account of the fact that each primary case prevented also prevents secondary and tertiary cases.** Now, while AIDS prevention programs are still in their formative stages, is the time to build in baseline data collection and subsequent monitoring activities, so that the cost per case prevented can eventually be calculated.

The Global Impact of AIDS, pages 137-144
© 1988 Alan R. Liss, Inc.

17. ESTIMATES OF THE DIRECT AND INDIRECT COSTS OF AIDS IN THE UNITED STATES

Anne A Scitovsky

Chief, Health Economics Division, Palo Alto Medical
Foundation/Research Institute, Palo Alto, California,
USA and Lecturer, Institute for Health Policy
Studies, School of Medicine, University of California,
San Francisco, California, USA.

INTRODUCTION

I want to begin with a very brief overview of the magnitude
and demographics of the AIDS epidemic in the United States as
background information for my discussion of the direct and
indirect costs of AIDS in the United States. According to the
Centers for Disease Control (CDC), there have been a
cumulative total of 51,916 cases of AIDS reported through
January 25, 1988 (CDC, January 25, 1988). This is about one-
third of all cases reported worldwide. Of the 51,916 cases,
28,965 - or 56% - have already died. By 1991, the CDC expect a
cumulative total of 270,000 cases of whom 179,000 - or 66% -
have died. The vast majority of cases - 99% - are **adults and
adolescents,** with pediatric cases totalling less than one
thousand.

By age, two-thirds of the cases are in the 20 to 39 year
group and almost 90% in the 20 to 49 year group. **By sex,** 93% of
the adult/adolescent cases are males. **By risk group,** 73% of the
adult/adolescent cases are homosexual or bisexual males,
including 8% who are also IV drug users. IV drug users who are
not homosexuals are the other major group of persons with AIDS
(PWA), accounting for 17% of the cumulative total. Of the
remainder, 4% are heterosexuals (in most cases individuals who
had sexual contact with HIV infected persons) and 3% are
hemophiliacs or persons who had received blood transfusions or
blood products. **By race and ethnicity,** minorities represent a
disproportionate share of the total number of PWA: Blacks are
25% of the adult/adolescent AIDS cases and 12% of the

population, Hispanics are 14% of the AIDS cases and 6% of the population, while Whites are 60% of the AIDS cases and 80% of the population. Looking at **risk groups by race and ethnicity,** 74% of homosexual and bisexual males with AIDS are White, while 80% of the IV drug users who have AIDS are Black or Hispanic.

Of the **children with AIDS,** 76% are the children of parents at risk, i.e., of women who are either IV drug users or partners of males at risk. The vast majority of these children - 78% - are Black or Hispanic.

To date, the epidemic has been concentrated in a number of **metropolitan centers,** with New York accounting for 23% of the total number of cases, San Francisco for 9%, Los Angeles for 8%, and Houston, Washington D.C. and Miami each accounting for about 3%. However, the epidemic is spreading to other areas. In 1984, areas other than these six centers accounted for 43% of all newly reported cases while by 1987 their share had grown to 58%. The CDC expect that in 1991, 63% of all new cases will be outside these six centers.

One final statistic: the distribution by risk group differs widely across the country. In New York City, only 61% of all PWA are homosexual or bisexual males and 31% IV drug users. By contrast, in San Francisco 97% are homosexual or bisexual males.

THE DIRECT PERSONAL COST OF THE AIDS EPIDEMIC

Despite the concern over the economic burden which the AIDS epidemic is imposing on the nation's health resources, hard data on the costs of treating PWA are still relatively scarce and incomplete. To date, only a handful of empirical studies have been published. Retrospective studies were conducted in Boston, (Seage et al., 1986), in San Francisco, (Scitovsky et al., 1987) and in Maryland, (Berger, 1985), where data were collected and analyzed for a number of cohorts of PWA. The California State Department of Health Services, using MediCal (Medicaid) claims data, has made two estimates of the lifetime costs of PWA in California (Kizer et al., 1986, 1987). The latest published study, by Andrulis et al., reports on a survey of 169 metropolitan public and private hospitals which treated PWA in 1985 (Andrulis et al., 1987). In addition, several other empirical studies are currently being conducted or have been completed but have not yet been published. Additional data on costs of treating PWA can be found in unpublished reports by state and local health departments, hospital associations and some individual hospitals.

Most of the data available to date have serious limitations. Most are limited to hospital inpatient services or at best hospital inpatient and outpatient services, and many of the studies also report data for fairly small numbers of AIDS cases.

In view of the scarcity and limited nature of the data on the use and costs of medical services of PWA, it is not surprising that to date only four estimates have been made of the medical care costs of PWA in the United States. The first was made early in 1985 (Hardy et al., 1986) at the CDC. They estimated the lifetime hospital costs of the first 10,000 patients with AIDS at about $1.5 billion, or $147,000 per PWA. A year later, in 1986, Dorothy Rice and I, at the request of the CDC, estimated the direct and indirect costs of the AIDS epidemic in 1985, 1986 and 1991. We made three estimates of direct personal costs, ranging from low to medium to high for each of the three years (Scitovsky and Rice, 1987). Our medium estimates, which we regard as the most likely, are $630 million in 1985, $1.1 billion in 1986, and $8.5 billion in 1991.

More recently, an estimate was made (Pascal, 1987) of the total costs of treating PWA in the five-year period 1986 to 1991, ranging from a low of $15.4 billion to an intermediate estimate of $37.6 billion and a high of $112.5 billion. The most recent estimate, by Andrulis et al., based on their findings from the hospital survey mentioned earlier, puts a total hospital inpatient cost of PWA in the United States in 1985 at $380 million. Converting the estimates of annual costs and total costs over a 5-year period into implied or assumed lifetime costs, we find that they range between $70,000 and $94,000 in later 1980s dollars. The exception is the Hardy estimate, which is now generally considered too high. In current (1987) dollars, lifetime costs of PWA most likely range between $60,000 and $70,000. The major factor which has determined costs to date is the number of days an AIDS patient spends in the hospital in a given year or over his lifetime. Data show that the average length of hospital stay per admission varies widely in different areas of the United States, while the other two variables determining hospital costs, average number of admissions per year or over a patient's lifetime and average costs of charges per hospital day differ considerably less. Length of stay per admission is lowest in San Francisco, where it averages about 11 days, compared to 19 days in Los Angeles, 21 days in Boston, and 20-25 days in New York City. As a result, the number of lifetime hospital days per

AIDS patient also varies by region, although it seems to be clustered in the 60 to 70 day range (over an average lifetime of 13 months). Hardy, for her early estimates of the hospital costs of PWA, has assumed an average lifetime use (over 13 months) of 168 days, but more recent data have shown that this was much too high.

To give our estimates some perspective, our medium estimate of direct medical care costs represents two-tenths of one percent of estimated total personal health care expenditures in 1985, three-tenths in 1986 and 1.4% in 1991.

The Impact of AIDS on Hospitals

Because at least to date, treatment of PWA has required substantial use of inpatient care, we have also estimated the impact the AIDS epidemic is likely to have on hospitals. Our best estimate of $8.5 billion in 1991 assumes **5.9 million hospital days.** This is equivalent to 2.6% of all hospital days used in 1985, almost four times the number of hospital days used in 1985 by patients with cancer of the colon (1.6 million) or cancer of the breast (1.5 million) and twice the number of hospital days used by patients with cancer of the lung (2.8 million). Only patients with acute myocardial infarction (who used 7.2 million days), pneumonia (6.8 million days), and women with normal deliveries (12.6 million days) used more inpatient days in 1985 than our estimate for AIDS patients in 1991 (US Department of Health and Human Services, 1985).

In terms of the number of beds AIDS patients will require, our estimate of 5.9 million hospital days translates into a requirement of just over 16,000 beds in 1991, which represents 1.2% of all hospital beds available in 1985.

Although there is an excess of hospital beds in the United States, the AIDS epidemic will impose a serious strain on the hospitals, especially the public hospitals, in the metropolitan areas with large numbers of PWA. For example, it is estimated that AIDS patients would require 25% of all public hospital beds in New York City in 1991 if they took care of the same percentage of AIDS patients as they do currently. In San Francisco they would require 10% - 20%. Clearly there is a limit to the number of beds public hospitals can provide for PWA since they have an obligation to provide many other essential services to their communities.

In addition to the strain on their **physical resources,** the public hospitals also face the most serious **financial problems** posed by the AIDS epidemic because of the high percentage of their AIDS patients who are either covered by Medicaid, which generally reimburses the hospitals for less than their costs, or who are self-pay, which frequently turns into uncollectible bills. For example, of the AIDS patients hospitalized in New York's public hospitals in a recent period, 70% were covered by Medicaid and 12% were self-pay; and at San Francisco General Hospital (the public hospital in San Francisco) 71% of the AIDS patients were covered by Medicaid and 8% were self-pay. By contrast 75% of the AIDS patients hospitalized in community hospitals in San Francisco had private insurance.

It is doubtful in view of the financial situation of PWA currently being treated by public hospitals that private hospitals are anxious to treat large numbers of AIDS cases. Thus unless the present piecemeal system of health insurance is drastically reformed, the AIDS epidemic will cause severe economic hardships for and place highly disproportionate financial burdens not only on many PWA and their families, but also on certain providers and local communities.

ESTIMATES OF THE INDIRECT COSTS OF AIDS

To date, only two estimates have been made of the indirect costs of the AIDS epidemic in the United States, that is, of the costs in terms of lost productivity resulting from illness and especially from premature death. Both estimates used the human capital method according to which morbidity cost are wages lost by people who are unable to work because of illness and disability, and mortality costs are the present value of future earnings lost by people who die prematurely.

Ann Hardy of the CDC estimated the indirect costs of the first 10,000 AIDS cases at $4.8 billion, or $3\frac{1}{2}$ times her estimate of the hospital costs of PWA (Hardy et al., 1987). Dorothy Rice and I estimated indirect costs in current dollars at $3.9 billion in 1985, $7.0 billion in 1986, and $55.6 billion in 1991 - or almost seven times the direct medical care costs (Scitovsky and Rice, 1987). Of the indirect costs, mortality costs represent by far the largest share, about 94%. Our estimates of the indirect costs of AIDS represent 1.2% and 2.1% of the estimated total indirect costs of all illness in 1985 and 1986; but by 1991 they are estimated to represent 12% of the estimated total indirect costs of all illnesses.

Mortality costs are high because PWA are concentrated among males in their most productive years. Moreover, just as the AIDS epidemic is not spread evenly across the country but is concentrated, at least to date and for some time to come, in certain metropolitan centers, the indirect costs are also concentrated in these areas. In 1986, AIDS was the leading cause of death for males aged 25 to 44 years in San Francisco and for males aged 30 to 39 years in New York. AIDS also exacts its toll on certain occupations, such as various branches of the arts whose ranks are being decimated in centers like New York, where few members of these professions have not had friends and colleagues who have died of the disease.

SUMMARY AND CONCLUSION

To sum up, current and estimated future costs of AIDS in the United States are high, especially the indirect costs of the epidemic. The direct medical care costs to date have been relatively small compared to the costs of all illnesses, and even the estimates for 1991 represent only a small percentage of total health care expenditures. However, the concentration of the disease in major metropolitan areas is already causing serious problems for the local governments and the public hospitals in these areas, and these problems will grow worse. We do not have a national health insurance system apart from a program for the elderly, and the Medicaid program for the poor consists of 50 different and widely varying state problems. As a result, large numbers of persons (estimated at 35 million) are without insurance or without adequate insurance. Thus we are ill-prepared for providing equitable financing for a catastrophic illness like AIDS.

In conclusion, I want to stress that the estimates of the costs of the AIDS epidemic made to date cover only reported cases of AIDS as defined by the CDC. But the costs of PWA are only part of the costs associated with what should more properly be referred to as the HIV epidemic. Thus costs estimates made to date do not include costs of persons with ARC nor those who are infected with HIV and have either very mild symptoms or no symptoms, but are worried and consult doctors in much the same way as other "worried well" members of the general population seek medical care and advice.

There are no hard data on the number of persons with ARC, but they have been estimated at two to ten times the number of persons with AIDS. Data on their medical care costs are totally lacking. Estimates of persons infected with HIV range from half a million to 1.5 million, but there are no estimates of the number of asymptomatic infected patients who seek medical care nor on their expenses for care. Furthermore, to the medical care costs and the indirect costs of HIV infected persons must be added the costs of testing for HIV antibodies, blood screening, research and education, for none of which we have hard data. Thus it is clear that the total direct costs of the HIV epidemic will far exceed the estimated $8.5 billion in 1991 and may well be twice or even more than twice as high.

REFERENCES

Andrulis D P, Beers V S, Bentley J D et al (1987). The provision and financing of medical care for AIDS patients in US public and private teaching hospitals. JAMA 258 : 1343-1346.

Berger R (1985). Cost analysis of AIDS cases in Maryland. Maryland Medical Journal 34: 1173-1175.

Centers for Disease Control. AIDS Weekly Surveillance Report, January 25, 1988.

Hardy A M et al (1986). The economic impact of the first 10,000 cases of acquired immunodeficiency syndrome in the United States. JAMA 255: 209-215.

Kizer K W, Rodriquez J, McHolland G F et al. A Quantitative Analysis of AIDS in California. California Department of Health Services, Sacramento, March 1986. And Kizer K W, Rodriquez J, McHolland G F. An updated quantitative analysis of AIDS in California. California Department of Health Services, Sacramento, April 1987.

Pascal A. The costs of treating AIDS under Medicaid: 1986-1991. A Rand Note N-266000-HCFA. The Rand Corporation, Santa Monica, CA., May 1987.

Seage G R III, Landers J D, Barry M A et al (1986). Medical care costs of AIDS in Massachusetts. JAMA 256: 3107-3109.

Scitovsky A A et al (1986). Medical care costs of patients with AIDS in San Francisco. JAMA 256: 3103.

Scitovsky A A, Rice D P (1987). Estimates of the direct and indirect costs of acquired immunodeficiency syndrome in the United States, 1985, 1986, 1991. Public Health Reports 102: 5-17.

US Department of Health and Human Services, National Center for Health Statistics. Detailed diagnosis and procedures for patients discharged from short-stay hospitals, United States, 1985. Vital and Health Statistics Series 13, No. 90.

The Global Impact of AIDS, pages 145–154
© 1988 Alan R. Liss, Inc.

18. THE IMPACT OF AIDS ON FOOD PRODUCTION
SYSTEMS IN EAST AND CENTRAL AFRICA OVER THE
NEXT TEN YEARS: A PROGRAMMATIC PAPER

Nick Abel, Tony Barnett, Simon Bell, Piers Blaikie,
Sholto Cross

School of Development Studies and Overseas
Development Group, University of East Anglia,
Norwich, United Kingdom

AFRICA'S ECONOMIES DEPEND ON SUBSISTENCE PRODUCTION

In Africa, a continent so exposed to food shortages, it is
vital that we consider the potential medium term impact of
AIDS on food production if we are to avoid the coincidence of
sickness and famine.

The Food Situation in Africa

African economies are based on subsistence rural
production. Relatively industrialised countries such as Kenya and
Zimbabwe have dominant agricultural sectors, providing a
livelihood for some 80% of their populations. Hence, the local
food/population balance is critical. Boserup (1985) stated that
"population increase will be rapid in Africa for many decades, so
a very large expansion in agricultural production is needed.
Agricultural production in many sparsely populated areas can be
multiplied, if long fallow agriculture and pastoralism are
replaced by more labour intensive systems". However, we may
now have to consider policy options which take account of falling
population in circumstances where overall economic viability
centres on rural household production.

We cannot assume that the population-land-food scenario
can exactly retrace its steps to a situation of land and food
surplus. In particular, it should be noted that ecological changes
associated with AIDS impact may result in land becoming
unusable through ecological changes associated with the
contraction of cultivation. Furthermore, changing relationships

between population levels, land use and food production, are not characterised by smooth transitions at the margin, they are often discontinuous.

Africa faces a "food crisis". It is the only region of the world where food production has been declining over the last twenty years (USDA, 1980). Per capita consumption in 1980 was 15% below that at the start of the 1970s and almost 20% below that at the start of the 1960s (USDA, 1981). In most of Sub-Saharan Africa, per capita calorie intake falls below minimal nutrition standards. Even if total food available were distributed equally and efficiently, in 18 countries where per capita calorie availability is less than 90% of the minimal requirements, serious nutritional problems are unavoidable, given present agricultural policies and patterns of income distribution. Although there were some indications of improved food output in certain areas of the continent in the period 1985-6, drought in north and central Africa suggests that the long term trend of decline may well continue.

One response to this situation has been to increase imports of staple foods, a strategy which has further weakened some subsistence and subsistence-market farming systems. In addition, increased cash cropping has meant increased labour demands, these crops being more labour intensive than traditional staples.

A General Method for Analysing and Monitoring the Impact of AIDS

Any strategy for coping with AIDS must include measures to support local farming systems if and when population declines. High priority should be given to the establishment of a monitoring system which will indicate the relative sensitivity of different types of farming system to the loss of labour and should include the development of an information network enabling the collection and sharing of such information within Africa.

Contingency plans can be developed so as to ensure continuing food production and the support of rural life in affected areas. We need to know more about the size and nature of the populations at risk, the consequences of the disease in terms of the modifications of economic and social behaviour, the possible adaptations of technology and farming systems, and the extent to which rural-urban linkages through common labour markets will extend the AIDS impact via both direct and indirect channels.

This information is crucial for the national economies of many countries, and we propose to undertake a detailed analysis, the goal of which will be to examine the socio-economic impact of AIDS on the rural economies of east and central Africa.

THE METHOD

Our method consists of sequential steps :-

(i)   description of rural production systems
(ii)   the diffusion exposure of a rural production system
(iii)   micro-analysis of rural production systems
(iv)   predicting AIDS impacts
(v)   policy implications

(i)   Description of Rural Production Systems Through the Concept of Labour Sensitivity

The essential task here is to measure the spatial and temporal aspects of labour application to different parts of the farming system together with the extent to which each part depends on the other. This task provides a logical framework for understanding the context within which farm labour decisions are made and resources allocated between different income generating activities. The key variable here is the concept of **labour sensitivity.** In using this concept, we are interested in a set of problems far wider than "labour intensity". We are looking at labour organisation as a social, cultural and economic decision process. "Labour intensity" implies that a system may be adaptable in purely neo-classical economic terms, either by capital substitution, or by labour substitution, or by downgrading from a labour intensive to a labour economising crop mix. This approach to the problem is satisfactory for some purposes but limited in the present context. The concept of labour sensitivity recognises that the impact of the disease is likely to be **cohort specific,** affecting some age cohorts, probably the most economically active, more than others. And, insofar as all societies are characterised by a division of labour, by age, status, gender, so measures of labour sensitivity must be able to differentiate between groups in the labour process.

The methods which can be used to describe a rural production system are fairly well established, and are described in more detail elsewhere.

Thus, we intend to classify and map rural production systems in terms of their sensitivity to labour loss. This will enable us to overlay various predicted spatial/temporal diffusion patterns of AIDS onto a map of rural production systems, and ultimately to chart in aggregate terms which **areas** will be vulnerable to AIDS because of differential labour sensitivity, and in what degree.

The differential exposure of rural production systems to increased mortality will also be influenced by the extent to which a particular system is spatially or culturally exposed to the diffusion of the disease. Thus we introduce the concept of **diffusion exposure.**

(ii) Diffusion Exposure

Although sophisticated spatial diffusion modelling of epidemics is at least twenty years old, its predictive performance has been disappointing. However, factors determining differential diffusion exposure to AIDS can be identified, and in many cases quantified. For example, rural areas have different intensities of contacts with urban areas. Urban-based civil servants in Kenya with shambas in Central Province may ensure the diffusion of AIDS to rural areas faster than , for example, in Western Province of Zambia where such urban-rural links do not exist, despite the possibly higher ambient incidence of AIDS in Zambia than Kenya. Urban-rural trade and labour movement paths may also determine the spatial pattern of diffusion. An additional set of risk factors might be proximity to rural dispensaries or ease of transport to larger medical facilities where infection can occur through blood transfusion or injection.

It is important to note that the conception of "diffusion exposure" includes cultural/functional factors as well as purely locational factors. We conceptualise these as **"socio-cultural filters"** to the transmission of the disease. Such filters may be located in child rearing practices, such as the practice of milk pooling among lactating mothers in Kenya (Panoscope, 1987) which may increase the risk of transmission through breast milk, or in the kinship system as in the case of the levirate in some societies, or in the ritual system, through the practice of scarification (Mann, 1986).

The "diffusion of AIDS" must of course be modelled in relation to the "impact" stage of AIDS, that is, the development of full-blown AIDS. Here the degree of uncertainty about the distribution of HIV-positive populations, of false positives, and the rate of development of AIDS, calls for robust rather than sophisticated modelling. Sensitivity analysis, and the development of diffusion patterns and rates under a number of different scenarios will form the core of this task.

If data accuracy allows, stochastic spatial diffusion models (of which many have now been developed) may be used. However, we do not intend to develop complex computer-intensive models for their own sake. Data availability and flexible and rapid turn-around of findings in a changing environment will be the two chief criteria that we are concerned to establish as the basis of a monitoring and information system which can enable and enhance rapid policy responses which may be developed and used locally within African administrations.

One important sub-component of this task will be to develop **life tables** for the population at risk. In this way, morbidity and mortality rates by gender, age and other distinguishing characteristics can be used to generate simulated changes in household size and composition - an important task given the cohort specific nature of the disease and the ways in which labour inputs to rural production systems are differentiated by gender and age. Such a model has already been developed by the Overseas Development Group to simulate the futures of "real" households under different assumptions of mortality, production and consumption. The output of this step will be indicative of the spatial-temporal spread of HIV-positive populations and full blown AIDS victims and of their mortality. As data become available, the life tables can be updated, made more accurate and disaggregated for different population groups and for different rural production systems.

(iii) Micro-analysis of Production at the Household and Individual Level

To complete the method, in-depth studies at the household and individual level will be necessary in order to understand the impact of AIDS within broad areas of different production systems.

Figure 1 outlines a conceptual model for predicting the impact of AIDS across a range of households within a rural production system. Basically an 'event', in this case AIDS (Box 1), impacts upon an array of households, each with a range of assets (Box 4) through the variables of morbidity and mortality (Box 2), food shortages, and possible re-arrangements of production,

150 / Abel et al.

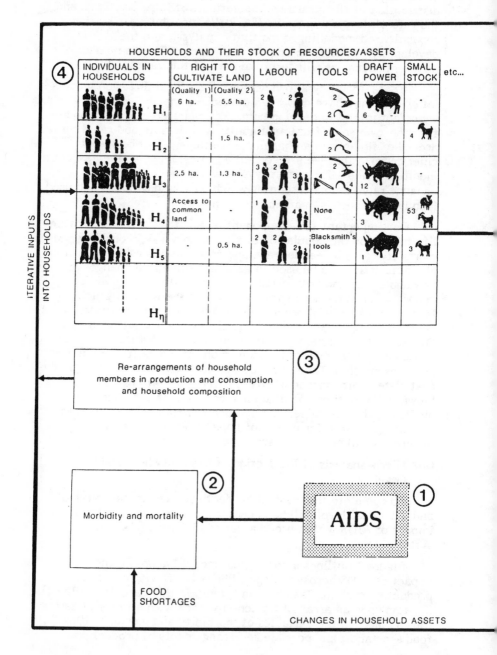

Figure 1.

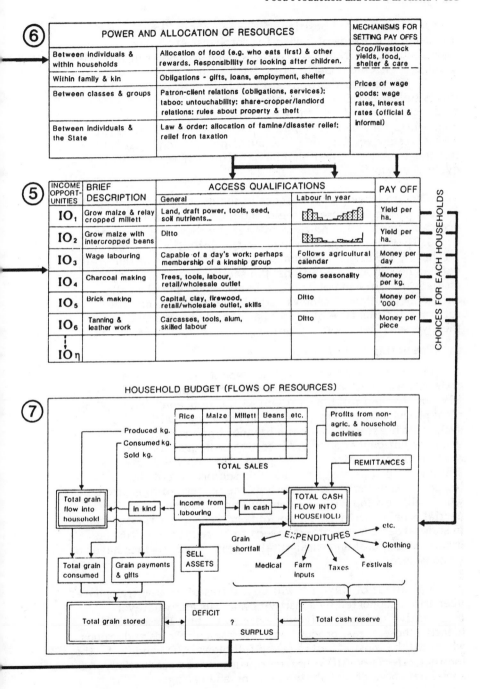

⑥ **POWER AND ALLOCATION OF RESOURCES** | **MECHANISMS FOR SETTING PAY OFFS**

Between individuals & within households	Allocation of food (e.g. who eats first) & other rewards. Responsibility for looking after children.	Crop/livestock yields, food, shelter & care
Within family & kin	Obligations - gifts, loans, employment, shelter	Prices of wage goods: wage rates, interest rates (official & informal)
Between classes & groups	Patron-client relations (obligations, services): taboo: untouchability: share-cropper/landlord relations: rules about property & theft	
Between individuals & the State	Law & order: allocation of famine/disaster relief: relief from taxation	

⑤

INCOME OPPORT-UNITIES	BRIEF DESCRIPTION	ACCESS QUALIFICATIONS		PAY OFF
		General	Labour in year	
IO_1	Grow maize & relay cropped millett	Land, draft power, tools, seed, soil nutrients...		Yield per ha.
IO_2	Grow maize with intercropped beans	Ditto		Yield per ha.
IO_3	Wage labouring	Capable of a day's work: perhaps membership of a kinship group	Follows agricultural calendar	Money per day
IO_4	Charcoal making	Trees, tools, labour, retail/wholesale outlet	Some seasonality	Money per kg.
IO_5	Brick making	Capital, clay, firewood, retail/wholesale outlet, skills	Ditto	Money per '000
IO_6	Tanning & leather work	Carcasses, tools, alum, skilled labour	Ditto	Money per piece
IO_η				

CHOICES FOR EACH HOUSEHOLDS

HOUSEHOLD BUDGET (FLOWS OF RESOURCES)

⑦

	Rice	Maize	Millett	Beans	etc.
Produced kg.					
Consumed kg.					
Sold kg.					

TOTAL SALES

Profits from non-agric. & household activities

REMITTANCES

Total grain flow into household ← In kind ← Income from labouring → In cash → TOTAL CASH FLOW INTO HOUSEHOLD

etc.

Grain shortfall — E:(PENDITURES — Clothing

Total grain consumed | Grain payments & gifts | SELL ASSETS | Medical | Farm inputs | Taxes | Festivals

Total grain stored ← DEFICIT ? SURPLUS ← Total cash reserve

consumption and composition of the household (Box 3) (e.g., break-up, new forms of caring for "orphans" etc.). The households with a range of assets defined at a point in time view a range of income opportunities, each with access qualifications (Box 5). These qualifications are crucially centred around labour (in its fullest definition as explained above). The choices that households make affect their household budget (Box 7). Sometimes they can accumulate, and sometimes be forced to sell assets to survive. Whatever the outcome for each household, it iterates back to the household asset situation at t + 1, and the cycle starts again.

Certain longer term changes in social organisation may also come about in response to the production system and the economic/material conditions of life, and these are suggested in Box 6. They may include changes in the definition and rearing of "orphans", the sexual division of labour, the nature of culturally defined behaviour prohibitions, the sanctioning of "theft", changes in rights and obligations between kin and clan, the autonomy position of widows and widowers, and so on. The software for this type of model has already been developed in the Overseas Development Group.

(iv) Predicting AIDS Impact

In the previous two steps, the impact of AIDS (under different assumptions of diffusion and development lags between HIV positive and full blown AIDS) will have been charted, (a) on rural production systems, and (b) on households within these systems. This step looks at the broader implications of AIDS upon the national economy. Since this project's data and analytical base centre on rural production, only indicative statements can be made outside this sector. One of the important sources of uncertainty is the pattern of migration which will develop with the depopulation of some areas. The partial breakdown of caring for old and young, shortage of labour in some areas but not others, needs to be recognised. Rural-urban, urban-rural and rural-rural migration will further have to be considered.

The output of this task will be a series of constantly updated 'scenarios', supported by sensitivity analysis and whatever quantitative and qualitative data are available. These will identify those areas, production systems, households and groups which will be most affected (a) by full blown AIDS and (b) by the indirect effects of AIDS through disrupted food production, and social networks of distribution, coping and caring.

(v) Policy Implications

On the basis of these techniques we will have a system for identifying the order in which rural production systems are most likely to be affected by decline in labour availability. This should enable policy measures to be developed, by government agencies, by NGOs, and by the communities themselves. In addition, the inclusion of this monitoring system within a wider information network from its earliest stages, should enable agricultural and social coping methods developed in one part of Africa to be tried very rapidly in another where farming practices and labour sensitivity may be similar.

Thus, questions such as how tenure systems are likely to respond to falling population, how methods of labour organisation are likely to respond, what changes occur in the mode of inter- and intra-household distribution of available products, might all be addressed, and experience shared across the continent.

Of particular importance will be the technological responses which are likely to occur both in terms of the recovery of "traditional" means of exploiting the environment (such as a switch in the balance between cultivation and hunting as animal populations increase in some areas as a response to falling human populations), and also the adoption of imported technologies as a response to falling labour availability. In the shorter term, the project will be able to identify vulnerable groups for immediate relief and targeting for reconstruction.

ECOLOGICAL CONTROL

An additional and very important implication of this project concerns the question of AIDS impact on rural production and some possible longer term ecological consequences.

Kjekshus (1977) and Ford (1971) are the main researchers providing outline accounts of the response of agricultural systems to falling populations in Africa. They show that the effect of falling population may have far wider implications than for the food system alone. Kjekshus (1977) says, "Ecological control is .... predicated on the presence of people. It can be maintained only by people who either expand or hold their own numerically; depopulation spells crisis in the control system and may initiate its total collapse". If this is so, then the failure of food production systems may well be followed by a more widespread collapse of the ecological control systems in parts of

Africa, leading to the expansion of other kinds of endemic diseases, trypanosomiasis for example, into areas where populations and domestic animals do not have any immunity. This will compound an already chronic problem, AIDS causing a fall in food production, and in the longer term and in some regions, leading to the expansion of the range of the trypanosomiases, resulting in a further contraction of land use, and thus food availability.

The development and use of a monitoring and information system based on a theoretical approach such as that outlined in this paper may go some way to reducing this impact.

REFERENCES

Boserup E (1985). Economic and demographic inter-relationships in sub-Saharan Africa. Population and Development Review 11.

Ford J. "The Role of the Trypanosomiases in African Ecology: a Study of the Tsetse Fly Problem". Oxford, Clarendon, 1971.

Kjekshus H. "Ecology Control and Economic Development in East African History". Heinemann, London 1977.

Mann J M, et al (1986). Human immunodeficiency virus seroprevalence in paediatric patients 2-14 years of age at Mama Yemo Hospital, Kinshasa, Zaire. Pediatrics 78: 673-677.

Panoscope. Aids and the Third World, 1, Panos Institute, London 1987.

USDA (United States Department of Agriculture). "Economic and Statistics and Cooperative Services, International Economics Division, Africa and Middle East Branch, Food Problems and Prospects in Sub-Saharan Africa - The Decade of the 1980s". Washington, September 1980.

USDA International Economics Division of the Statistical Service, World Food Aid Needs and Availabilities, Washington, 15 March 1981.

The Global Impact of AIDS, pages 155-160
© 1988 Alan R. Liss, Inc.

19. THE IMPACT OF HUMAN IMMUNODEFICIENCY VIRUS
INFECTION AND AIDS ON A PRIMARY INDUSTRY:
MINING (A CASE STUDY OF ZAMBIA)

Benjamin M Nkowane

Consultant Epidemiologist/Lecturer, Department of
Community Medicine, University of Zambia School of
Medicine, University Teaching Hospital, PO Box
50110, Lusaka, Zambia

INTRODUCTION

The impact of the human immunodeficiency virus infection
on a primary industry such as mining in a developing country will
be shaped by numerous factors that are different from what is
known in the industrialized countries that have mining industries.
In the developing countries, the virus has been introduced into a
whole adult population that is sexually active and not
subdivisions of it; the disease is a family disease in that those at
risk if infected will spread it to their spouses or any other sexual
partners. The impact on the primary industry will therefore be
no different from that of the general population except that
there may be significant consequences for the industry and its
employees.

I shall discuss the possible impact of HIV infection and AIDS
on a primary industry (i.e. mining) in a developing country, in
this case Zambia, a southern African country.

The Country Zambia

Zambia is a landlocked country in southern Africa covering
an area of 300,000 sq. miles. Its population is estimated at about
7 million (5.5 million 1980 census). The country is divided into
nine provinces or administrative regions. The Copperbelt region
which is 70 miles by 30 miles is the most important mineral
region of Zambia. In 1980, it was estimated that the mineral
resources of copper were about 34 million metric tonnes, the
fourth largest content after Chile, USA and USSR. In addition to
these there are coal fields, lead and zinc deposits in the country.

The economy of the country is heavily dependent on copper mining, with the industry accounting for almost 20 percent of the Gross National Product, while the other major industry (agriculture) accounts for 17 percent. The country is highly urbanized, with almost 50 percent of the population being urban. The areas of greatest density of population are the Copperbelt and Central Provinces.

The Copperbelt and its Population

The Copperbelt region has a population of 2 million persons. This represents about one third of the total population of Zambia. Twenty-two percent of this population is in the rural areas of the Copperbelt Province. Like most parts of the country, the population is young, with 50 percent being less than 15 years of age and about 42 percent being aged 15 to 44 years. The Copperbelt Province also has the smallest proportion of the population over 65 years of age. This is no surprise since the majority of those who are formally employed in the mining industry are young. In fact most of the persons aged over 65 years are retirees who have settled in the rural areas and are mainly involved in subsistence farming activity.

The Mining Industry

Copper mining in Zambia is a labour intensive industry, employing the young and healthy component of the population. This industry employs at the moment a total labour force of 56,100. Of these, about 67 percent or two thirds are labourers or equipment operators, obvious jobs that obviously require healthy persons. Although the labour force of the mining industry only comprises 6 percent of the total work force of Zambia (and 13 percent of the urban work force), it is a vital portion of the economy of the country. The large majority of the labour force is male, with the females making up only 15 percent. The female employees are almost exclusively in secretarial jobs and administration.

In general almost 80 percent of the male miners are married and almost all miners aged above 35 years of age are married. In about 80 percent of the mine employees households, the husband is the sole or major breadwinner. The miner's wife is typically 10 years younger than her husband and the average household size is about six. The number of dependents rises with the miner's age and duration of service in the industry.

It is therefore not unusual to find a miner with seven or eight children and other dependents. The dependency ratio is therefore high, with over 4 dependents for every working adult. Marriages are typically very stable in these areas as they are in all urban areas of the country.

The mining industry provides services for its employees and their dependents. These services include health, education, housing, and social services. These are free to the employees and their dependents. In addition to these, there are government services that are also freely available to all.

The industry provides training for all its recruits in most of the skilled jobs on the mines. It also has a scholarship program under which graduates with high school diplomas are sponsored for professional studies at technical colleges and the University. On completion of training, these individuals are retained as employees. It is through this program that the industry has Zambianized most of its technical and professional positions. This is naturally a well planned human resources investment by the industry. The industry also has developed a retirement program where retirees are encouraged to go into farming and are allocated pieces of land for this purpose.

In summary therefore, the typical Zambian miner is young, probably in his mid-thirties, married to a twenty-six year old woman with five children and two other dependents.

HIV INFECTION AND AIDS IN ZAMBIA

There are a number of factors relating to HIV infection and AIDS in Zambia that will have a bearing on the population at risk:-

1. HIV transmission is primarily through heterosexual intercourse.
2. All persons who are sexually active and have more partners than one mutually faithful sexual partner are at risk of infection.
3. Infected persons are likely to transmit infection to their spouses and any other sexual contacts.
4. HIV infection and AIDS is a family disease that will take both the breadwinners in the family through premature deaths. Almost all cases of infection or disease in infancy are a result of vertical transmission.
5. The true seropositivity in the community is not known.

However, it can be expected to rise until there is a dramatic change in behaviour.

IMPLICATIONS FOR THE MINING INDUSTRY

The primary implications for the mining industry will be related to efforts to maintain mining as a viable and important component of the country's economy. Naturally, being labour intensive, the health of the miner will be paramount to achieve this. It follows therefore that any conditions that will reduce the efficiency of the labour force, such as low individual productivity, absence from work due to ill-health as well as social commitments will have a significant impact on the industry. In addition, if there is need for additional services to be provided, this would reduce the overall profits.

The secondary implications will be those that will dictate the role of the industry in providing extra or special services such as those that will be a result of early and forced retirement that will become common with an increase in the numbers of HIV infected employees.

Recruitment of Miners

Although up to now, as long as you were medically fit you could be employed as a miner, it will become necessary for the industry to review their procedures of recruitment. Since every new employee is considered an investment and will have to undergo some training whether formal or informal, screening for HIV would have to be introduced as a mandatory exercise. The implications of this are numerous. For those who are seropositive but asymptomatic, it will mean denial of job prospects and career in the industry. What will probably be more significant will be the likely denial of scholarships for specialist training of university graduates on the basis of being infected with HIV. The big question that will continually have to be asked will be "Can the industry afford to continue to invest in terms of training in persons who are infected with HIV?". On purely economic grounds the answer is no.

HIV Infected Employees

What will happen to these? Naturally, those who are infected and sick will be forced to retire on grounds of poor health. However, for those who are asymptomatic, if confidentiality of HIV screening or testing is not maintained,

there will be discrimination. The proportion of the labour force
that will probably be affected will be significant unless the
current trends are arrested. Early retirement will lead to many
man-days of service lost, while at the same time the industry
will be obliged to provide terminal benefits prematurely. If the
affected labour force is even as low as 3 to 5 percent, the cost
to the industry would be substantial. The industry will have to
employ more persons to take over the positions due to premature
retirement. All these new employees will need training.

Families of Infected Employees

The Spouse. These will also be infected. As the majority are
female, there are risks to the unborn as well as poor maternal
health when pregnancy occurs. There can be an expected strain
on the health services if the number of infected women rises.

The family. With the eventual death of the breadwinner, the
meagre retirement benefits will not be able to sustain the
remaining dependents. Choices will have to be made for
relocation to other areas and the bereaved would eventually have
to leave the town or look for alternative housing. This will entail
more costs. Since many persons on the Copperbelt towns have
been in the urban areas for long periods of time, relocating to a
rural area under these circumstances will not be an attractive
proposition.

Forced or Early Retirement. The industry will have to invest
in systems that will have to cater for the welfare of such persons
and their families. Questions will have to be asked on what the
criteria will be for retirement. Will those who are HIV positive
but are in the early stages of the disease be retired, or will it be
only those who are so sick that they cannot work? Discrimination
will eventually arise. Questions regarding the right of the
employee to refuse testing will have to be resolved.

Social services. Social services will therefore have to be
expanded to take care of issues such as counselling for the HIV
infected and their spouses and families, services for the care of
dependents, services to support the health education initiatives
aimed at changing the behaviour of the young at risk in the
community. The mining industry will have to make investments
into this as well to support the work of the government.

Emergence of disease. Although infectious respiratory
disease has been completely controlled in the mining industry

employees, it is conceivable that there may be an increase in the incidence of tuberculosis, as may be the case with the rest of the population. The chances of spread will have to be reduced by vigilance in detection or investigation of all suspected employees. This will require more investment into the preventive aspect of health in the mining industry.

Impact on the economy. The impact on the economic contribution is difficult to quantify. However, the mining industry will definitely have more expenses to take care of in terms of health, and social services for its miners. The only possible way to avoid this would be to recruit only those who are free from HIV and to routinely screen all miners at frequent intervals and terminate the services of all who are infected - clearly a solution that is not acceptable.

CONCLUSION

The impact of HIV and AIDS on the primary industry of mining, which is labour intensive, will be significant. Many issues relating to the health of the employee will have to receive serious and critical consideration if the industry will be expected to remain a viable and important component of the economy of the country.

REFERENCES

1980 Population and Housing Census of Zambia. Analytical Report, Vol. II. CSO. Lusaka, 1985.

Situation Analysis of Children and Women in Zambia. GRZ/UNICEF, Lusaka, 1986.

Biggar R J (1986). The AIDS Problem in Africa. Lancet i: 79-83.

Third National Development Plan 1979-1983. GRZ. Lusaka, 1979.

Van der Hoeven R (1982). Zambia's economic dependence and the satisfaction of basic needs. International Labour Review. 121: 217-231.

Bygren L O. Health and Health Services in Zambia. Ministry of Health, Lusaka. 1982.

Selected Socio-Economic Indicators of Zambia. CSO. Lusaka.1987.

Melbye M, Njelesani E K, Bayley A C et al (1986). Evidence for heterosexual transmission and clinical manifestations of HIV related conditions in Lusaka, Zambia. Lancet ii: 1113-1115.

The Global Impact of AIDS, pages 161–165
© 1988 Alan R. Liss, Inc.

20.   AIDS : ITS IMPACT ON DEVELOPMENT PROGRAMMES

Timothy S Rothermel

Director, Division for Global and Interregional
Programmes, United National Development
Programme, 1 UN Plaza, New York.

The topic that I have been asked to address is the impact of
AIDS on development programmes from the perspective of
UNDP - the United Nations Development Programme. Although
its budget is now over $1 billion annually, UNDP may not be a
well known institution to all of you, so a brief remark on what
we do. As the world's largest voluntarily-funded international
technical assistance organization, UNDP operates in all
developing countries and territories with field offices, headed by
Resident Representatives, in 112 developing countries. In the
countries we serve, UNDP seeks to provide interdisciplinary
assistance to governments in planning and helping to achieve
overall development priorities. While most of our funds are
allocated to individual countries based on their population and
per capita GNP, a small portion of UNDP's resources are set
aside for basic and applied research of an interregional or global
character. This latter aspect of UNDP's work, which principally
involves agriculture, health, water, trade and energy, is my
responsibility.

In recent months, as the implications of the global spread of
AIDS have been more sharply perceived, it has also become
quickly apparent that AIDS is a social, economic and political
issue, just as much as a medical and scientific one. Since AIDS
has no respect for national frontiers, the consequences of AIDS
already have become a special concern for virtually all
developing countries. With the likelihood of five to tenfold
increases in the number of AIDS cases in some countries within
five to ten years, there are serious development implications.

There are good reasons - many of which we have heard

here - for concern about the relationship between AIDS and development. We face the grim and sobering prospect that in some of the poorest developing countries, based on present HIV infection levels, the death rate from AIDS could equal or exceed the number of deaths from all other causes by the early 1990s. And excluding the increasing number of children who will succumb to AIDS, the men and women who die will generally be in the 20 to 40 year age group, depriving countries, already desperately lacking in human resources, of their most productive citizens. In all likelihood this group will include many of those who have the most to contribute to their country's development. Added to this is the yet undetermined but doubtlessly enormous future cost of health care for governments which today face extraordinary health constraints. These costs will include not only the provision of direct hospital care to AIDS victims, but the related costs of counselling, blood screening, medical supplies and training. Taken together these costs can be expected to exceed by far current health expenditures, resulting in an enormous drain of resources. Finally, and on top of the diversion of human and financial resources as a direct result of AIDS, the poorest in the world will face indirect economic costs as a result of lost years of production. Here again, precise data for developing countries are not yet available, but the predicted indirect economic costs of AIDS in the United States alone, is estimated at over $55 billion for 1991. The result can be devastating, resulting in declining GNPs, the necessity to rethink development priorities, and the deferral or possible elimination of vitally needed development programmes, just to cope with the AIDS crisis.

The United Nations system, consisting of some forty international organizations, sometimes appears to be unwieldy and slow moving. It has, however, responded, in my judgement, remarkably quickly to meet the challenge presented by AIDS, especially in developing countries. It is working together with bilateral and other development organizations to achieve two overriding objectives for AIDS protection and control. They are **first,** the development and implementation of strong national AIDS prevention and control programmes since the sole and prime responsibility for AIDS programmes rests with governments. The **second** objective required is for international leadership, co-ordination and co-operation. The WHO Global Programme on AIDS is the lead directing and co-ordinating organization in combatting AIDS. In other parts of the United Nations system, international organizations in their respective fields of competence, are assisting and complementing WHO's leadership role. UNICEF is bringing its expertise to bear on childhood immunization and breast feeding and the impact of AIDS on mothers, children and family life. The World Bank has begun studies on measuring the direct and indirect costs of AIDS in developing countries. The UN Population Fund is collaborating in the interaction between AIDS and family planning programmes and envisaging demographic studies to be carried out in collaboration with the United Nations Secretariat. And UNESCO is assisting in the educational aspects of AIDS.

I am pleased to note here that the collaboration between UNDP and WHO in assisting developing countries in the field of AIDS has never been stronger in our work at both the country level and between the respective Headquarters. Later this month the Director-General of WHO and the Administrator of UNDP will formally announce the creation of a unique joint agreement called the WHO/UNDP Alliance to Combat AIDS. Under this agreement UNDP's Resident Representatives in the 112 field offices I mentioned earlier, will bring together UNDP's experience in multi-sectoral socio-economic development with the health policy and scientific expertise of WHO to support governments of developing countries in initiating, implementing, monitoring and evaluating national AIDS prevention and control plans. We will also be involved in seeking to ensure that these AIDS plans are integrated into countries' overall national development policies and priorities. Although the Alliance has not yet been formally launched, in developing countries UNDP and WHO officials have already begun to give expression to this new relationship with positive results. In Zaire, for example, as a result of co-ordinated assistance through the United Nations system, that country's National AIDS Committee includes not only officials from the Ministry of Health but also the Ministry of Planning. In recent days a similar result was achieved in Senegal which augurs well for ensuring that governments are preparing for the broad economic and social implications of AIDS control as well as its health and biomedical aspects. Another aspect of the Alliance has been the provision by UNDP of a modest revolving fund which will enable national AIDS plans to be set in motion as soon as there are firm indications of financial support from the international donor community.

At the international level, the UNDP Governing Council three weeks ago approved a global project entitled The Global Blood Safety Initiative. The intent of this project is to set in motion the steps required to make blood supplies safe throughout the world in order to stem the spread of AIDS and other diseases.

Specifically, UNDP is providing seed money - $700,000 in this case - to establish a consortium of organizations beginning with the League of the Red Cross and Red Crescent Societies, the World Health Organization and the International Society of Blood Transfusion to be joined within the next two months by an expected number of national and international organizations. Working together with governments this consortium will seek to ensure that blood supply systems are fully sustainable and that comprehensive safe blood banks and transfusion mechanisms are in place in every country. It is our hope that the Global Blood Safety Initiative will attract financial support from private sector groups as well as from traditional supporters of public health efforts. If successful, in a few years, the spread of diseases through this mode of transmission, such a hepatitis B and malaria, as well as AIDS, can be stopped.

In contemplating the potential economic and social impact of AIDS for the poorest countries, it seems inevitable that those least able to afford the consequences of AIDS will be the hardest hit. In light of what seems to be a consensus among scientists that a cure for AIDS is not yet in sight, the outlook at the moment for developing countries is bleak. Nevertheless, in an heretofore unprecedented manner, activities at a variety of levels have given rise to some hopes. Rarely, if ever before, has co-operation among national and international development institutions been as intense as in the fight against AIDS. Thanks in particular to the United Kingdom Government, the World Health Organization and World Ministers of Health, as witnessed here in January through the London Declaration on AIDS Prevention, this disease has been recognized as a global threat requiring urgent action. Similar resolutions have been adopted in recent months by the United Nations General Assembly, by the World Health Assembly and by numerous other international and non-governmental organizations. Virtually every country in the world, developed or developing, now has a national AIDS committee and has begun to take concerted action to seek to control the spread of AIDS or to prevent its spread in countries which currently have a relatively small number of cases. The international machinery to assist governments at their request in coping with AIDS is basically already in place and is consistently being fine-tuned and strengthened. The WHO/UNDP Alliance to combat AIDS is a good example of this process. In addition, financial resources to combat AIDS and to carry out research have increased geometrically. And finally, the political commitment to the health sector in general and to health education and preventive health care in particular, especially in developing countries, is growing.

Obviously, more resources and greater commitment and co-operation will be required, especially if the aspirations of developing countries are not to be denied or deferred, but the resolve to begin to slow the spread of AIDS can mean that today's predictions of economic, social and cultural disasters can be made less severe for the poorest. To achieve this it is vital for all of us who are concerned about AIDS throughout the world to turn resolutions into action and to be prepared for a long term struggle. In UNDP, the Administrator clearly, and at an early stage, charged all of my colleagues to put our financial, intellectual and managerial resources at the disposal of developing countries in combatting AIDS. And in doing so, we will need the contributions and commitment of all assembled here today. We firmly intend to spare no effort in assisting governments to meet this challenge.

The Global Impact of AIDS, pages 167–169
© 1988 Alan R. Liss, Inc.

21. THE ECONOMIC IMPACT ON FAMILIES OF CHILDREN WITH AIDS IN KINSHASA, ZAIRE

F Davachi[1], P Baudoux[1], K Ndoko[1], B N'Galy[2], and J. Mann[3],

Department of Pediatrics, Mama Yemo Hospital[1]; Ministry of Health, Kinshasa, Zaire[2]; Global Programme on AIDS, World Health Organization[3].

INTRODUCTION

The concern over the financial burden of Acquired Immunodeficiency Syndrome (AIDS) on the patient and on the society at large has prompted a number of studies on medical care costs of patients with AIDS. In the metropolitan centers of the United States, estimates have varied from $7,000 to $9,000 per hospital admission (Scitovsky, 1986) and from $27,000 to $100,000 lifetime costs (Groopman, 1983; Kizer, 1986; Landesman, 1985; Scitovsky, 1986; Seage, 1986). Hardy estimates an average hospital expenditure, including inpatient professional charges, for the first 10,000 patients with AIDS at $1,473 billion or $147,000 per patient. This estimate was based on an average initial hospitalization of 31 days, (data from New York, San Francisco and Philadelphia estimates a lifetime use of 168 hospital days and an average survival time of 392 days), (Hardy, 1986). Reports coming from all these centers indicate that medical care costs of patients with AIDS in the United States is indeed very high.

To our knowledge, estimates for medical care costs of children with AIDS in Africa are not yet available. Therefore, we have studied 33 families of children with AIDS in Kinshasa, Zaire to determine the economic impact of the disease on these families, their employers and the State.

METHODS

We collected data on 33 families whose children were hospitalized with AIDS at the department of pediatrics at Mama

Yemo Hospital in Kinshasa, Zaire. This is a 2,000 bed metropolitan hospital which offers primary to tertiary care and which serves the less fortunate segment of the population. The hospital is partially subsidized by the Ministry of Health. Patients pay a hospitalization fee according to their income. Government employees and the poor who can produce proof of indigency are exempt from payment. All others pay according to their income which falls into three categories (low, middle and high income).

The hospitalized children range in age from 2 years to 12 years. There was a 1.1 to 1 male/female ratio. All children were symptomatic at the time of admission and the clinical diagnosis of AIDS was confirmed by HIV ELISA and Western Blot tests in each case. In addition to presenting a variety of symptoms related to AIDS, they also manifested associated diseases peculiar to the region such as malaria, anemia and intestinal parasites.

The average length of hospitalization was 25 days with 7 (21%) hospital mortality. This study is based on the cost of a single hospital admission for each child. It is noteworthy that many services such as HIV ELISA and Western Blot tests and physician daily rounds are free of charge.

RESULTS

The average hospitalization cost for 25 days was 3,000 Zaires, cost of drugs and I.V. treatment was 6,500 Zaires and laboratory tests were 2,000 Zaires, thus making an average total cost per patient of 11,500 Zaires ($90).

Although the cost of hospitalization for AIDS patients in Zaire ($90) is not comparable to the cost in the United States (approx. $9,000) yet compared to the average monthly income, it is quite impressive.

In our study, 17 fathers were employed (8 by the State and 9 privately), 14 were unemployed and 2 had died. Of the 17 who were employed, all held low-income jobs. The average monthly income was 3,750 Zaires ($30). The cost of one hospitalization, therefore, was 3 times the average monthly income. Normally those employed by the government or by private companies have their hospital and funeral expenses paid by their employer. For those who are self-employed or unemployed, the burden falls on relatives and friends. In cases where there is proof of indigency, some help may be obtained from the State.

DISCUSSION

Twenty-one percent of our cases died during hospitalization, thus adding the burden of funeral expenses to the already heavy hospitalization and treatment costs. Traditional African beliefs, which demand a great show of respect for the dead, require that the funeral ceremony lasts from two to seven days. During this time the bereaved family must bear the expense of feeding the multitude of family and friends who come to give moral support and who gather to ensure that the deceased is given a respectful farewell. A casket, a clean sheet, transportation for the casket and guests to the ceremony all are necessary to fulfill the minimum funeral requirements. The average total cost of a funeral and wake in Kinshasa is 40,000 Zaires ($320). This is the equivalent of 11 months of salary.

CONCLUSION

A single hospitalization of a child with AIDS equals three months of a father's salary and the child's demise equals eleven months. Therefore a minimum of 14 months of salary must be paid by the family, the employer or the State for each child with AIDS. We conclude, therefore, that a single hospitalization of a child with AIDS and his eventual death can have an immense economic effect on the immediate and extended family and friends, on the employer and on the State.

REFERENCES

Groopman J E, Detsky A (1983). Epidemic of acquired immunodeficiency syndrome: a need for economic and social planning. Ann Intern Med 99: 259-261.

Hardy A M, Rauch K, Echenberg D et al (1986). The economic impact of the first 10,000 cases of acquired immunodeficiency syndrome in the United States. JAMA 255: 209-215.

Kizer K, Rodrigues J, McHolland G F et al (1986). A quantitative analysis of AIDS in California. Sacramento, California Department of Health Services, p.13.

Landesman S H, Ginzberg H, Weiss S H (1985). The AIDS epidemic. N Engl J Med 312: 521-525.

Scitovsky A A, Cline M, Lee P R (1986). Medical care costs of patients with AIDS in San Francisco. JAMA 256: 3103-3106.

Seage G R, Landers S, Barry A et al (1986). Medical care costs of AIDS in Massachusetts. JAMA 256: 3107-3109.

The Global Impact of AIDS, pages 171–174
© 1988 Alan R. Liss, Inc.

22. AIDS - THE GRANDMOTHER'S BURDEN

Christopher Beer, Ann Rose, Ken Tout

HelpAge International, St James' Walk, London
EC1R 0BE

A continuing burden of AIDS will fall most heavily upon the grandmothers in many countries. This assertion, probably contrary to received wisdom on AIDS, needs some justification.

Commentators on the global impact of AIDS, particularly those in the Western media, seem to suppose that it is persons of the sexually active generations who will constitute the population at risk. Epidemiologically, and certainly in terms of mortality statistics, this is a sustainable view. As full blown AIDS is fatal, sociologically the main impact will be felt by the survivors. Although we consider survivors as secondary victims it will be these survivors upon whom the full weight of sustaining a decimated, confused and demoralised community will fall.

Perhaps we should consider a scenario which, at the moment, is largely notional but the tragic inevitability of which is already discernable in some developing countries. Let us focus on a small community, along one of the main routes of AIDS transmission, in a country where medical and social services are already deemed to be inadequate. Let us further focus upon a particular family in that community. The father, head of the family, has been in contact with the virus during a casual relationship. He goes on to develop full blown AIDS. In a relatively short time the wife becomes infected. The unborn child becomes infected. Within this family therefore the situation arises, and persists over a relatively long period, that both parents and one or several infants are dying of AIDS.

In this instance the surviving responsible person in the family is likely to be drawn from the older generation. In most countries longevity rates indicate that in the over sixty generation the woman survives longer than the man and sometimes the survival rates of women are significantly superior to those of men. In many cultures the elderly man plays little part in domestic affairs and might also be only marginally involved in economic production. The grandmother is likely to be the most active and competent person, though not necessarily the most physically fit, to manage the family affairs.

Where both parents and some infants are terminally ill in a society where there are no adequate medical, hospice or counselling facilities, the grandmother will be required over a long terminal period to nurse patients suffering from a disease which is unfamiliar, and whose symptomatology is still unaccounted for, and for which local traditional remedies have no application and no effect. It is a disease for which the grandmother may have no access to advice on treatment or prognosis. She will herself be at risk and perhaps afraid. She will have little or no knowledge of prophylaxis, either for herself or the surviving infants.

It is likely that the family resources of income and the family's ability to produce or procure food supplies will have been cut off. The grandmother will have to become the wage earner or food producer.

The present knowledge of AIDS leads us to suppose that it could have the effect of annihilation of a parent generation in a close community where the virus prospers through heterosexual transmission, and where male promiscuity is traditional and sometimes even deemed meritorious. It would follow that, in the community upon which we have focused, the cohort of elderly women could find themselves sustaining at least the major share of economic survival as well as the hierarchical and organizational burdens of the entire community and family structure.

A further negative factor which must be taken into account is that in many developing countries the unforeseen effects of educational improvements, industrialisation and urbanisation have tended both to dislocate the traditional extended family and to damage the traditional roles and skills of elders. Many developing country communities will therefore be less well equipped to counter the socio-economic impacts of AIDS than they might have been twenty years ago.

This scenario is at the moment evident only in individual families and in relatively few villages but the nature of the spread of AIDS and its associated socio-economic effects requires that these very serious considerations be put forward before such a situation develops on a community or national scale. Rather than to wait until such a tragic problem is fully developed before rousing public and professional concern, we should attempt to plan and prepare adequate responses.

What then can be done? The resources likely to be available, compared with the rapidity of the spread of the disease and its widespread effects, suggest that the methods of relieving the family burden will not be found in widespread construction of centers, or in a massive provision of sophisticated drugs, or in a large scale programme of placements of qualified specialists. This will continue to be, at base, an individual family burden, to be tackled at family level and in terms of family comprehension by the methods capable of the most basic application and the widest diversity.

The first obvious method would be the provision of counselling and family training in basic terminal care. Yet taking into account the large numbers of families likely to be involved, no international plan is likely to provide sufficient numbers of trained counsellors or community health visitors. The appropriate level of input would be the provision of trainers able to instruct and advise the grandmothers directly so that they may undertake the necessary duties in emergency conditions. Considering even this method an international plan could probably only contemplate providing 'trainers of trainers'. That would mean specialist trainers who would then rapidly and intensively train unskilled community volunteers (possibly with some small remuneration) in only the most basic, immediate and essential elements of knowledge required by the individual family carers.

Allied to this, a planned programme of development for hospice methods of care needs to be instituted in those countries of higher incidence. This need not involve the institutionalized establishment of hospice care. Care of the dying needs to be integrated into PHC systems which will reach into village structures and assist the family. An imaginative programme of home based care has been developed by the Salvation Army at the Chikankata Hospital in Muzambuka, Zambia. The hospital has set up an AIDS care unit, consisting of a social worker, clinical officer, nurse and supported by a laboratory assistant. The team conducts home visits on a regular basis to assess and meet needs. This type of initiative needs to be encouraged elsewhere and more pilot schemes funded.

Beyond this programme we also have to look urgently at alternative means of family income and production. Some experience of programmes exists which suggests that older people are able to be trained in alternative skills but only if considerable capital and some revenue costs are supplied from outside the local community. In such an emergency, a small developing country community cannot quickly discover a novel system of economic production without external aid in both skills and material resources.

"Alternative" cottage and rural industries for the elderly, with which HelpAge projects have had some success in various cultures and environments, include the raising of chickens, rabbits and other immediate animal sources of food; fish-farming; weaving and sewing; the manufacture and sale of local handicrafts. But many more resources need to go into identifying and promoting such opportunities. Other agencies involved in appropriate agriculture and technology must be called upon to lend their skills in this sector in the countries profoundly affected. This will necessitate a move towards village-based development and training and a greater awareness of the welfare and family implications of development programmes. Can we make a plea for the training of elders - who in many societies have been marginalised in recent decades - by the very development agencies which will now need to support AIDS affected communities?

Ironically, one ray of hope in this gloomy scenario lies in the fact that some of the socio-economic effects of AIDS upon the surviving grandmother generation have already been simulated in developing countries as a consequence of previous development and urbanisation. In some remote rural villages, in some newly established shantytowns and in some transitory refugee camps HelpAge and associated agencies have already encountered the phenomenon of the abandoned grandmother left to care for a family or small infants in a community whose population profile has been distorted by migration of the current parent generation. Lessons learned and models proven in such communities can now be utilised for the family and community tragedies caused by AIDS.

Should the scenario which we have presented develop, it is imperative that support to the individual grandmother and to groups of surviving family carers should be efficient, and backed by adequate financial resources and political will. Only then will we ensure the survival of remaining infants until they are old enough to fend for themselves in a world where hopefully the worst effects of the AIDS virus will have been eliminated.

The Global Impact of AIDS, pages 175–182
© 1988 Alan R. Liss, Inc.

23.   AIDS : CONSEQUENCES FOR FAMILIES AND FERTILITY

Isaac W Eberstein, William J Serow and Omar B Ahmad

Center for the Study of Population, Florida State University, Tallahassee, Florida, USA.

Since its discovery, substantial effort has rightfully been devoted to the basic research necessary for AIDS prevention. Although much remains to be accomplished on this front, and, additionally, along curative lines, it is becoming increasingly important to expand discussion of AIDS (used here to refer to all sequelae of HIV as well as to AIDS proper) to include its more general social consequences. There has been essentially no consideration of the impact that AIDS morbidity and mortality might have on the most fundamental of social and economic institutions, the family.

One reason for this inattention to the family and household consequences of AIDS might be the presumption that AIDS is first and foremost an individual disease; that is, the chain of HIV exposure, infection, disease, and death is obviously an individual-level phenomenon. Nonetheless, at least three reasons suggest the potential significance of family or household level observation. First, although evidence suggests that "casual" contact within household settings is not even a secondary means of HIV transmission, the primary avenues of HIV exposure do occur in a family context: sexual relationships, pregnancy and childbirth, and, although to a lesser extent, breast feeding (Fischl et al, 1987). Second, although Western countries delegate much responsibility for care and support to a highly monetized and technologically-based system of formal medical institutions, health resources are relatively limited throughout the Third World, so that the responsibility for care and support rests to a greater extent on the family and kin. Third, in all societies the family or household is the important interface between the individual and society. Medical care, if purchased, is typically paid for by the family rather than exclusively by the individual. Further, if individuals are shunned or ostracized, either socially and/or economically, the family bears the brunt of this stigma and its consequences. The widely cited instance in the USA of the three young boys in Florida who were forced by arson to leave their home following exposure to HIV through blood transfusions, attests to the general relevance of this point. Clearly, adopting a family (ties of kinship) or household (co-residence without regard to kinship ties) frame of reference adds an important perspective to assessing the social consequences of AIDS.

More specifically, AIDS will have important consequences for families and households. These range from problems of physical survival of family and household members to demographic structure (e.g., fertility rates and numbers of surviving children, patterns of marriage and divorce, household headship/living arrangements, youth and aged dependency, orphanhood) and to economic functioning (e.g., income; labour force participation rates for women, children, and the aged; the extent of pauperization due to medical care costs; and patterns of intergenerational inheritance), as well as to more social-psychological factors such as socio-emotional support and patterns of interpersonal interaction within the family unit as well as with members of the larger society, as referred to above. To our knowledge, the only information available on these issues is at best anecdotal. We focus specifically on several demographic characteristics of families and households, although the point of the paper is more widely applicable.

Our purpose here is not to offer polished research empirically demonstrating particular links between AIDS and specific family or household characteristics but, rather, to propose the significance of this general area of study. What is necessary is basic data collection on the family and household characteristics of infected persons and members of their households as they progress through each stage of the exposure-infection-disease-death chain, as well as analogous information on comparison households, in order that basic research can be undertaken along these lines. In what follows, we highlight some basic points and substantive areas which might be fruitfully explored for hypotheses which could inform such inquiry.

AIDS and Family

Knowledge of the long-term consequences of AIDS at the

family or household level is solely anecdotal. At present, data are simply not available that would permit us to state with any confidence whatsoever those outcomes which might be anticipated, their probabilities of occurrence, or how these might vary by household type or social context. In essence, we need to develop both research paradigms and data sets to address these issues. This paper is an initial effort along these lines.

In assessing the consequences of any medical, social, economic, or other event for families and households, it is necessary to begin with a recognition of the diversity that exists in family structure and living arrangements, internationally as well as subnationally among racial/ethnic groups or social classes. Most discussion of family and household variability is based on a simple contrast between the prototypical nuclear and extended families, in line with both the widely cited hypothesis that long term convergence in family structures is occurring along the lines of the nuclear model. However, in order to take into account recent increases in living alone and in divorce within industrialized countries, it may be more useful to recognize five distinct family and household living arrangements: single adult, single parent family, married couple (no children), nuclear family, and extended family or household (depending on the presence of non-kin). Obviously marriage and kinship should be defined in de facto rather than de jure terms, following the normative patterns in the populations of interest.

Superimposed on this diversity in household and family arrangements is the fact of AIDS. What might its consequences be for important family and household characteristics, and how might these consequences vary across different family and household types? Two properties of the AIDS pandemic are relevant here. First, the age pattern of AIDS means that disease and death is more likely among those in the prime working years and among infants and young children. While there is likely cross-sectional variability in this pattern internationally according to whether AIDS is spread primarily through heterosexual contacts (e.g., Africa, some parts of South America, Caribbean) or through homosexual ones as well as behaviours linked to drug abuse (e.g., USA, Europe), these differences should reflect variability in the degree, rather than the fact, that AIDS is unevenly distributed by age.

Second, in speculating about particular effects which AIDS morbidity and mortality might have, it is useful to begin with a "simple" pattern of a single infected individual within the household or family. However, this may not be a plausible scenario in many cases, although data to address definitively this question are not presently available. Indeed, the long asymptomatic period means that HIV transmission to a spouse through sex is probable and, further, it is clear that infants born to seropositive women have about a fifty percent chance of developing AIDS. Moreover, transmission through breast milk is apparently possible, although less common than perinatal transmission. Alternatively, no evidence suggests that transmission to other household members is likely from normal household contact, including the sharing of lavatory and kitchen facilities.

Following from the above, we would suggest that a reasonable basis for the development of a research paradigm is by "analogizing" - considering the observable consequences of other diseases which are also disproportionately concentrated among the younger segments of the population and which are associated with exceptionally high levels of premature mortality (cf. Brandt, 1988). While no condition may be viewed as being perfectly analogous with AIDS in terms of these factors as well as the possibility of transmission to a spouse through sexual contact, or, moreover, the morality connotations which the disease may reflect within the population at large, we would hypothesize that the observed family and household consequences of conditions such as cancer (especially leukemia) or sickle cell anemia might be at least indicative of the manner in which AIDS might influence the pattern of household functioning and relationships. These hypotheses remain to be explored.

In terms of a strategy for data collection, information is needed on both an immediate and long-term, continual basis. In the short term, we need to initiate a data collection program which provides a cross-sectional view of households, arrayed by type. The sample of households must be drawn in such a way that it includes infected persons at all stages of the disease, from asymptomatic seropositive through clinically confirmed diagnoses of the presence of those opportunistic conditions associated with "full-blown" AIDS. It would be essential that the position of the infected person(s) in the household be clearly specified as well as information, where available and relevant, on race/ethnicity and those risk behaviours which might have introduced the infection initially. By insuring that this sample is representative of the larger population, we will immediately be able to develop point estimates of the prevalence and, with follow-up, incidence by age, household type, stage of disease and other appropriate variables. This would enable interpretation of the representativeness of reports such as one where roughly 5.5% of a sample of married couples in Kinshasa, Zaire were found to have at least one person seropositive (Ryder, 1988).

It will also be necessary, for control purposes, that any sample include additional households, all of whose members would be currently seronegative. Ideally, the distribution of these control households would be similar to those of the study households in terms of type, size, age of parents and children, income level, occupation and other appropriate variables. Ideally, this data collection operation would be conducted in as many different national settings as possible and with maximal possible conformity to standardized data collection instruments. In this way, cross-national comparability would be assured (see for example, Zoughlami and Allsopp, 1985 on the World Fertility Survey). Obviously, standard sampling methods are not appropriate to the study of AIDS; a case-control rather than a random approach is necessary. Similarly, issues of confidentiality and counselling require careful consideration in any data collection effort.

Cross-sectional data collection will satisfy short-term information needs regarding current prevalence levels and will permit some initial assessment of the role played by household type and national setting. However, the collection of data for a single point in time does nothing to enhance our understanding of the dynamics of AIDS within a household. It is essential to consider not only the epidemiology of disease transmission, but also the degree to which the deterioration of the health status of infected person(s) impacts upon household functions and responsibilities of non-infected members, upon the nature of relationships between and among infected and non-infected persons, and upon the social and economic well-being of all members of the household. In order to accomplish this goal, it is vital that the households and household members included in the initial sample be followed and re-interviewed over time.

Demographic Effects of AIDS

One demographic characteristic of families and households is their complexity or, more specifically, the pattern of living arrangements. Clearly, living arrangements would be expected to vary with the presence and stage of the AIDS disease process. For instance, taking AIDS-related mortality first, it is obviously the case that a death occurring in a single adult household would mean that the household would cease to exist; however, in all other cases the effects are not so straightforward.

In the case of a married couple, death of a spouse leaves the surviving partner, who may or may not remarry depending, among other things, on their own seropositivity. For a single parent family, death of the adult means that children become orphans (if the other parent is dead) or, at a minimum, are residentially displaced. If alternative housing is available with kin or close non-kin, the surviving children might be able to maintain household-base residence in a more complex extended family; if not, institutionalization or state-administered adoption or referral programs might be their only option. This is now proving problematic in those cases where the children are themselves seropositive (McIntosh, 1987).

When one adult in a nuclear family dies, the impact on surviving family members might vary. If the surviving spouse is economically able to maintain an independent living arrangement, then the single parent family might continue. If not, then some form of dependent arrangement in an extended family or household or, perhaps, dependence on institutional resources would be the only alternatives to homelessness and/or family separation. In an extended family or household, the death of one adult might have fewer consequences on living arrangements *per se*.

The death of a child would seem to have fewer direct consequences for living arrangements than does the death of an adult, in any family system. However, both child and adult mortality can affect the extent to which typical transitions among household types occur at all and/or at the timing appropriate to the normative family life cycle. Although less clear than in the case of AIDS-related mortality, morbidity might also affect living arrangements insofar as infected individuals might be excluded from family relationships and/or may be forced by others to leave their typical place of residence.

Living arrangements are complex. Other, more "elementary" household and family characteristics also serve to illustrate the potential impacts of AIDS. For example, consider patterns of marriage and divorce. It seems likely that seropositivity in one spouse/partner or potential spouse/partner will reduce the probability of marriage and increase that of divorce, if this is known to the other, and a similar if not stronger effect might occur for ARC and AIDS. In the extreme, AIDS mortality might affect mate selection through attrition from the marriage market. Alternatively, to the extent that families exercise control over marriage timing as well as spouse selection, the possibility of AIDS may reinforce early marriage because this may be perceived as an effective strategy for reducing the risk of HIV exposure. Apart from this general hypothesized relationship, though, it is difficult to predict *a priori* how this behaviour might vary across family and household types.

Further, consider fertility. There is little or no reason to believe that seropositive individuals will limit their fertility, although to the extent that the fecund period is shortened by premature morbidity or death, completed family size may decline. Further, there may be a reason to hypothesize an increase in the tempo of fertility as infected adults try to compensate for lost opportunity for childbearing in relation to their normal life expectancy or to "replace" children who have died. Even a consideration based only on the concept of exposure to the risk of conception - marital duration - is ambiguous as to direction, since younger marriage ages in some societies would increase the duration of exposure to the risk of pregnancy and thus fertility while higher divorce would reduce both. While the possible impact of AIDS on the number of surviving children may be more complex than that on fertility in general, it seems likely that this number will decline.

One final demographic characteristic of families and households which might vary with the pattern of AIDS-related mortality involves dependency, both aged and youth. At the societal level decreases in the number of adults due to AIDS seems to be effectively balanced with decreases in the number of infants and children such that aggregate dependency ratios show little change (Bongaarts, 1988; McLean, 1988). This is particularly the case where AIDS is largely a disease of the heterosexual population. Shifts in the extent and pattern of dependency are apt to be more striking at the family and household level. AIDS-related mortality will likely have more of an impact on the extent of dependency within families in those societies where the elderly are cared for in an extended family arrangement and without outside help. Clearly, these consequences are more striking for families with one as opposed to two wage earners, and with some children as opposed to none. Similar observations are suggested concerning youth dependency.

SUMMARY AND CONCLUSIONS

Overall, we have argued in favour of viewing the social and economic consequences of AIDS from the point of view of families and households. After a brief overview of the rationale behind such a paradigm, we provide some initial direction to research efforts by focusing on basic issues of family and household types and the utility of analogizing from other diseases. In addition, the paper proposes certain questions covering the specific demographic implications of AIDS and suggests a research design to collect the kinds of data which are necessary to answer them.

While our treatment of these issues has been necessarily abbreviated, the significance of the topic should be evident. More generally, we assert that in order to understand and deal in policy terms with the social consequences of the AIDS pandemic, it is absolutely essential both to understand its impacts on families and households and to recognize the role of families and households in mediating linkages between the individual and society. The intent of our contribution to this symposium is to stimulate efforts along these lines.

REFERENCES

Bongaarts J P. Modelling the demographic impact of AIDS in Africa. 1988. Paper at the Annual Meeting of the American Association for the Advancement of Science.

Fischl M A, Dickinson G M, Scott G B, Klimas N, Fletcher M A, Parks W (1987). Evaluation of heterosexual partners, children, and household contacts of adults with AIDS. J Amer Med Assn 257: 640-644.

McIntosh J. Prepared statement. In US House of Representatives Select Committee on Children, Youth and Families: "Aids and Young Children: Emerging Issues", Washington: US Government Printing Office, 1987, pp 97-107.

McLean A, May R M (1988). Transmission dynamics of HIV infection. Paper at the Annual Meeting of the American Association for the Advancement of Science.

Ryder R (1988). Heterosexual and perinatal transmission of HIV infection. Paper at the Annual Meeting of the American Association for the Advancement of Science.

Zoughlami Y, Allsopp D (1985). "The Demographic Characteristics of Household Populations", Voorburg: International Statistical Institute, (WFS Cross-National Series, no. 45).

The Global Impact of AIDS, pages 183–190
© 1988 Alan R. Liss, Inc.

24. HIV-INFECTION, AIDS, AND FAMILY DISRUPTION

Gary A Lloyd

Professor and Coordinator, Institute for Training and
Research in HIV Counselling, Tulane University
School of Social Work, New Orleans, Louisiana, USA.

INTRODUCTION

Although exceptions have been recognised, it can be
assumed that discovery of a person's HIV status or diagnosis of
AIDS has profound and disruptive effects upon other family
members and their capacity for problem-solving. This disruption,
while expressed differently, occurs in all cultures. It is evident in
traditional, extended families; small, nuclear and basically urban
family units; and alternative, or affiliated family structures.

The extent and duration of family disruption are influenced
by history and strength of family bonds, previous experiences
with illness and loss, and attitudes about HIV and AIDS. The last
is a most important determinant. Shame about HIV infection and
AIDS, and concern about the reactions of other people, are
virtually universal reactions.

Shame is a powerful emotion, and a central aspect of
disruption, experienced by both the HIV infected person and
members of his or her family.

Disruption in customary activities, intra-familial
relationships, and patterns of family maintenance and caring
occur because of (1) stigma attached to HIV and those infected
with it; (2) disrimination directed toward them and members of
their families; (3) revelations of previously unknown
homosexuality, prostitution, infidelity, promiscuity, or drug use;
and (4) shame and guilt about behaviours and practises known to
be linked to transmission of HIV. The young age of persons
afflicted and the need to plan for the future of their own young

children, and heavy burdens placed upon family caretakers also
contribute to family disruption.

FAMILY FORMS AND RESPONSES

Positive HIV-status shocks and changes the life of the
infected person, and disrupts both Traditional and Affiliated
families.

Traditional monogamous or polygamous families are
comprised of parents and children (the "nuclear" family),
frequently living in proximity to grandparents, siblings and other
relatives (the "extended" family or kinship group). Such families
have formal standing (and responsibilities for caretaking) in law
and tradition. The modern, smaller "nuclear" family has become,
or is becoming, the norm in urban areas throughout the world.
Economic and emotional resources for taking care of AIDS
patients are often quite limited in traditional, nuclear families.

Particularly in Europe and North America, an alternative to
traditional and socially sanctioned family structures is the non-
traditional, **affiliated** family made up of friends or same-sex
partners who live together. These families do not have standing
in law or tradition. Affiliated families experience the same
stress as traditional families. They may face additional stress
from the fact that they are not recognised as "real" families, and
partners are not entitled to resources and benefits available to
traditional families.

In either family form, the infected person and family
members experience a post-diagnosis process of **shock, blow,
recoil and recovery.** If the family and the HIV infected person
can pass through all the steps in this process ambivalence will
remain, but the prospects are good for mutual support,
expression of love and acceptance, appropriate handling of
various and often quickly changing emotions, and reflection and
grieving. Families who become fixated at some point in this
process will tend to ignore or reject the infected or diagnosed
member.

DISRUPTION IN ACCEPTING AND REJECTING TRADITIONAL FAMILIES

Positive HIV-status and AIDS creates a family disruption
which is pervasive and enduring. It is felt at all levels of
individual and collective life within the family. **Whether the**

family accepts of rejects the person is irrelevant: disruption will be experienced.

The first disruption for all families comes with recognition of the social and personal implications of HIV status or diagnosis. Knowledge of HIV status invariably leads to revelation of behaviours or practises which heretofore were unknown or were denied and not discussed by family members. Once HIV-status is known to a person, he or she must undergo the stress of deciding when or if to tell the family. When family members know, they face the stress of deciding to accept or reject caretaking responsibilities.

When the **accepting** family agrees to care for the infected member, emotional and material resources of the family are immediately affected. Routines are disrupted, particularly as disease progresses. Stress is experienced by the entire family or household, and is not limited to a primary caretaker.

If a parent or sibling must stop working outside the home in order to provide care, loss of income and reduced standard of living will be a critical concern. Resentment toward the ill person may follow. Resentment may also develop as physical weakness becomes more pronounced and the demands upon the caretaker are more extensive and tiring.

Family disruption also occurs because of the reactions of the infected or ill person to his or her HIV status or diagnosis. Depression, mood swings, anxiety, and projected hostility onto caretakers are rarely understood by the family. Particularly if the HIV-infected person has put a spouse or children in jeopardy, signs of self-punishment will appear. Self-punishing behaviours, which will be viewed as ingratitude by caretakers, include causing arguments with caretakers, failing to follow through on medical procedures or advice, refusing to take medications, and self-destructive abuse of drugs or alcohol. Arguments, threats, and tensions between patient and family can build to a point of rejection even though there had been acceptance previously.

Some families do not agree to offer care at the time they learn of diagnosis. In these **rejecting** families, disruption in another form is apt to occur. Not all family members will agree with the decision to reject, and there will be internal (usually covert) dissent. Rejecting families are likely to maintain traditional sex role behaviours and standards of morality, rigid division of power and authority between parents, and views of "proper" family life supported by traditional and fundamentalist religious beliefs. Families who reject are also apt to be highly sensitive to the opinions of the extended family, kinship groups, or neighbours. Concerns about being viewed in a good light by outsiders is a major factor in the decision to reject.

Ambivalence about their decision is found in both **rejecting and accepting families.** Where acceptance is given, for example, the family may truly want to provide support and care. Yet, at least some members may fear negative reactions from other people, and loss of relationships which are valuable to them. They may feel and express love for their ill relative, but at the same time resent the nature and cause of his or her disease, and the impact it has on the family.

For similar reasons, ambivalence is also present in rejecting families. Not everyone will want to reject. If the situation becomes known to others, some people outside the immediate family may support the decision to reject, while others will criticize it as an uncharitable act.

FAMILY DISRUPTION AND THE CYCLE OF ANGER

Knowledge of HIV status creates ambivalence and a complex mixture of sometimes volatile emotions in everyone involved. Families of all kinds often experience intense anger which is cyclical in nature.

In rejecting families, anger is related to ambivalence about the decision to reject, and takes the form of covert quarrelling or passive-aggressive behaviour.

In accepting families there are at least two discernible cycles. They have different origins. The end result of each is the same: alienation, stress, regret and emotional distance.

The first cycle starts when the **patient** resents his or her dependency and at the same time fears abandoment from those who are caring for him or her. Acting upon this fear, he or she begins to make demands on the caretakers which are viewed by them as unreasonable. When the demands are resisted, the patient responds with anger and emotionally withdraws or exhibits self-punishing behaviour. Caretakers conclude that their efforts are not appreciated and themselves withdraw. The fear of abandonment which initiated the whole process is then perceived by the patient to be well-founded. The patient and the caretakers retreat from one another, often into silence and mutual feelings of loss that will not be spoken of before death ends the impasse.

The second cycle begins with the **caretakers.** It is particularly observable in families who have not had access to support and information through counselling. Because of ambivalence about accepting the illness and previous risk behaviours of blaming the person for them, caretakers begin to withdraw emotionally. This withdrawal usually takes place through action; it is not expressed verbally. The patient may comment on this change but usually will not directly acknowledge what is happening, particularly if he or she feels intense guilt. Caretakers experience feelings of shame and sorrow about their actions which are then frequently transformed into anger directed toward the patient. As with the first cycle, the result is isolation and alienation for all concerned.

Because cycles of anger are fuelled by resentment, distress, remorse and shame, it is probable that families and patients affected by HIV and AIDS will not share feelings openly, and will not communicate honestly and directly. As a consequence, the patient may die feeling alone and unloved. The family is left to sort out unspoken and unresolved feelings of guilt and anger. The disruption caused by HIV status and AIDS may continue, therefore, to have a disrupting influence on family relationships long after the AIDS patient is gone.

FAMILY THEMES

Families must come to terms with the fact that relationships between generations will be markedly changed. Persons afflicted with HIV and AIDS are usually young. They are not of an age at which death is expected. Rather than children caring for ailing parents, the situation is the other way round.

Once the shock is felt and dealt with initially, and some decision is made on the family's position about providing care, certain themes will emerge in all affected families, and are factors in family disruption.

The **stigma** and shame associated with HIV and AIDS is widely noted in the literature. Infection or disease indicates that the person has had a secret life and has engaged in behaviours and practises which are illegal or culturally unacceptable, be it drug abuse, homosexuality, promiscuity or infidelity. Stigma is so powerful in some cultures that it, and fears about individual and familial contamination, can be generalised to the entire family.

Stigma and **social attitudes** are closely linked. Because of perceived or actual social pressure, the family might deny the reality of condition or diagnosis. They will avoid talking to outsiders (such as counsellors) or each other about the person's illness and condition. A "conspiracy of silence" creates strain for everyone in the household and disrupts family bonds. Not being able to talk openly about HIV and AIDS - the symptoms, the course of disease, the heartbreak of caring for a child, spouse or sibling who is going to die - is a heavy burden for all family members. If someone breaks silence, he or she will become a source of further disruption because the family secret has been revealed.

Family members must come to terms with their felings about the way the infection was contracted, and with their own and society's view on **homosexuality, prostitution, drug abuse, promiscuity and infidelity.** If the family cannot overcome negative attitudes about past risk behaviour, denial, resentment and alienation are inevitable. Some families come through this process of examination of attitudes with a quasi-accepting position. This is felt by the patient as false and patronizing.

In some cultures, the family will also have to cope with a view of AIDS as **retribution.** Although there is nothing the infected person can do to change his or her present status or past behaviours, the theme of retribution can be powerful enough to forestall acceptance of the current condition. The retribution belief reinforces shame and guilt in the patient or infected person, and creates for caretakers feelings of helplessness, remorse and anger.

A final and universal theme for families is **loss.** Infected people and AIDS patients experience many losses; status, physical mobility, independence, strength, and appearance to mention but a few. Families experience loss too. Members know that the person they love, and who has AIDS, is going to die. If they are ambivalent about the illness or past behaviour, the sense of impending loss may be particularly acute.

DISRUPTION FOR THE NUCLEAR FAMILY AND CHILDREN

Discovery of infection or diagnosis of AIDS creates severe

levels of stress in couples when one partner is diagnosed as infected or ill. As in all instances, it is likely that previously hidden behaviours will become known. The most common and expected reaction of the spouse/partner is a keen sense of betrayal by a partner who has jeopardized the health and life of the innocent partner and children. Separation and estrangement may take place immediately. Social isolation is strongly felt by all involved. This isolation has extremely negative effects on children who are not told about what is wrong with their mother or father, but warned not to tell others about the illness at home. Their relationships with relatives and playmates may be drastically changed. Although not yet documented, it is probable that the incidence of physical and emotional abuse increases.

Previous feelings of intimacy and trust are diminished or denied. Decisions must be made about continuing sexual relations - with condom use or other means of protected sex - or celibacy. In cultures where women are expected to follow orders from their husband, the possibility of forced sexual relations and thus further transmission must be considered.

Provisions for taking care of children is a major concern when one or both parents are infected or ill. When a single parent is infected, early planning for provision of care for self and for children is particularly necessary. In all instances, if the extended family will not or cannot take in children, their future care is problematic. Prospects for finding adequate child care may not be very good in many parts of the world. Even where there are traditions for adoption and foster care, the HIV status of the parent may lead potential caretakers for the children to shun them because of fear of contamination.

DISRUPTION IN AFFILIATED FAMILIES

Affiliated families affected by HIV are usually made up of homosexual men living together in a couple relationship, and involved with a circle of friends who serve as family members. Even if parents and relatives are accepting of sexual orientation, there is high probability that a homosexual man will look to his affiliated family, more than to his family of origin for support. (This may be perceived as rejection by the family, particularly if they have maintained close emotional ties.)

Because affiliated families are not legally sanctioned, the partner of the HIV infected person may not feel any compulsion from law or family to stay and provide care. Some men have left at once, while others have stayed and nursed the partner to the very end.

Especially if the affiliated family is dissolved, a critical task for the person is to seek support from the family of origin. If there has been a continuing relationship between the person and his family, the task of the person (and of HIV counsellors) is to **reinforce** family ties. If there has been some degree of tension and estrangement, the goal is to **reconnect**. Where the alienation is total and irrevocable, **replacing** the family support is essential.

SUMMARY

Regardless of the form or structure, families with a member discovered to have HIV infection or diagnosed with AIDS will experience high levels of stress, and disruption in all areas of family life. Powerful feelings of ambivalence, resentment, denial, guilt, and anger are characteristically found. Rejecting families cut themselves off completely from the affected person. Accepting families provide care. Both types of family experience strong, personal, emotional and social impact from their decision.

Because of the stigma attached to HIV and its modes of transmission, and the shame which is characteristically felt by both the AIDS patient and his or her family, bonds of loyalty and love in even the most supportive families are stretched when infection or disease appears. Cycles of anger are both creations and results of feelings of hurt, rejection, and regret about broken family ties. Those feelings often remain with the survivors as a persisting cause of family dissension and disruption, long after the death of the family member.

The Global Impact of AIDS, pages 191-199
© 1988 Alan R. Liss, Inc.

25. SOCIAL AND CULTURAL ASPECTS OF THE PREVENTION OF THE THREE EPIDEMICS (HIV INFECTION, AIDS AND COUNTERPRODUCTIVE SOCIETAL REACTION TO THEM)

Ronald Frankenberg

Centre for Medical Social Anthropology, Keele University, Staffordshire, UK ST5 5BG

Technical Reasons for International Nature

It cannot be overemphasised that the problems raised by AIDS are international. The long period before effects of the virus are manifest, the speed of modern travel, the impossibility of global quarantine even if it were desirable, the virus's lack of class, race or wealth consciousness, the imperative but infinitely diverse nature of sexual desire and practice combine to impose international co-operation. AIDS may achieve a renewed acceptance of health promotion and prevention as the main resources.

Prevention of HIV (epidemic 1) : the three epidemics and the institutional framework of change

The usual relative cost effectiveness of preventive health care is absolute and will remain so in each of the three epidemics namely :-

(1) HIV infection,
(2) the development of the AIDS syndrome and related diseases and,
(3) the social difficulties to which both give rise.

Preventive measures related to each must be seen in separate social contexts.

We are fortunate that it was in the social environment of the western United States, whose public health infrastructure enabled recognition of a new set of diseases, the infective agent and its mode of transmission that AIDS appeared. The culture of the US public health social institutions was however forced to change (Shilts, 1987). The National Institutes of Health and The Centers for Disease Control were forced to relate to each other in new and more constructive ways. Eventually in Britain, the government was constrained, or used the opportunity, to take health education under central control. They were also persuaded, in contradiction to other policies, grudgingly to accept the importance and fundability of some gay organisations and education in sexual relationships. Other countries were obliged to overlook the racist, self righteous language in which the metropolitan power revealed their problems and themselves acknowledge the reality of their needs. Those who work within and are constrained by (normally useful and necessary) institutional culture still have to consider alternatives to accepted, quasi-instinctive reactions before alternatives are forced upon them (Douglas, 1987; Burns and Stalker, 1961).

Community Culture and Culturally Self-induced Change

Gay men, first recognised as infected by the syndrome, also included some who were rich and many who were well organised, and were experienced in combating unpopularity and overt hostility and highly politically and above all culturally self conscious as a group. The gay community had values and a style of organisation which also constrained if they did not determine the actual, fantasised and self reported behaviour of those within it. The out-of-closet gay male activist had translated his desires into practices and, socially and in interaction with others, friendly and hostile gays, hostile and friendly straights, constructed his own individual identity within sub-culture and overarching culture. To change practices was to reconstruct identity and re-form culture. They succeeded in doing this helped by a hard won solidarity, encouraged by compassion and concern for comrades, and hindered but at the same time challenged by the often violently aggressive and viciously alienating straight world. What AIDS had brought about then was in a very real sense only secondarily a change of individual behaviour. Primarily an already relatively coherent group, even if its coherence came from the agreement on the topics they thought important to disagree about, collectively chose to change the way of life that characterised their culture, without abandoning that culture in its entirety. Gay sex gave way not to no sex or to "backsliding" repentance but to safer sex and perhaps deepening relationships.

Desire, Behaviour, Identity-Culture

We can learn much from this. First while it is true that prevention of transmission of HIV involves changing sexual behaviour, researchers and health promoters, in preventive medicine and the media, must recognise for others as they do for themselves, that accepted behaviours, especially those related to life style and identity, are socially arrived at and not merely autonomous individual or dyadic choices. "What will others think?" is not an indication of a subservient mentality but an essential and necessary feature of social life even or especially for those who wish to shock those thought of as respectably conformist.

Second it is not for the observer to predict how diverse sexual behaviour could change. In the past history of pandemics, some of the threatened fled, some repented and some, in joyous despair, gave themselves up to riotous living while there was still time. Within the general framework of WHO's global strategy some countries' campaigns are arguing not for fewer sexual acts but for richer, more equal and safer personal relations and others for tighter moral, and even legal, control and monogamy or abstinence. What is advocated is not directly related to what is going to be effective but rather to the social and ideological background of the advocates. If rhetoric and reality coincide, then people with the same cultural background will be influenced. By and large, however, if the message of what has to be avoided is made clear and the options open are explained, then members of groups who are convinced will adapt their own socially determined culture and sense of identity to the new biological situation. The grave problem of a long latent period emphasises the need for prevention of epidemics two and three as well as direct transmission of the virus.

The "Deviant" and the "Innocent Victim"

In earlier centuries, the rich had painfully to learn that diseases aided by poverty made no distinction between deserving and undeserving poor and the rich themselves. HIV infection in intravenous drug users, whether stigmatised as addicts or not, and in prisoners, either injecting drugs or practising anal intercourse, is no less in need of treatment or prevention than in those passively infected through blood transfusion or more legitimately regarded intercourse. This requires the overt recognition that such "deviant" activities exist and a change in attitude of institutions towards them. Unfortunately, those who

see themselves as having nobly resisted such "deviations" may
need to be persuaded where their real interests lie.

Prevention HIV to AIDS : Living with Infection or Dying from it

Whether and how fast HIV-positive move towards AIDS,
AIDS-related complex or other pathology or towards death,
complicated or uncomplicated by such syndromes, appears at
first sight to be a purely medical (even individual clinical) rather
than a social issue. The number of studied cases is still too small
and the history of the condition too short for there to be clear
indications of the factors involved. Disease has always however a
social component sometimes distinguished as sickness, - the way
biological disorder is culturally performed: how it is diagnosed
and by whom, what it is called and why, whether patients are
hospitalised and when, whether they are treated and what for,
when the struggle to keep them alive ought to be or is abandoned
because it is seen as futile, impossible, too painful for patient,
for relatives in the broadest sense, or for health workers or
perhaps prohibitively expensive. Consciously or unconsciously,
overtly or secretly, honestly or less honestly, choices and
decisions are made and social factors like age, perceived quality
of life, marital status, dependent children, responsibility for self
and others, "willingness to fight" are taken into account.

HIV infection here presents both challenge and opportunity
that have only been partly met and, significantly, to a much
greater extent from within the gay community and by the
directly affected rather than by medicine.

(In Britain, compare Tatchell's (updated 1987) **AIDS : A
Guide to Survival** on the one hand and Miller, Webber and Green,
The Management of AIDS Patients. The latter title reveals
institutional publishing imperatives - "Helping AIDS patients to
help themselves" would bridge the cultures of patients and health
workers.)

Already in Britain the prescription of expensive, rare drugs
which may prevent the development of AIDS in the HIV-positive
and are known to slow the process of AIDS itself have not been
authorised for the former perhaps for fear of side effects or of
expense. How are such decisions going to be taken in poorer
countries where even serum tests for those "at risk" would
exhaust available health budgets?

Death and Social Acceptance

Death, dementia and the process of dying in western industrial society have become the prerogative of the old. In the less industrially developed poor nations, death often comes very early in childhood. Although AIDS strikes down people in their procreative and productive prime it does not do so suddenly but, especially if serum testing were to become widespread, with ample but uncertain warning. Medicine, social services, even family structure are not well organised to deal with the material, spiritual or social consequences of such a change in death patterns. Outside hospice and geriatric ward and especially in teaching hospitals, doctors are trained to cure, and nurses to care for, the acutely sick. Even before the advent of HIV infection, this was inappropriate, certainly as a model for the developing countries (King, 1966) but also in very advanced industrial countries with a pattern of recurrent acute episodes of chronic disease and high technology care (Strauss et al., 1985). Primary health care practitioners find difficulty in meeting more than the surface needs of the chronically sick and the dying (Cartwright et al., 1973).

Many patients with cancer and other diseases already discover that their days are numbered. Few are offered general counselling on how to live their dying days, or specific advice on nutrition, exercise, staying fit and independence. They may in fact be worse off than in those countries where townsmen return to their villages to end their days. Those diagnosed HIV-positive are in an even worse position, condemned not to a reasonable and more or less measured certainty but to an uncertain certainty, complicated perhaps by ostracism, unemployment and lack of funds (and in some cases mental decline). Uncertainty is widely recognised as one of the major pains of chronic disease and disability (Locker, 1983). Uncertainty in detail with perceived certainty of a not distant ultimate terminal outcome, related to guilt and mortal lack of control, is a recipe for misery which, in the absence of support may lead to suicide or wilfully anti-social and infection spreading behaviour.

The nature of AIDS as supervulnerability rather than specific disease puts people with it on a roller coaster of a possible rapid succession of ups and downs, ins and outs in relation to hospital, transitions from patient to person and back. Just the kind of situation which on a slower and smaller scale even the most developed hospitals have found most difficult to deal with both in terms of patient welfare and their own economies.

The Family as Answer?

In societies of all kinds the traditional solution to this kind of problem has been the family in its various forms. In countries such as Britain, the term community care is used as a euphemism for the family and to conceal the burdens placed on married women who at the age of 50 plus may well be cooking, cleaning and mending for their husbands, their grandchildren, remaining own children, own or husband's widowed parent, and doing a part time job for wages within or outside the home (Phillipson, 1982). Such a pattern may result in middle aged illhealth (re-labelled menopausal problems). Could it be sustained where AIDS was widespread or if the woman herself had HIV or AIDS related pathology? Other countries with different labour market patterns present this kind of problem in different ways. It is not only the most productive but the most procreative who are at risk, special problems are likely to arise for children, seropositive or not, already living on the edge of malnutrition whose parents are dead or too debilitated to provide for them.

Restructuring of Old Institutions and the Creation of New

Failure to check additional HIV infection and the seropositive developing AIDS will require the allocation of funds to providing drugs, hospital and home care, as well as the retraining of health workers and aides or the mobilisation and social support of friends, neighbours, the wider family, traditional or alternative healers; or the creation of totally new social institutions as has already happened in the buddy system and other forms of self help. There is no society where it is easy for the dying or for the survivors to deal at the level of meaning or economic survival with the deaths or rapid mental and physical decline of young women and men at the height of their physical and mental powers.

The Third Epidemic - Discrimination, Ostracism and Civil Rights

The social ostracism of the sick or potentially sick is of course no new phenomenon to history. If disease is a biological disturbance of the individual body leading to social disruption and disorder in the body politic, a human social reaction is to turn back on the biological. In the search for meaning "Why has this disease struck them now?" there is a rapid transition to a search not merely for guilt or guilt-laden behaviour, but for a guilty group. Social and especially individual behaviour is hard to identify, to make precise and to observe. Social groups are easier to pinpoint particularly by more or (usually) less relevant visible biological and therefore surface characteristics. We are familiar with this social process in the various forms of racism and sexism. Thus, in presecond world-war Germany, Jews saw themselves as bearers of culture and religion: the Nazis characterised them by their noses and lisps. In Britain Afro-Caribbeans and South Asians seek to identify themselves by their respective historical and cultural heritages; racists by colour of their skin. Women's claim to equality is based on what they can do; this is rarely disputed. What is put in question is what they are, biology is once more selectively translated into totality.

The boundary between biological disease and social sickness overlaps the boundary between life and death, the consciousness of human mortality and ultimate uncertainty and lack of social control over life at the moments of both potential conception and actual dying. HIV infection and subsequent AIDS (and more poignantly HIV-induced dementia), lend themselves to being caught up in this socially symbolic emotional maelstrom as gays, the "seropositive" and persons with AIDS have already suffered on a grand scale.

This presents us with the problem of distinguishing between measures which are genuinely likely to be effective in reducing high risk behaviour and those, the superficial rationality of which conceal deeply held prejudices and the apparent (but ineffective and short lived) social convenience of blaming an easily identified and unpopular group.

In the history of sexually transmitted disease, women have been ascribed this role, either because as mothers they "failed" to educate or as wives they "failed" socially to satisfy and control the "naturally" overwhelming forces of male sexual desire. Alternatively, because by practising prostitution they at once undermined the family and its health by providing an illegitimate social outlet for these natural forces. Past epidemics or periods, usually of military origin, when the social consciousness of STD and especially syphilis has been high, have led to the persecution and imprisonment of prostitute women and proposals for tighter social control of all women (Brandt, 1987; McNeill, 1976). Seeing prostitution in this way in the present pandemic is misleading and diverts attention both from risk behaviour in all sexual relationships and one of the most effective areas for health promotion. Furthermore, for all women in whatever social context they are sexually active, HIV and AIDS have created a situation in which control over the use of their own bodies, already a moral imperative, has become not merely a health issue but a necessity for individual and societal survival. The personal is the political. The implications of this for social organisation of the world's diverse societies are enormous and complex and it is by no means obvious that the result must be a new, politically, coercively or technologically imposed puritanism. This has already become contradictorily apparent in national health promotion strategies.

Much modern medical thinking is presented in terms of quasi-military analogies of excluding or killing organisms invading the body from outside. It is not surprising that ancient notions of quarantining, expelling the so-called "carriers" of disease from society should be revived and that groups deserving of such treatment should be seen in quasi-biological terms. This is particularly tempting to countries where HIV infection is as yet rare and provides a potential source of conflict. Are the results of such actions likely to prevent transmission of the biological agents of epidemics one or two or merely to constitute the social causes of epidemic three? The virus does not necessarily infect the politically least powerful or guarantee that those most likely to be infected are the most likely to be expelled.

Social relations at an international level, between ethnic groups within nations, social control of the supposedly deviant within neighbourhoods, family and household relationships, control over women as individuals and as members of groups, attempts to monitor and control personal life in one place or through travel brings us back full circle to where I began and makes clear that the three epidemics have profound effects at every level of social action and experience.

The social consequences of the advent of HIV do not necessarily have to be entirely bad. They present difficulties but also challenges and choices. They enable us to see that racism, sexual oppression, gross economic and health inequalities within and between nations, are threatening to individual, social, national and international survival and require concerted and co-operative action.

Bringing most nations together to formulate a global strategy is one of the few areas of hope in the future of a world where the consequences of technology so often run ahead of their social control.

REFERENCES

Brandt A (1985). "No Magic Bullet". New York: Oxford University Press.

Burns T, Stalker G M (1961). "The Management of Innovation". London: Tavistock.

Cartwright A, Hockey L, Anderson J L (1973). "Life Before Death". London: Routledge.

Douglas M (1987). "How Institutions Think". London : Routledge.

King M (1966). "Medical Care in Developing Countries". Nairobi: Oxford University Press.

Locker D (1983). "Disability and Disadvantage". London: Tavistock.

McNeill W H (1979). "Plagues and Peoples". London: Penguin Books.

Miller D, Webber J, Green J (1986). "The Management of AIDS Patients". London: MacMillan.

Phillipson C (1982). "Capitalism and the Construction of Old Age". London: MacMillan.

Shilts R (1987). "And the Band Played On". New York: St Martins Press.

Strauss, Anselm, Fagerhaugh, Shizuko, Suczek B, Wiener C (1985). "Social Organization of Medical Work". Chicago: University Press.

Tatchell P (1987). "AIDS: A Guide to Survival". London: Gay Men's Press.

Part III: THE RESPONSE

The Global Impact of AIDS, pages 203-205
© 1988 Alan R. Liss, Inc.

26. AIDS PREVENTION AND CONTROL

Jonathan Mann

Director, Global Programme on AIDS, World Health
Organization, Geneva, Switzerland

Epidemics, chronic health problems, illness and death have
been a characteristic of human society since the beginning of
time. Historically man has found many ways of dealing with and
adapting to health problems. To be conscious and aware of the
need for health and disease prevention and to generate social
commitment for health is a continuing challenge. We know that
particular types of behaviour are related to disease, yet we are
surrounded by examples of persistence of those behaviours.

For a variety of reasons AIDS may be different :-

* it very quickly achieved public prominence;
* it has received extensive and detailed coverage by the
  world's media;
* it has received more attention by national and international
  policy makers than any other epidemic we have known;
* it was the first disease reviewed and discussed by the United
  Nations General Assembly;
* it brought together more health ministers than any other
  single health concern has ever done, at the London Summit
  meeting in January of this year.

All this has happened in the space of seven years. During
that time we have seen numerous examples of how national and
international resources can be mobilized. The virus has been
isolated and described. Epidemiologic surveys have pinpointed
the modes of transmission and the behaviours that can transmit
the virus. Within a period of fifteen months the World Health
Organization has helped bring the global AIDS strategy to
national Governments in over 120 countries. It has helped bring

planning and coordination into the worldwide fight against AIDS and has demonstrated the need for a United Global Effort.

In many countries and certainly for many individuals and families, however, the last seven years have been replete with human tragedies. But we should not forget that those seven years have also shown what can be done when we set our minds to it, and when national and international communities are willing to commit themselves to dealing with a social and health threat of this kind.

To date, most of the emphasis has been placed on the biomedical aspects of the problem. This Conference has helped to mark a new phase in our global effort. It has been organized to define the magnitude of the third epidemic, to which we have referred many times in the past; namely, the social, cultural, economic, legal and political implications of AIDS and the response that it has generated.

This third epidemic, perhaps less easily quantifiable than the second epidemic, less dramatic in some ways, is nevertheless, the one that will govern not only our lives but the lives of our children. This epidemic has the ability to change the face and nature of human society, the way we interact with each other, organize our lives, conceive of health, illness and commit ourselves to working with those who are most affected and most in need of support.

AIDS is pushing us to question and explore aspects of our world that we have never systematically confronted: the design and function of our health care and social welfare systems; our approach to health planning and disease prevention; and the role that all people have to play. AIDS, in the space of seven years, has pushed us to consider the symbiotic intimacy of individual health, public health, and human rights, and in so doing recognize the needs, expectations and hopes of all concerned.

There is no doubt that the AIDS epidemic will force us to confront deficiencies in these areas, problems that we have learned to live with and have accepted in the past. The AIDS epidemic provides us with one of those opportunities to reassess our world and to take up what historians will call a unique biomedical, biosocial and social development challenge.

As we move forward in dealing with this problem we must learn to acknowledge the cultural diversity of our societies and of the unique interests of different peoples within those societies. We must involve them in ways that we have rarely done in the past recognizing that their experience·and their empirical knowledge is fundamental to the design of effective control and prevention strategies.

AIDS is sexually transmitted. It is among the most democratic of diseases. It potentially affects all of us. It affects us through a part of our lives which is both basic and among the most difficult to change.

The World Health Organization's Global AIDS Plan has therefore focussed on the prevention of transmission, the helping of those persons already infected with HIV, and the unification of national and international efforts to control AIDS.

Jointly, with countries, developed and developing, the World Health Organization's Global Programme on AIDS is providing support to national AIDS programmes, as well as leadership and coordination in biomedical, behavioural and epidemiologic research, in health promotion, surveillance, and in the forecasting and assessment of the impact of AIDS. For these activities to fulfil their potential, a degree and type of resource mobilization unprecedented in international health will be required. Social and political will are needed.

We would like to take this opportunity of thanking the London School of Hygiene and Tropical Medicine for its initiative in organizing this Conference and for the Corporation of London for so graciously hosting it.

Above all, we would like to thank the participants - those representing National Committees on AIDS around the world, those representing people who are HIV-infected, the non-governmental organizations and the scientists - all of whom will need to work even more closely toegther if we are to learn to dominate the social, cultural, political and economic impact and challenge of AIDS.

HIV infection can be prevented. We believe it will be prevented. We believe that the steps already being taken are moving us towards effective prevention. Yet the next 10-20 years will be the telling years. Our responsibility is to make sure that for this and future generations human society is not dominated by a disease, but rather that human society learns and commits itself to the domination of AIDS and, through AIDS, many of the other social problems that have characterised and, in different ways, plagued society until now.

The Global Impact of AIDS, pages 207–214
© 1988 Alan R. Liss, Inc.

27. GLOBAL STRATEGY FOR THE PREVENTION AND CONTROL OF AIDS

D Tarantola

Global Programme on AIDS, World Health
Organization, Geneva, Switzerland

The WHO Global Programme on AIDS (GPA) was launched on 1 February 1987, with two objectives in view :-

(1)   To prevent HIV transmission; and
(2)   To reduce morbidity and mortality associated with HIV infection.

As a global programme, GPA calls for the creation of strong national programmes in every country, both developing and industrialized, in the world. It calls for cooperation and collaboration in research, prevention and control efforts at the scale of the planet.

As a global programme, it fosters the simultaneous and coordinated participation of multiple sectors through governmental and non-governmental organizations under the emerging leadership of the health sector.

As a global programme, GPA is directed to all population groups irrespective of demographic, behavioural or any other personal characteristics. The society as a whole, in its most exposed and vulnerable groups, is being threatened. The society as a whole will stop AIDS.

As a global programme, GPA requires leadership and coordination, for which a mandate has been given to the World Health Organization on the basis of a universal concensus.

This presentation will briefly review the six elements of the global strategies and describe the main steps that have been taken to give the programme its intended global scale.

The first strategy, prevention of sexual transmission, relies on the strong belief and emerging evidence that changes in sexual behaviour can be induced through information and education.

The major constraints facing national programmes in this regard include the very limited knowledge of sexual behaviour available in industrialized or developing countries,the low priority and scarcity of resources allocated to health education programmes in the past, and the resulting present scarcity of skilled manpower and adapted infrastructure for effective health promotion and education.

The ingredients for success are not self-evident, yet there are early signs of significant progress. In most countries, sexual issues are being addressed with more openness, and there is a noted increase in the scientific skills and resources allocated to this area.

In less permissive societies, such as in countries of the Eastern Mediterranean Region, there has been a significant positive change in the last two years in the attitude of national authorities to the AIDS problem. Collaborative plans drawn up by these countries and WHO now include education on AIDS and sexually-transmitted diseases. This is a striking phenomenon given the initial reluctance to acknowledge AIDS as a problem, let alone to speak about its modes of transmission and methods of prevention. In other countries the policies on promotion and use of condoms have been reassessed and adapted to the new situation. In a number of societies, the discussion of sexual behaviour and practices are taboo. Recently, the development of a national plan for the prevention of AIDS in Polynesian island countries met with difficulties in that the local language included no words for genitals or for common patterns of sexual practices.

The global strategy for health promotion and education on AIDS received a major boost in January this year, when delegates at the World Summit held in London declared that all countries in the world needed to devise national programmes, the single most important component of which should be "information and education because HIV transmission can be prevented through informed and responsible behaviour". An important statement made by Ministers of Health at that meeting said that **sectors other than health** should be involved to the fullest possible extent in the planning and implementation of national programmes.

Already, 151 of the 182 countries and territories in the world have established national advisory committees on AIDS. Initially, these committees were heavily dominated by health professionals, in particular clinicians and laboratory specialists. Today, as medium-term plans on AIDS are being formulated, countries are restructuring their committees, so as to expand their membership and scope outside the health sector. A noted trend has also been the increased participation of non-governmental organizations in programmes, not only in their traditional role of providers, but also in the planning process.

In line with a resolution of the United Nations General Assembly in October 1987, the Global Programme on AIDS has fostered an alliance between WHO and the United Nations Development Programme (UNDP). The Alliance will enable the Global Programme to take full advantage of the communication, administrative and logistic support available within UNDP and collaborate more effectively with all sectors concerned, other UN agencies and NGOs.

The prevention of transmission through blood, **the second strategy,** necessitates strengthening the blood transfusion system and monitoring the preparation of blood products and promoting the safe use and re-use of skin-piercing and dental instruments. Many countries are showing considerable interest in this approach, which offers the possibility of doing something rapid, visible and popular in a non-controversial area. The moral, ethical and legal commitments on the part of the health system to provide safe medical care are additional motivating factors.

"Over-prescription of blood transfusion" is a contributor to HIV transmission. The application of criteria for transfusion, abiding by the principle that "any blood transfusion which is not strictly indicated is strictly contra-indicated" requires sustained educational efforts among health professionals and the public. In addition, developing countries are facing difficulties in the procurement of blood substitutes. Local production of these, together with efforts to minimize instances in which blood transfusion is required, for example when malaria, thalassemia and sickle cell patients are concerned, represent a new dimension of AIDS prevention and control activities. Industrialized countries have promptly introduced HIV testing as a routine measure in blood banks. In South-East Asia and the Western Pacific Regions, the preferred approach is to develop blood bank capabilities in both HIV and Hepatitis B screening. In Latin America and Africa, all capital cities and a good proportion of large cities will have HIV-screened blood available by the end of 1988.

With the emergence of a new strain of HIV, countries are faced with the dilemma of deciding at what point HIV 2 screening should be added to that for HIV 1. The rapid multiplication of tests available for large-scale use and the concurrent plummeting cost of these tests, constantly change the parameters for cost-benefit analysis. Again, the critical decision is the threshold of HIV 2 prevalence beyond which screening becomes justified, knowing that once initiated it will have to be maintained for an indefinite period.

The global needs in the area of blood transfusion are such that WHO, UNDP, the Red Cross and several NGOs are embarking on a global "safe blood" initiative, under which technical and financial resources will be mobilized in support of national blood transfusion schemes.

Transmission of HIV through blood can also occur if unsterile needles, syringes, lancets and other skin-piercing instruments are used. Information and education directed to both health professionals and in the government, private sector and the general public will promote the use of "one sterile needle, one sterile syringe, for one injection". The message has already found its way through many health systems, either as a result of basic training or of promotional and educational efforts developed by Expanded Programmes on Immunization. The number of vaccinating injections represents only a small proportion of all injections performed. Proper sterilization of equipment, on which WHO is about to publish guidelines, should be expanded to the entire spectrum of medical care. A reduction in the number of injections (which can often simply be omitted or replaced by oral prescriptions) will result from increased awareness among health staff and pressure from an educated community. The logistic implications of this strategy are quite complex, for example, the choice between sterilization (but not always sterilizable) and non-reusable (but often re-used) injection equipment.

The association of HIV infection with drug abuse was initially thought to be a concern of only developed countries, but new markets are opening in developing countries, particularly those which serve as transit points. A technical meeting held last January in Geneva concluded that traditional approaches to the prevention and control of injecting drug behaviour called for strong multisectoral approaches, all sectors providing support and services through comprehensive programme policies. In particular, care must be taken to ensure the involvement of persons with injecting drug behaviour in designing and implementing intervention programmes.

The third strategy is the prevention of perinatal transmission. In some urban and periurban areas where seven to eight percent of the young sexually active population are already infected with HIV, the vertical transmission of infection emerges as an important cause of early childhood morbidity and mortality. In fact, this increase in mortality is likely to offset the mortality decline anticipated from major efforts developed under primary health care to immunize, prevent malaria, treat dehydration and acute respiratory infections.

In order to prevent perinatal transmission through HIV infected women, both men and women should be informed about the consequences of HIV infection in relation to pregnancy and birth, and voluntary testing should be encouraged. An increasing number of countries have included HIV testing among the tests routinely performed during pregnancy. The issues of informed consent, confidentiality, and the provision of counselling are particularly complex here. In many societies, the inability or unwillingness to bear children may lead to the rejection of the woman by her spouse. Such instances have catastrophic consequences on individuals, the family and the society as a whole.

The fourth and fifth strategies concern the development, testing, production and delivery of therapeutic agents and vaccines which are still very much at the research stage. The global strategy is to facilitate the development of these products, coordinate research, establish mechanisms for scientific collaboration, and guarantee social and ethical acceptability of field trials. Furthermore, in the area of vaccine development, the strategy calls for the establishment of a WHO coordinated international bank for HIV and related retroviruses, sera and reagents.

Should therapeutic agents and vaccines become available and affordable, the experience that has been gained in recent years, worldwide, in the area of expanded immunization, community-based treatment and the execution of schemes for the delivery of essential drugs will be most valuable.

The sixth and last strategy is the reduction of the impact of HIV infection. This impact on individuals, communities and the society as a whole raises the immediate concerns of human suffering, family disruption and social unrest. The legal, financial and political implications of this disease threaten the notion of human rights in creating an antagonism between the right of the individual and the rights of the society. This antagonism is exacerbated in the eyes of the public and professional groups as a result of ignorance and fear. While enhancing medical and social support to those infected with HIV including AIDS cases, the global strategy addresses a wide variety of research issues. Of immediate priority are the development of improved surveillance mechanisms, the assessment and forecasting of trends and impact, the development and advocacy of sound policies.

Finally, I would like to describe how countries are implementing the global AIDS strategy and how WHO supports them in this effort.

The attainment of a concensus on the strategies to be promoted globally, and on WHO's leadership and coordinating role was achieved in 1987 with the endorsement of the Global Programme on AIDS by the World Health Assembly, the Economic and Social Council of the United Nations and, for the first time in its history concerning any health issue, by the U.N. General Assembly. The recent summit meeting held in London reiterated this consensus.

National policies and plans, consistent with those endorsed globally, are being formulated. Starting in January 1987, the Global Programme on AIDS developed a capacity to respond to government requests by sending teams of consultants and staff to countries for short visits. These visits resulted in quick assessments of AIDS situations and of ongoing prevention activities. Their immediate outcome was the formulation of short-term plans of action. Support was made available to countries within an average of 4 to 6 weeks of the visit. While the short-term plan was being implemented, a second mission was organized to review the progress made and problems encountered and, in collaboration with national colleagues, to formulate a medium-term plan. These plans cover a three-to-five-year planning period. They are designed so as to represent a sufficiently detailed but flexible framework for government sectors, multilateral, bilateral and non-governmental agencies.

In order to reach an agreement on the role that each of these participating parties will play within the scope of the national plan and coordinate the financing of these plans, Donor meetings are held in countries. Resources required to supplement national funds and staff are mobilized either through WHO, or bilaterally between the country and a third party. As of today, 136 countries have requested collaboration from WHO and, in response, 115 assessment visits have taken place, leading to the formulation and financing of 78 short-term plans. Of these, 42 are in Africa, 8 in South-East Asia, 10 in the Eastern Mediterranean, 8 in the Western Pacific, 7 in the Americas and 3 in Europe. Twenty-one more visits are planned to take place in March and April this year. Training courses and workshops have been organized in the areas of laboratory diagnostics, clinical aspects, counselling and epidemiological surveillance. Twenty-two medium-term plans have been formulated. In the last 12 months, over 350 consultant missions have been conducted - consultants are drawn from multiple professional groups and geographic areas. Altogether, more than 150 consultants have been prepared for these tasks in seminars held in Geneva, Sydney and Washington. More of these consultant orientation seminars are planned to be held in Africa, Asia, the Eastern Mediterranean and Canada. Seven Donor meetings have been organized in African countries where the funds required for first-year implementation, which ranged from two to eight million US dollars, were fully pledged by donors. It is anticipated that by the end of 1988, collaboration will have been established with all countries in the world needing support for their national programme. This number will be close to 140. Medium-term plans will have been formulated in 100 countries:-

*   specific efforts are currently made to describe in more detail in the plans the integration of AIDS activities with other primary health care initiatives in order to make maximum use of available resources and expertise and avoid creating vertical structures;

*   by the end of 1988, effective coordinating mechanisms will have been established in the 75 or so countries which will have a medium-term plan under implementation by the end of the year;

* resources will have been mobilized for these countries either through on-site Donor meetings or, for smaller countries, through Donor consultations; in this process, caution will be applied to ensure that resources allocated to very important programmes such as those under primary health care are not diverted in support of AIDS programmes;

* five programmes will have undergone their first comprehensive evaluation.

The budget foreseen to be channelled through the Global Programme on AIDS in 1988 in **direct support of country programmes** is estimated at 34.5 million US dollars, representing approximately one-third of all resources directed to developing countries to combat AIDS.

In implementing the global strategy, difficulties are encountered in formulating plans which should first and foremost suit country needs and also the donor community while remaining consistent with globally agreed objectives and approaches. It is also difficult to maintain the required degree of coordination in countries without creating delays. The international selection, recruitment and deployment of staff continues to be a critical issue. The need to implement the strategy while developing guidelines and technical documents has compelled the programme to "build the ship while sailing it", often in stormy waters. The paramount concern of those involved in the programme was whether, with available resources, **more** could be done **more quickly.**

1987 will be remembered as the year of global mobilization against AIDS. 1988 should be remembered as the year when as many battle fronts against AIDS are opened as there are countries in the world.

The Global Impact of AIDS, pages 215-218
© 1988 Alan R. Liss, Inc.

28. EPIDEMIC CONTROL THROUGH PREVENTION

Maria Paalman

Director, Dutch Foundation for STD Control, member
of National Committee on AIDS Control in the
Netherlands, Catharijnesingel 56, 3511 GE Utrecht,
Netherlands

Different Forms of Prevention

It is without much dispute that diseases are generally better
prevented than cured. Three forms of prevention can be
distinguished. Primary, secondary and tertiary prevention.
Primary prevention means preventing disease or infection
altogether. Early diagnosis and treatment is referred to as
secondary prevention, in order to prevent the infection from
being spread to others, and cure the patient. The term tertiary
prevention is reserved for preventing complications, or
preventing a disease from getting worse.

In the case of AIDS, **tertiary preventive medication** so far
has not yet fully succeeded in preventing the patients from
dying, although promising drugs are being tried out that prolong
life and alleviate symptoms. As for **secondary prevention,**
treatment of seropositives is still further away. Warning
contacts of seropositives can have some preventive effect on the
spread of the epidemic, but difficult ethical questions have to be
answered. Thus the most powerful tool in the control of AIDS at
this moment is **primary prevention.**

The development of vaccines has made great contributions
in wiping out several epidemics, but for AIDS a **vaccine** will not
be available for years. In many countries the **screening** of blood,
organ and semen **donations** has been implemented. The
preventive effect of these measures depends on the
sophistication of the health care delivery system and on
available resources. The cost-effectiveness of screening
donations depends primarily on the prevalence of infection in the

population and the costs of patient treatment. Another technological form of primary prevention is the sole use of **sterile skin-piercing equipment** in the (para) medical professions. The vast majority of infections though can only be prevented through **changes in behaviour,** i.e., safer sex and safer use of needles and syringes by intravenous drug users.

Factors Influencing a Prevention Strategy

In designing a prevention strategy for a specific country several factors have to be taken into account :-

1. First of all the stage of the epidemic. Through surveillance the **prevalence** of disease and, more importantly, of infection can be estimated. Obviously a low prevalence implies that a lot of infections can still be prevented, but cynically enough, a San Francisco study showed that a high prevalence ("knowing someone with AIDS") might be the most important factor in motivating people to actually behave safer.

2. To direct prevention efforts effectively it is no doubt important to know **which people in the population are particularly at risk.** Prevalence studies can be done to estimate the spread of the epidemic among groups that might be potentially at risk because of their behaviour.

3. A prevention strategy should match the **social context** in which it is to be implemented. Norms and values towards sexuality, especially homosexuality, promiscuity, IV drug use, fertility and death vary enormously among different cultures. In most societies several taboos are entangled around these issues, contributing to the complexity of prevention efforts.

4. The **political situation** can also be influential. Whether a country stresses individual freedom and responsibility or adheres more to principles of collectivism will be reflected in political decisions about the strategy of choice.

5. Many **religions** proclaim restrictions on sexual behaviour. If such a religion is a powerful factor in a society and is not very tolerant it will have a profound influence on the prevention message.

6/7. Besides the already mentioned prevailing ethical views, the **existing laws** pertaining to public health, especially infectious diseases or sexually transmitted diseases, will supply a framework by which also an AIDS control programme will be measured. On the other hand, AIDS has such an impact on society, that it seems possible that AIDS will lead to a re-evaluation of existing health laws.

8. The **level of education** of the population sets limits to the means of communication. A brochure for instance is clearly not very useful if a substantial percentage of the population is illiterate.

9. The same applies to the **technical communication possibilities.** Although it is well known that television is a powerful medium, it looses impact when only a few people have a TV set, or when the group to be reached does not watch it.

10. Similarly the **existing health services system** limits what can be done, especially when there are other competing health priorities. It is of no use to call up everybody to be tested when there is not enough personnel to explain to them what a test and its result mean.

11. A last, but important, factor on which a prevention strategy is dependent is the amount of **available resources.** When dividing the AIDS budget it is wise to keep in mind that each case that is prevented pays itself back in less health care costs, but above all in less sorrow.

Starting Points for Prevention Strategies

1. From the above the first starting point follows logically. Each country should conceptualize an **overall prevention programme,** addressing stategies, target groups, technological inventions, resource allocation, behaviour information and behaviour modification, taking into account all the above mentioned factors.

   Even with all the differences in countries, it has been proven at several meetings that about certain principles concensus can be reached. The following starting points are such principles :-

2. It is recognized that **screening of donations** is a priority in all countries with a high or mediocre seroprevalence rate. It

is tragic that some countries with the highest prevalences lack the resources to implement such a screening programme.

3. Another principle is that **individual HIV antibody testing** must be accompanied by counselling before and after. Such testing should be voluntary and confidential. Mandatory testing of specific groups does not seem to serve a preventive purpose.

4. Everybody has a right to **information** about this disease. But information alone does not make people change their behaviour. **Education** efforts should be focused on target groups, be tailored to their needs and speak their language. Small scale interventions with an opportunity to deal with emotional aspects are apt to be more effective in bringing about safer behaviour in the long run than mass-media campaigns. In general one could also argue that the more explicit the information and education can be, the more effective the communication will be.

5. To implement such education strategies **engaging the target groups** in planning and implementation is indispensible, including people with HIV infection and AIDS.

6. Strategies to **destigmatize HIV infection** and those perceived to be at risk of infection should be encouraged. There are great dangers in creating a split society with seropositives and seronegatives ("them" and "us"). Discrimination and stigmatism are better replaced by solidarity and concern.

7. A **pragmatic approach,** also called risk reduction, that emphasizes and encourages safer and responsible behaviour is likely to be more effective than a negative approach which emphasizes the consequences of unsafe behaviour.

8. Education efforts should be **evaluated** for both short and long term effects on knowledge, attitudes and practices, as well as for cost-effectiveness.

9. Incorporating the above activities into existing structures/organisations is to be preferred above creating new ones.

One global strategy for AIDS prevention is neither possible nor desirable. But the more underlying principles we agree on, the less destructive the global impact of AIDS will be.

The Global Impact of AIDS, pages 219–228
© 1988 Alan R. Liss, Inc.

29. EFFECTIVENESS OF THE AIDS PREVENTION CAMPAIGNS IN SWITZERLAND

Dominique Hausser, Philippe Lehmann, Francoise Dubois-Arber, Felix Gutzwiller

Institut Universitaire de Medicine Sociale et Preventive, Bugnon 17, 1005 Lausanne, Switzerland

INTRODUCTION

With a cumulated incidence of 55.8 AIDS cases per million, Switzerland has the second highest AIDS rate after the United States: as of 31 December 1987, 355 cases and 184 deaths. 61% of those affected are homosexuals or bisexuals (100% more than at the end of 1986), 19% are drug addicts (up 230%) and 10% are people with whom it is presumed the virus was transmitted heterosexually (up 250%). The estimated prevalence of HIV carriers in the heterosexual population is between 0.003% (prevalence with blood donors) and 1% (prevalence with heterosexuals with risk-prone behaviour as found in anonymous AIDS screening centres). In the homosexual population the same rate is about 15%. The main risk of blood infection is associated with intravenous drug injection: there have only been 5 cases of blood infection from other sources in haemophiliacs and blood receivers (1).

The STOP-AIDS prevention campaign is part of a strategy for fighting AIDS as defined by the Swiss Federal office of Public Health (OFSP), including epidemiological surveillance, public information, and support given to those affected by the illness or the virus (2).

The first large scale prevention operation undertaken in the spring of 1986 was the distribution to every Swiss household of an information booklet containing essential information about AIDS epidemiology, HIV transmission and prevention (3). This operation was evaluated and confided to the University Institute of Social and Preventive Medicine (IUMSP) based on variables in the fields of knowledge, beliefs and attitudes towards the subject of AIDS, as inspired by the "Health Belief Model". It was shown, by means of a telephone survey of representative samples of the population, questioned both before and after the distribution of the booklet, that it had been well received, was read by over half the population and that knowledge about AIDS and its prevention were quite clearly improved for its readers (4). With basic knowledge about AIDS being acquired, there was a noticeable reduction in the occurence of false beliefs concerning the risk of transmission of the virus through acts of everyday life. The first phase of information prepared a favourable terrain for the campaigns to follow.

In February 1987, a press conference marked the launching of a multi-media national prevention campaign, under the slogan of "STOP-AIDS" by the Swiss AIDS Foundation (ASS) and the OFSP. This campaign is based on the following themes: the use of condoms in sexual relationships with multiple or casual partners, the need to stop syringe exchanges in the case of drug addiction, and mutual faithfulness between partners. The form of the messages is simple, clear and undramatic. The means of exposing the public to the information are varied and include posters, advertisements in the press, radio and television. Much educative material, created for the diverse target groups (the young, women, teachers, social workers) is progressively complementing the media campaign. These operations are designed for the long-term, come in successive waves, repeating and complementing the previous ones, and diversify the messages, the means of influence and forms of action.

The OFSP asked the IUMSP to continue its evaluation of the totality of the prevention process being undertaken (5). The evaluation has several objectives:-

* to measure to what degree the campaign's objectives have been attained
* to contribute to its success by making the necessary adjustments possible by the detection of areas of resistance or of areas where effects are amplified.

The group of evaluators binds itself to supply results every six months to the OFSP, STOP-AIDS campaign managers and other interested parties.

TABLE 1. Studies and Variables

Results	Variables	Studies
Use of condoms	Sales	Condoms (1)
	Risk-prone behaviour Protection behaviour	17-30 years (2) (representative phone study)
	Risk-prone behaviour Protection behaviour	Sentinella (3) (single adults by their doctor)
Knowledge	Knowledge	Young Ticinese (4) (19 years old interviewed at the time of recruitment for military service)
Attitudes and behaviour (target groups)	Knowledge	Teenagers (5)
	Beliefs	Multiple sexual partners (6)
	Attitudes	Homosexuals (7)
	Behaviour	Drug addicts (8)
Process		Sex tourists (9)
Stop AIDS Campaign	Diffusion Audience	Diffusion (10)
	Repercussions in press	Argus/Media (11)
	Audience of messages	Studies 5 to 9
Multiplyings	Repetition of the new STOP-AIDS messages	Argus/Media
	Informal actions Institutional actions	Informal leaders (12) Cantons (13) Argus/Media

METHOD

Based on behavioural change model adapted from McAlister using social learning and communication theory (Figure 1) (6), the evaluation is made up of thirteen studies (Table 1) using both quantitative and qualitative approaches. More than 5500 people have been interviewed in this research programme. The **dependent variables** used were : (i) preventive behaviour in respect of AIDS (use of condoms, not exchanging syringes, etc.), (ii) attitudes (of fear, of stigmatisation, of denial of AIDS' existence and towards prevention), (iii) beliefs (images) concerning AIDS, (iv) knowledge. The **independent variable** is: the action of the prevention campaigns in its largest sense (preventive actions of all sorts and sources).

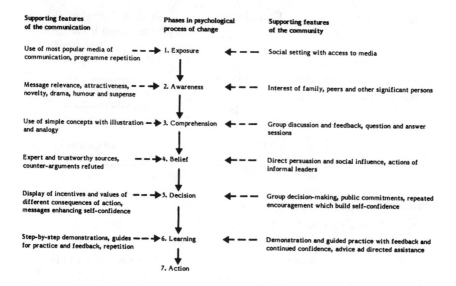

Figure 1. Model of Changes of Behaviour

All these variables are made up of several factors which evolve with time. Therefore, it is not always possible to confirm a cause and affect relationship between the efforts made in the way of prevention and behavioural change. This is all the more the case, in that behavioural change is as much influenced by the social and cultural environment and the effect of AIDS in its own right as the theory model shows.

All the studies furnish answers which tend towards the same direction, thus giving us a reason to suppose that the results obtained are valid. It has therefore been possible to identify the main existing tendencies in society in relation to the AIDS problem.

MAIN RESULTS

Changes in Knowledge

All the studies show that the resident Swiss population has a good level of knowledge of AIDS. The repetition of information concerning the nature of the illness and the means of contamination have made this knowledge become more and more precise (studies 2 and 4). More than 90% of those questioned knew of the means of contagion through sexual relationships and through infected injection equipment, and denied the risk of contagion through everyday contacts, mosquitoes etc. They were aware of the means of prevention (use of condoms, not exchanging syringes, mutual faithfulness). Unfounded beliefs concerning the means of infection are gradually disappearing except in regard to receiving blood transfusions (more than half those questioned mentioned it). It is difficult however to interpret this data as it is possible that a certain number of people regard the residual risk (which is very slight in Switzerland) as a real risk. This error has probably very little effect in regard to the adoption of preventive behaviour, as the behavioural categories concerned have very little to do with blood transfusion.

Changes in Attitudes

More and more people feel concerned by AIDS, even if the idea that "it can only happen to others" is still present. 53% of 17-30 year olds (study 2) consider themselves personally concerned by AIDS prevention. For instance, adolescents (study 5) are sure they will have several partners before they find their "other half" and that this situation constitutes a risk. We can conclude that even if the risk of AIDS is still generally associated with the notion of social groups outside the norm, quite a number of people seem to be convinced that the risk of contamination by the HIV exists in the normal course of their life.

In the different groups studied, similar attitudes concerning AIDS and the preventive messages can be found, that pave the way to a positive attitude towards the need for prevention :-

* Rejection, negation of the problem ("AIDS doesn't concern me"), an attitude which holds the seeds of ostracism in respect of the groups of people affected, but which diminishes if information and open discussion increase.

* Fear is linked to the proximity of AIDS: it's with homosexuals and drug addicts that it is the most widely spread. It seems to be progressively evolving from the panic-stricken fear with all its inherent dangers in terms of irrational behaviour, to a more worried fear, which is rather helpful in confronting the questions like "how do you protect yourself from it?", "how can you accompany the ill and seropositives?"

* The relativity of the AIDS situation is expressed with drug addicts (study 8) by reactions like: "AIDS is yet another problem to be dealt with" or with the young (study 5), who find for example, that the dying forests is a more important problem. Despondency confronted with an illness that is so threatening incites some people to reject any form of self-protection (study 7 and 8).

* Bargaining and conspiring are attitudes that are also to be found and which express themselves by means of some sort of magical protection, such as in the case of drug addicts, desire to become pregnant in spite of their seropositivity, or in the case of adolescents the possession of condoms without necessarily using them.

The phenomenon of resistance to behavioural change is often linked to the non-perceiving of one's own risk, associated with the contradictory and discordant effects of information in the press and rumour. For example, how can one protect oneself from HIV by using condoms, when contamination can take place while kissing or shaking hands.

Although cynicism (willful infection of others by seropositives) is an attitude that exists in the population's imagination, it has not been encountered in the studied groups.

Even if we accept that the press gives quite a positive image to preventive action, that cantonal policies do not develop discriminatory actions, that the theme of solidarity is mentioned more and more frequently, and that we are fairly confident in a continuing positive climate in Switzerland in the future, there are sometimes appearances of other attitudes which evoke *de facto* ostracism at a personal level and in certain circumstances of everyday life.

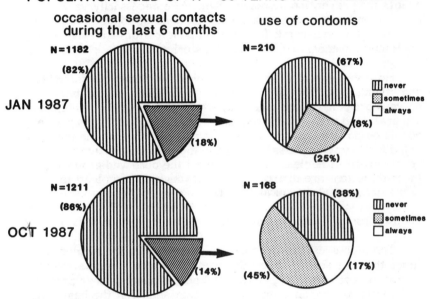

POPULATION AGED OF 17 - 30 YEARS IN SWITZERLAND

Figure 2. Occasional Sexual Relationship and Use of Condoms.

Behavioural Change

Almost 18% of the 17-30 year olds (study 2) had had casual sexual relationships in the six months preceding the interview (Fig. 2). In January 1987, 67% + or - 7% of them did not use condoms, 25% + or - 6% used them occasionally and 7% + or - 8% used them systematically; in October 1987, the figures were 38% + or - 7% never, 45% + or - 8% sometimes and 17% + or - 6% always. The total number of condoms put on the market during the first nine months of 1987 (about 9,200,000 articles) was increased by almost 60% compared to the same period of the previous year. This increase was most noticeable (up to 140%)

just after the launching of the "STOP-AIDS" campaign.

These results show changes, which are still modest, concerning acceptance of the condom. The qualitative studies confirm these data and show a great diversity of other changes. Their degree (and probably their efficiency) are variable in the different groups under observation and depend upon a number of factors. Behaviour patterns are orienting themselves towards an individual management of the risks involved; each individual adapts the prevention messages, which are necessarily very general, to his/her own situation. This mode of conduct is clearly visible with homosexuals (renouncing penetration) and with adolescents (reconstituting sexual histories).

However, the fact of being in love, the influence of alcohol and other drugs, a pressing urge, improvised orgies, holidays, nervous breakdowns, or places where furtive and consumable sex are practiced are some of the exceptional circumstances where people do not protect themselves. It is apparent that the more individuals experience safer sex, the more the exceptions become rare. It is clear however, in all the observed groups that these situations are difficult to live through and can lead to renewed fear and discouragement.

The Process of Exposing the Public to the Prevention Message

The messages' exposure can be measured by the number of times they are repeated and the proportion of the population the messages reach. In 1987, almost 100 poster panels, three posters wide, were permanently billed in Switzerland. If in the beginning only urban and suburban areas benefited from poster billing, country areas were reached from the end of the spring. It is difficult to estimate how many people have seen these posters, but it can be taken for granted that the virtual totality of the population saw them. The advertisements included in the weekly and Sunday newspapers represent, over the year, an accumulated circulation of over 25 million copies spread over 150 appearances. The television advertisements have been seen one to four times by viewers, depending on the linguistic region. The difference is due to the ratings and not to the rate of showings, as they were similar in the three regions (study 10).

The campaign and the preventive messages were echoed by the media to a very large degree all year long and have certainly had a "reminder" effect. The regional newspapers played the most important part in reinforcing the messages in that they are perceived closest to the reality of the readers' daily life. 64% of articles published on AIDS in the regional papers were about concrete events, whereas in the major dailies this figure was only 49% (study 11).

The STOP-AIDS campaign counts on the multiplying effect that can be played, particularly in respect to the young, by parents, teachers, doctors and church men. These groups were interviewed at three different occasions throughout the year (study 12) and they showed quite a favourable disposition towards the fight against AIDS. It is apparent however, that spontaneous discussion of the subject is less common than replies to questions asked by the young, and this applied to the four groups studied. The experience gained here shows that the young are very thirsty for information and need to be listened to.

In the nine cantons studied, which represent 3/5 of the Swiss population (study 13), local expert resources contributed to the concept of preventive action and the care to be taken of those affected by the illness or the virus. In the school context, in particular, many operations intended for children and adolescents have been established or are in the process of being so.

These studies show the great diversity of operations and means of exposing the public to prevention messages. The messages and operations appear to have reached the entire population whatever people's interest in one or another of the means of communication employed. It has not been possible to find any counter-productive operations which have prejudiced the STOP-AIDS campaign.

CONCLUSIONS

The conclusions that can be drawn after ten months of an intensive prevention campaign are the following :-

* the campaign's messages reached the general public and the groups with high-risk behaviours, due to the messages' wide exposure and the amplifying effects of the media.

* little opposition or resistance were expressed in regard to the campaign.

* multiplying phenomenon were numerous and, in themselves contributed to the campaign's effect.

*   the behavioural change observed is tending towards better individual protection both in the general public and in the studied groups. These groups were chosen specifically for their greater probability of having high-risk behaviour, thus giving us reason to suppose that this tendency will generalise itself, for as long as the campaign continues without let or changing its tone.

ACKNOWLEDGEMENTS

The smooth running of this evaluation could not have taken place without the great amount of work furnished by all of our colleagues (Blaise Duvanel, Felix Gurtner, Mauro de Grazia, Jean-Blaise Masur, Marie-Claire Mathey, Inge Schroeder, Mathias Stricker, Hughes Wulser, Peter Zeugin). There would be nothing to say had not many people co-operated in accepting to participate in the different studies, some of whom have had to overcome their fears and their anguish in order to be able to speak of their difficulties, their illness and their death. All of this was done in the aim of fighting AIDS, so that others will not have to be confronted with the same problems they face. We thank them sincerely.

REFERENCES

1.   Bull, OFSP, No. 3, 28 January 1988.

2.   OFSP, Concept de lutte contre l'épidemie du SIDA en Suisse, Bern, 8 April 1987.

3.   Office fédéral de la santé publique, AIDS/SIDA., Bern, March 1986.

4.   Lehmann Ph, Hausser D, Somaini B, Gutzwiller F (1987). Campaign against AIDS in Switzerland: evaluation of a nationwide education programme. Brit Med J, 295: 1118-1120.

5.   Hausser D, Lehmann Ph, Dubois-Arber F, Gutzwiller F. Evaluation des campagnes de prévention contre le SIDA en Suisse -sur mandat de l'Office fédéral de la santé publique. (Rapport de synthèse) December 1987, 1988, p.96. (Cah Rech Doc IUMSP, No. 23)

6.   Hausser D, Lehmann Ph, Dubois F, Gutzwiller F. Evaluation des campagnes nationales de prévention contre le SIDA: Modèle d'analyse. Soz-Präventivmed, 32, 207-209, 1987.

The Global Impact of AIDS, pages 229-232
© 1988 Alan R. Liss, Inc.

30. PUBLIC HEALTH ORGANIZATION IN BRAZIL

Lair Guerra de Macedo Rodrigues

Director of the National Division of Sexually
Transmitted Diseases and AIDS, Ministry of Health,
Esplanada dos Ministerios, Bl. 'G'- Annexo A,
Terreo-sala 52, Brasilia DF, CEP 70058, Brazil

AIDS presents a growing challenge to public health
throughout the world. The HIV epidemic will only be controlled
by developing a national strategy that combines public
education, health care, legal, educational, public health and
financial wisdom available.

The Brazilian public health services were unprepared to
address the complex issues raised by the HIV epidemic, and to
develop and implement control strategies rapidly. Most of the
problems were due to : (1) the inadequacy of the public health
system; (2) multiplicity and excess of decision-making bodies;
(3) difficulties in managing the public health services.

Health policies are jointly formulated by four ministries,
namely: Ministry of Health, Ministry of Social Security and
Welfare, Ministry of Labour and Ministry of Education. The
function of the Ministry of Health is the formulation of health
policies with emphasis on standardization, planning, control of
endemic diseases, epidemiological surveillance and sanitary
surveillance, drug supplies, among others. The Ministry of Social
Security and Welfare handles the provision of medical assistance
and social security. The Ministry of Education handles the
formulation of all health professionals and the administration of
universities and hospital-based research facilities. The Ministry
of Labour is responsible for the occupational health policies.

The health policy, as proposed by the 8th National Health
Conference, recommended the unification of the system.

Created by law in July 1987, the unified decentralized health system is based on three principles. First, **Institutional Unification** which requires integrated actions in planning, budgeting, articulation of preventive and patient care actions, among others. Second, **Decentralization of Services,** implying the delegation of health services to the State, Municipal and District levels. Third, **Democratization,** that is the provision of free health services to all citizens.

Where are we so far as the organization of the AIDS Program in Brazil today? The complexity of issues surrounding the HIV epidemic, the multiplicity of information sources, the increasing individual and collective anxiety attendant to the growth of AIDS urged the Ministry of Health to develop strategies to face these challenges in the following areas: Health Promotion; Infection Control and Surveillance; Research; Medical Assistance; Training; and Planning, Supervision and Evaluation.

As I have said, organization of services plays an important role in our strategy. Its importance derives from two reasons: First our action needs to be decentralized; Second, our services need to be delivered to every individual.

Now I would like to describe the seven channels constituting our network of services.

1. **The National AIDS Committee.** Made up of 19 members, the committee represents a broad spectrum of the society. Its function is three fold: consulting, technical and normative.

2. **The Macro-Regional Reference Centers.** The peculiarities marking the distinct regions in the country make it difficult for the Ministry of Health - and specifically the AIDS program - to maintain homogenous actions. The five Macro-Regional Centers constitute and attempt to bridge this gap. Each center should reflect the social, cultural and economic characteristics typical of its region.

3. **The States Program.** Each state has its own committee formed also by representatives of the different segments of society. AIDS cases are reported by the state to the Ministry of Health monthly.

4. **National Reference Centers, Universities and Hospital-Based Activities.** Research and training related to

AIDS in Brazil are carried out by three type of institutions. One is the National Reference Centers funded by the Federal Government. The others are the Universities, also funded by the Federal Government and International Institutions. The third are the foundations, such as Oswaldo Cruz, funded by both national and international institutions.

5. **Community Based Organizations.** Across the nation, community based organizations are providing primary assistance to the individual seeking information about AIDS and also providing care to individuals who may otherwise be left without assistance.

    These organizations are typically staffed by volunteers. Some religious groups have also been leaders in providing assistance for terminal patients. One area in which community-based organizations are beginning to provide assistance is in developing home care facilities. Many of these organizations serve specific population groups such as haemophiliacs.

6. **The Private Sector.** The private sector has made contributions, specially in the areas of patient care and education. The Ministry of Health is particularly interested in partnership with this sector.

7. **International Cooperation on AIDS.** The last channel is the international cooperation. AIDS is no respecter of national boundaries and we need a global response to it. Brazil has acquired substantial experience that it is willing to share. Brazil is aware that actions by government must be complemented by that of other groups such as voluntary organizations and non-governmental agencies.

    Finally, I would like to give a brief review of the epidemiological profile of AIDS in Brazil.

    As of 31st January 1988, a total of 2,651 cases were officially reported to the Ministry of Health. Twenty-five states have reported cases and the estimated prevalence of infection by region is - the North Region 0.41%; Northeast Region 0.41-0.83%; the Middle West 1.25-1.67%; South 0.83-1.25% and Southeast Region 1.67-5.55%. Regarding the patients' age and sex, 80% of the reported cases occurred in patients between 20 and 40 years of age and 5% occurred in females. With respect to sexual preferences, 50% of the cases occurred in homosexual,

23.84% bisexual and 6.74% heterosexual.

14% of the cases were due to blood, blood products and IV drug abuse. 78 pediatric cases were reported which represents 2.9% of the total, distributed this way: less than one year, 13; 1-4, 20; 5-9, 28 and 10-14, 17.

An interesting clinical finding was that a significant number of these patients contracted tuberculosis, especially the generalized type, which makes the pattern different from that of the United States and European countries.

Since the disease AIDS occurs years after the virus infection, the number of AIDS cases occurring in Brazil today does not tell us about the present level of infection in the population. We estimate that for each AIDS case, there are likely to be an additional 50 to 100 HIV-infected people. Therefore, we can expect between 12,000 - 16,000 people with AIDS-related complex and 200,000 - 400,000 infected people.

As we look towards the future, we recognize that the AIDS situation in Brazil will likely become more serious during the next few years.

We are here, searching for new and useful information and very much in the spirit of cooperation ask for help to fight the AIDS virus.

The Global Impact of AIDS, pages 233-239
© 1988 Alan R. Liss, Inc.

31. INTERNATIONAL CO-OPERATION IN THE NATIONAL AIDS CONTROL PROGRAMME

Philip R Hiza

Chief Medical Officer, Ministry of Health, P O Box 9083, Dar Es Salaam, Tanzania

ABSTRACT

Tanzania is one of the countries of the Third World to report the occurrence of AIDS and HIV infection since 1984. The Ministry of Health immediately established a task force to monitor the disease and advise the Ministry of control measures. Soon it became evident from epidemiological studies that the main mode of transmission was through heterosexual contact. Appropriate public education campaigns were initiated by the Health Education Unit. A number of international agencies became interested in assisting, and the Swedish Agency for Research Co-operation in Developing Countries (SAREC) were the first to assist with screening using both ELISA and western blot techniques. WHO, however, assumed the leadership in both assisting the Ministry of Health in organising its AIDS control programme and organising a successful donors meeting held from 23rd - 24th July 1987, where pledges amounting to US dollars 4.0 million were made to cover the programme activities for the first year. Such international co-operation is, I believe, a prerequisite to global efforts in eradicating the pandemic which has so far spared few countries of the world, if any.

Background Information

Early in 1984 information was received from community leaders from villages bordering Uganda in Kagera Region of Tanzania that young people were suffering and many of them dying from a mysterious disease akin to "slim" in Uganda. It was noticed that most of the culprits were young and that dispensary or Health Centre treatment was not effective. The disease was immediately named juliana because it affected a section of the population, both male and female, that was in the habit of wearing fashionable T-shirts with JULIANA inscriptions brought into the area by long-haul vehicle drivers.

In October 1984, the Regional Hospital in Kagera began to notice increase in admission of patients with extensive genital ulcerative disease coupled with severe weight loss, diarrheoa, prolonged fever and oral ulceration. The local surgeon (1) was the first to become suspicious and reported this new disease as suspected AIDS at local clinical meetings. Consultations with the Microbiology Department of the University Teaching Hospital in Dar es Salaam resulted in local experts visiting the area and confirming the suspicion. Retrospectively, similar cases had been reported in late 1983 from nearby hospitals in the Region.

Through joint efforts between the Ministry of Health, the World Health Organization, the Microbiology Department of the Muhimbili Medical Centre and the Centers for Disease Control in the United States of America, AIDS was confirmed serologically in the Kagera Region in August 1985 (2) and it can be said that the disease surfaced in Kagera as early as late 1983.

An analysis of laboratory-confirmed patients admitted to the Muhimbili Medical Centre in Dar es Salaam between 1st July 1985 and 31 August 1986 shows that 27 per cent of these cases originated from Kagera Region, followed by Dar es Salaam 15 per cent and Coast region surrounding Dar es Salaam 10 per cent. Moreover, the remaining 17 regions of the country were each a source of less than 5 per cent of cases admitted to Muhimbili Hospital. Moreover, 6 other patients originated from neighbouring countries, namely Zanzibar (two), Malawi (one), Kenya (one), and Uganda (two). While Kagera Region was the source of 72 per cent of all AIDS cases reported in the country by the end of December 1986, the population in all the other regions has been exposed to HIV infection as indicated by notification of AIDS from different parts of the country (3).

Modes of Transmission

The Ministry of Health in Dar es Salaam instituted information system of notification of cases throughout the country and an analysis of these cases in the Epidemiological Unit provided an idea on the possible modes of transmission. It was apparent the majority of cases had heterosexual relations with multiple partners, 63 per cent males and 46 per cent females, hence heterosexual promiscuity was identified as the major risk factor. Other factor was blood transfusion. Nearly 50 per cent of the male and 36 per cent of the female patients were married. Blood transfusion alone without any additional risk behaviour constituted 2.6 per cent of cases and all of them were children.

Up to the end of December 1987, 1,608 cases had been reported, (Table 1) the majority originating from Dar es Salaam and Kagera Regions.

TABLE 1. The Spread of Disease in Tanzania

Year	Number of regions notifying	Number of cases
1983	1	3
1984	1	16
1985	7	266
1986	20	654
1987 up to October	20	715

Of the analysed 232 cases (Table 2), 181 (78 per cent) belong to the 20-39 year age group. There was a preponderance of males to females 14 : 9 (Table 3).

International Cooperation

AIDS is pandemic. No country is spared. Even countries that have not reported cases have no reason for complacency. As such, therefore, the problem is global and requires concerted effort from all of us whatever our health or economic status. In developing countries it threatens the attainment of Health for All by the year 2000 (HFA/2000) through diversion of manpower and financial resources from established programmes, and by the very nature of the sensitivity it creates, puts high demands on Ministries of Health as a result of pressure from the public. It creates confidence crisis on the medical profession and panic in

Ministries of Public Health. In developed countries it creates
frustration because, having attained HFA, and having eradicated
infectious diseases and found solutions to most chronic life-
threatening diseases, AIDS, with no known remedy or cure should
suddenly surface.

TABLE 2. The Distribution of AIDS Cases by Age-groups and
Sex (1984-1986)

Age - Group	Cases	%	Male	Female
0-5	7	3	3	4
6-14	-	-	-	-
15-19	8	3.4	2	6
20-24	27	11.6	11	16
25-29	53	22.9	32	21
30-34	53	22.9	32	21
35-39	48	20.7	32	16
40-44	14	6.0	10	4
45-49	7	3.0	4	3
50+	10	4.3	9	1
Age not mentioned	5	2.2	5	-
Totals	232	100.0	140	92

As such therefore, international effort is all the more called
for. There is need to gather information from all the world over
and use such information to our mutual benefit. The setting up of
the Global AIDS Control Programme by WHO is in the right
direction, especially as it provides the necessary leadership.
WHO is also working with member States to assist them form
their own AIDS Control Programme.

TABLE 3. Distribution of AIDS Cases by Sex and Marital Status

Marital status	Males Cases	%	Females Cases	%	Total Cases	%
Married	70	50.0	33	35.9	103	44.4
Single	49	35.0	19	20.7	68	29.3
Widow(er)	1	0.7	3	3.3	4	1.7
Divorced	6	4.3	20	21.7	26	11.2
Unspecified	11	7.9	12	13.2	24	10.4
Children	3	2.1	4	4.3	7	3.0
Total	140	100.0	92	100.0	232	100.0

The Tanzania Experience

Since the formation of AIDS Task Force in 1984, we have
tried to co-operate with WHO by regular reporting of cases. The
collaborative efforts between the Ministry of Health with WHO
and the Centers for Disease Control in the USA was the first
step in international co-operation which enabled us to
serodiagnose the disease in 1985. It was through bilateral co-
operation between the Government of Tanzania and SAREC that
we were able to perform research and acquire screening
facilities for patients and blood for transfusion. We were,
therefore, able to set up an AIDS Reference Centre at the
Muhimbili Medical Centre. SAREC has provided screening
facilities too at Bukoba Hospital in Kagera and instituted a
multiple study research programme for Kagera to determine
prevalence of HIV infection and behavioural patterns related to
transmission of AIDS. Research is also continuing in Dar es
Salaam and other parts of the country to determine different
parameters of HIV infection. Non-governmental organisations
(NGOs), through the Lutheran Church are currently equipping 14
hospitals in various parts of the country with ELISA screening
facilities for blood donors.

The Tanzania Episcopal Council is formulating a strategy

for participating in the National AIDS Control Programme and has so far equipped five hospitals with screening facilities. The Church organisations are engaged through their medical wings to provide printed educational materials in the most affected parts of the country. The WHO has helped us formulating and evolving a National AIDS Control Programme which has annual action plans covering a 5-year period and has also helped us in organising a very successful Donors meeting on 23rd - 24th July 1987 to solicit financial, manpower and material resources required for the Programme.

We were able at that meeting to get pledges for donations amounting to US dollars 4.0 million, enough to finance the activities for the first year of the Programme. The bulk of this money will be used for information, education and communication, and a great deal will be used for screening blood and expectant mothers, while the remainder will be used for research on epidemiology and behavioural patterns of transmission.

The international community that were represented at the Donors meeting include, among others, USA (USAKID), DANIDA, SIDA, NORAD, ODA, EEC, FINIDA, WHO, Canada, Federal Republic of Germany, Netherlands, UNDP, UNICEF and AMREF.

WHO has continued to offer consultancy services which have culminated in finalising plans for the National AIDS Control programme and Action Plan with budgeting for the activities of the National AIDS Control Programme for the first year.

The Tanzania experience on international co-operation is, I am sure, no different from that in many other Third World countries that have recognised AIDS as a major threat. I know that similar efforts have been done in Uganda, Kenya, Burundi and Ethiopia, just to mention a few of our neighbours.

It is my hope that through these efforts we shall realise our goal of ultimately containing the pandemic through international co-operation.

REFERENCES

Corrado B, Nyamuryakunge K. AIDS in Kagera Region, Proceedings of Fourth Meeting organised by Italian Medical team to Tanzania, March 1985.

Forthal D, Mhalu F S, Dahoma A U et al. AIDS in Tanzania, 2nd International Conference on AIDS, Abstract No. 517F, p105. Paris, June 1986.

Mhalu F S et al. Some aspects of Human Immunodeficiency Virus in the United Republic of Tanzania, 2nd International Symposium on AIDS and associated Cancers in Africa, 7-9 October, 1987, Naples, Italy.

The Global Impact of AIDS, pages 241-250
© 1988 Alan R. Liss, Inc.

32. ACQUIRED IMMUNODEFICIENCY SYNDROME (AIDS) AND OCCUPATIONAL HEALTH IN UGANDA

D K Sekimpi

Occupational Health and Hygiene Department, Ministry of Labour, P O Box 4637, Kampala, Uganda

INTRODUCTION AND BACKGROUND

AIDS in the World

AIDS is now a worldwide problem with some common but also some differing epidemiological patterns in different parts of the world.

Everywhere, the AIDS virus, HIV, is transmitted sexually, through contaminated injections (including blood transfusions) or from infected mother to baby. The sexually and economically active age group of 15 to 49 years is universally the most affected while children 0 to 4 years are also affected due to mother-to-baby transmission. Adult victims, worldwide, are therefore likely to be workers who could be occupationally predisposed, exposed or just socially so. In all cases however their economic productivity will either be grossly reduced due to sickness absence or halted by death with negative effects on the family, enterprise and the nation.

Expatriates and travelling businessmen who stay away from home for long without their spouses are universally occupationally predisposed groups (Tauris and Black, 1987; Mann, 1987), whereas health workers handling AIDS patients or their blood are occupationally exposed, as are prostitutes. In Africa some occupational group specific HIV seroprevalence studies and occupational group specific AIDS control measures have been reported, Kenya being an example (Plummer et al, 1987; Ngugi et al, 1987). In Africa there is a consistently higher prevalence in urban than rural areas (Okware, 1987; Saracco et al, 1987;

Delaporte et al, 1987).

In difference are the predominantly male homosexual and intravenous drug abuse modes of transmission in the Western World as opposed to heterosexual transmission supplemented by transmission through contaminated intra-muscular injections in Africa (Bouvet and Vachon, 1987). As a result the male to female ratio differs with the ratio tending to unity in Africa as opposed to massive male predominance in the Western World. In a study in the UK this ratio was 1.75:1 for cases with infection related to Africa as opposed to 41.7:1 for non-Africa related cases (Marasca et al, 1987). In a study in Uganda the ratio was 1:1.2 (Berkley et al, 1987), whereas in a Zairean sero-survey no sex difference was noted.

AIDS in Uganda

The epidemiology of AIDS in Uganda is typical of the African pattern. About 90% of cases are in the 15-49 years age group, while 10% are children below 5 years (Table 1). There is almost equal male and female prevalence due to the heterosexual transmission while urban prevalence is much higher than that in rural areas. Whereas prostitutes, long distance drivers and businessmen have been observed as high risk groups because of having a large number of sexual partners and contracting sexually transmitted diseases (Berkley et al, 1987; Okware, 1987), the role of occupation in predisposing to HIV infection and AIDS are yet to be explored.

The AIDS Control Programme - ACP - in Uganda's Ministry of Health, supported by WHO and other local international agencies, has done commendable work through a national health education campaign, screening of blood for transfusion and supporting AIDS Research. Research has been done on risk factors, seroprevalence, analysis of morbidity and mortality records, standardising and evaluating case definition, defining the natural history and exploring the pathological features of HIV infection and AIDS.

Operationally ACP has prompted the safe handling of blood and blood contaminated instruments in health facilities and has encouraged high risk groups to use condoms. There is however, little as yet in way of occupational health contribution to this noble struggle against AIDS in Uganda.

TABLE 1. Age Distribution of 139 Cases (AIDS) in Uganda 1987

Age(Yrs)	Number of cases	%
0-4	14	10
5-14	1	0
15-19	10	7
20-39	96	70
40-59	18	13
60+	0	0
Total	139	100

From : Okware (1987)

Occupational Health Care in the World

In the world today occupational health care should cover workers in all occupations, as opposed to industrial workers only as was the practice earlier this century. The health or ill-health of the worker is now considered in totality irrespective of cause because his health status also affects his environment in total. An occupational disease will cause as much suffering as a general disease or injury and so both types need to be primarily prevented, for the benefit of the worker, his family, his workplaces and his community. Technological advancement and automation in developed countries may mask the relationship between the health of workers and the health of the economy. In Africa where direct human manual or intellectual contribution to the economy is paramount, the importance of this relationship must be recognised so that occupational health care is no longer considered a luxury.

Workers' health services usually provide limited curative care before referring patients to general health facilities. In Africa workers' health services may be the only accessible services for communities where workers live. These services can be centres for health education to workers and also to the rest of the community, either directly or by multiplier effect through workers.

Therefore, occupational health care services should play a role in AIDS control in the world.

Occupational Health Care in Uganda

Workers' health services in Uganda are mainly curative and usually limited to large workplaces. However diversification to have mainly preventive occupational health care for all workers in all occupations is a goal being pursued by the supervising Occupational Health Authority.

While many employers provide curative care for their employees on humanitarian grounds, they are being constantly encouraged to appreciate the economic importance of preventive and promotive health care for the advantage to production. Workers' health services are encouraged to serve workers, their families and the communities where they live. This is the position in a number of workplaces. Most services are run by nurses during the day only although in the last two years or so more doctors are being employed. Very large workplaces may have doctors, nurses and other support staff working around the clock.

Health statistics from workplaces are primarily returned to the Occupational Health and Hygiene Department, Ministry of Labour, but also to the Ministry of Health.

Most of the groups considered at risk from AIDS have as yet no organised workers' health services. Due to limited specialist manpower, and other resources at the disposal of the occupational health care system, it is presently a weak link in Uganda's national health care system. However, because of the threat AIDS is posing to the health of Uganda's workers and therefore her economy, the place of occupation health care in the struggle against AIDS and other diseases in Uganda needs to be defined and strengthened.

OCCUPATIONAL HEALTH IMPLICATIONS OF AIDS IN UGANDA

Age and Sex

About 90% of AIDS cases in Uganda are in the economically active age group of 15 to 59 years. Their ill-health is most likely to be first noticed at their workplaces when their performance deteriorates or when they attend the workers' health service. Because men and women are affected equally, working parents dying of AIDS are likely to leave behind helpless orphans, since the parents are likely to die in pairs. The workers' health service is likely to provide subsequent health care for such orphans. The loss of persons in the working age group has direct negative economic effect on the family, enterprise and nation, while deaths of children below 5 years robs the nation of potential manpower.

Urban - Rural Difference

Most urban adults are employed "migrants" from within or across Uganda's national borders. The urban population is therefore culturally amorphous, lonely but "rich" and thus predisposed to casual sexual behaviour as many workers leave their spouses in the rural areas. The health consequences of this behaviour include AIDS and are likely to be first noted by workers' health services. A number of workplaces are foci of communities so that workers' health services may be the first to receive cases of AIDS from such communities. The implications for the occupational health care system are self-evident.

Occupational Groups at Risk and the Effect of Occupation on HIV Infection and Spread

Among Ugandan workers there are two risk groups. The occupationally exposed, such as health workers and prostitutes can be directly infected in course of their work. In turn these can infect their clients. The second group, the occupationally predisposed, include urban labourers and members of the forces, who leave their wives behind in the rural areas for long periods, and are therefore likely to succumb to prostitutes. Long distance drivers, who make long and frequent journeys without their wives, may have multiple sexual partners along their routes, hence increasing the risk of infection and spread of the AIDS virus. High income or glamorous occupational groups, such as businessmen, executives, doctors, students and successful entertainers, attract the opposite sex, and with the urban sexual liberalism could be victims and then instruments of HIV spread. The urban rich businessmen frequently travel to rural areas so that with the cash on them they could fuel the HIV spread in rural areas as well.

Loss to Economic Production

AIDS attacks adults who are already employed or are being prepared for employment, for example students, and the very young children, the potential workforce of tomorrow. At the victim's workplace, the AIDS patient works very little and later stops completely up to the time of death. The employer, on the other hand, has to pay sickness benefits, treatment costs, for burial arrangements and for support of the "orphaned" family. The rural areas suffer too because whoever dies in an urban area has to be buried in his rural area of origin. Mourning takes many days for the whole village and many weeks for the extended family. Agricultural fields remain unattended for that time. The rich victims leave behind many "orphaned" economic projects both in rural and urban areas and these tend to wither, thus adversely affecting the national economy.

The Need for Occupational Health Care

The foregoing discussion implies that there is a need to make Occupational Health Care more relevant so that workers in all types of economic activities can be provided the necessary preventive care against AIDS and other diseases while continuing with curative care as well.

POSSIBLE ROLES OF THE OCCUPATIONAL HEALTH CARE SYSTEM IN THE CONTROL OF AIDS IN UGANDA

Ascertainment of Occupational Health Implications in AIDS

The occupational health care system in Uganda should take part in scientifically validating or excluding the implications observed above. Thereafter, there can be defined roles for occupational health care in the control of AIDS. Even now, however, some roles are already quite clear.

Provision of Health Care for AIDS Cases

In workers' health services there can be occupation specific HIV screening especially for groups at risk. Health professionals running workers' health services should be able to identify AIDS and the related diseases and provide supportive care before referral to larger health units. The importance of record keeping and returning of AIDS morbidity and mortality statistics in workplaces to both the Occupational Health Department and the Ministry of Health cannot be over-emphasised.

Preventive Care Programmes in the Occupational Health Setting

At national level the Occupational Health Department in conjunction with ACP could work out health education and screening programmes relevant to specific occupational groups.

At the workplace level, workers' health services could be advised and supervised to implement health education and screening programmes for workers and the communities in which they live. Workers should work as messengers against AIDS in the Community.

Prostitutes could be encouraged to stock condoms and insist that their clients use them, while long distance drivers could be encouraged to use condoms always, while all other workers should be encouraged to "zero graze". Hospital workers would be required to adhere to strict hygiene and use personal protective devices when at work. Better work schedules, reducing periods workers stay away from their spouses and the provision of housing and food adequate for a worker's family in an urban area are also possible preventive occupational health measures against AIDS.

Alerting all the Concerned about the Socio-economic Implications of AIDS

Generally in Uganda health care is taken for granted with little attention paid to its socio-economic necessity. In the occupational health setting where enterprises always aim at maximising production at minimum cost, even the cost of health care is assessed in terms of contribution to production. AIDS especially among workers disrupts socio-economic harmony from individual up to national level. The occupational health care system could therefore contribute to the fight against AIDS by highlighting the negative socio-economic effects of AIDS, so that the necessary preventive measures are considered by all as a positive contribution to the economy at all levels. The fight against AIDS need not be considered to be just against a disease, but rather a contribution to national development.

POSSIBLE OCCUPATIONAL HEALTH STRATEGIES IN AIDS CONTROL IN UGANDA

It is clear that the occupational health system should participate in AIDS control in Uganda. I would suggest the following strategies for such participation: Research; Health Education; Strengthening or starting occupational health services for workers and lastly, the Strengthening of the now weak occupational health link in the national health care system.

Research

Occupational health research on AIDS should be geared at confirming, or otherwise, of the occupational health implications discussed above and at comparing the effectiveness of various AIDS control measures in the occupational health setting. Occupational groups' contribution to AIDS morbidity and mortality can be worked out from records and from serological and clinical surveys, while the occupational risk can be investigated by Knowledge, Attitudes and Practices (KAP) studies. The direct cost of AIDS among workers, the loss to economic production caused by AIDS and the social effects of AIDS among workers should also be important areas of basic research to fill in our gaps of knowledge. Operational research comparing the effectiveness of alternative preventive or control approaches in the occupational health setting should also be carried out.

Health Education

The Occupational Health Care system should initiate or participate in workers' health education programmes against HIV infection and AIDS in conjunction with the national AIDS Control Programme (ACP). The two areas to consider should be developing occupation specific health education measures, at national level, for each of the occupational groups at risk such as health workers, businessmen, drivers and prostitutes, and secondly, the facilitation of health education activities against AIDS at the workplaces.

Strengthening or Creation of Occupational Health Services for Groups at Risk

Many of the workers at risk of HIV infection have no access to workers' health services or at best they may have only weak curative services. Therefore the strengthening or creation of workers' health services especially for those at risk should be initiated by the Occupational Health and Hygiene Department as a matter of urgency in order to stem the AIDS scourge among workers and in the community.

Strengthening the Occupational Health Link in the National Health Care System

While the occupational health implications of AIDS and the possible occupational health roles and strategies in the control of

AIDS have been discussed, occupational health is not yet well coordinated with the general health care system. Therefore in the context of this paper the strengthening of the now weak occupational health link in the national health care system should be considered a crucial step in the fight against the AIDS epidemic in Uganda.

REFERENCES

Aktar L, Larouze B, Mabika wa Bantu S et al (1987). Distribution of antibodies to HIV 1 in an urban community (Aru, Upper Zaire). Abstracts, 2nd International Symposium, AIDS and Associated Cancers in Africa, Naples, 7-9 October 1987, p.89.

Berkley S, Widy Wirski R, Okware S, Downing R, Linnan M, Sempala S (1987). Risk factors associated with HIV infection in Uganda. (A survey report).

Bouvet E, Vacnon F (1987). Non-tropical and tropical AIDS are not so paradoxical. Abstracts, 2nd International Symposium, AIDS and Associated Cancers in Africa, Naples, 7-9 October 1987, p.138.

Delaporte E, Dupont A, Merlin M et al (1987). Prevalence rates of Antibodies to HIV 1 and HIV 2 in population samples from Gabon. Abstracts 2nd International Symposium, AIDS and Associated Cancers in Africa, Naples, 7-9 October 1987, p.87.

Mann J. AIDS and the Traveller, World Health, December 1987, pp.14-15.

Marasca G, McCormick A, Hostler E (1987). AIDS cases and HIV infections related to Africa in the United Kingdom. Abstracts, 2nd International Symposium, AIDS and Associated Cancers in Africa, Naples, 7-9 October 1987, p.99.

Ngugi E N, Plummer F A, Cameron D W, Bosire M, Ndinya Achola J O et al (1987). Effect of an AIDS education programme on increasing condom use in a cohort of Nairobi prostitutes. Abstracts, 2nd International Symposium, AIDS and Associated Cancers in Africa, Naples, 7-9 October 1987, p.65.

Okware S (1987). The epidemic of AIDS in Uganda. Paper presented at the 2nd International Symposium, AIDS and Associated Cancers in Africa, Naples, 7-9 October 1987.

Plummer F A, Simonsen J N, Cameron D W, Ndinya Achola J O, Piot P, Ngugi E N (1987). Risk factors for HIV infection in a cohort of East African prostitutes. Abstracts, 2nd International Symposium, AIDS and Associated Cancers in Africa, Naples, 7-9 Ocotber 1987, p.65.

Saracco A, Galli M, Zehender G, Uberti Foppa C, Lazzarin A, Norom M (1987). Low prevalence of HIV antibodies in a remote area in Kenya. Abstracts, 2nd International Symposium, AIDS and Associated Cancers in Africa, Naples, 7-9 Ocotber 1987, p.91.

Tauris P, Black F T (1987). HIV positivity among Danish professionals returning from Africa. Abstracts, 2nd International Symposium, AIDS and Associated Cancers in Africa, Naples, 7-9 October 1987, p.99.

The Global Impact of AIDS, pages 251-262
© 1988 Alan R. Liss, Inc.

33. COST-BENEFIT ASPECT OF AIDS PREVENTIVE
PROGRAMMES: ITS LIMITATION IN POLICY MAKING

Gen Ohi[1], Ichiro Kai[1], Hiroaki Terao[1], Yasuki
Kobayashi[1], Wataru Hirano[1], Tomonori Hasegawa[1],
Kenji Soda[2], Kazuo Fukutomi[3]

Department of Environmental and Community
Medicine, Teikyo University School of Medicine[1];
Department of Public Health, Yokohama City
University School of Medicine[2]; Department of
Public Health Statistics, The Institute of Public
Health[3]

INTRODUCTION

The first officially registered case of AIDS among Japanese
was reported in March 1985. At the start of 1986, some 15 cases
had been recorded, about one half of them were haemophiliacs,
the other half homosexuals and all males. Information regarding
the spread of HIV in various high risk groups was scanty and
fragmentary. Even the population size of homosexual males was
unknown.

In the spring of 1986, we attempted to estimate the
imminent growth of AIDS epidemic through Delphi technique
based on an assumption that no effective therapy nor vaccination
would be made available in the 10 years to come. Fourteen
experts representing AIDS related disciplines made predictions
as to the annual incidence of AIDS patients for the years 1988,
1991 and 1996: their estimations for respective years were 100,
450 and 950 (Ohi et al, 1987a).

With this background data, it becomes important to
appreciate the efficacy of preventive programmes in relation to
costs in order to make the most of our limited public health
resources. We analyzed the cost-benefit aspect of preventive
programmes which included education, surveillance and provision
of safe supply of blood and its products (Ohi et al, 1987a). The
analysis suggested that the implementation of blood screening

programme which covers major metropolitan or wider areas would yield a net loss. However, this analysis did not include intangible benefits such as placating public unrest. Subsequently, in the end of 1986, a blood donor screening covering entire Japan was implemented and at the end of 1987 the prevalence of HIV antibodies was as low as 0.0002% (22 out of 11,200,000).

In January 1987, a female prostitute in Kobe was reported to have AIDS and Japanese society was immediately stricken by a panic. Within the following 2 months, some fifteen thousand people came forward for blood testing in Kobe and adjacent areas alone (Ohi et al, 1987b). Several thousand prostitutes were estimated to have taken tests, but not a single case of seropositivity was uncovered. The absence of seropositive individuals among the prostitutes as well as drug abusers was quite encouraging in planning AIDS control programmes. Thanks to strict drug control regulations, the population of drug abusers in Japan is distinctly small (e.g. in 1984 five heroin addicts were treated in Japan, 13,335 in USA).

At the end of 1987, the cumulative number of AIDS patients was 59, two thirds being haemophiliacs and one third male homosexuals. With the available data and some assumptions, a study team under the auspices of the Ministry of Health and Welfare including two of us (Soda et al, 1988) made an epidemiological prediction regarding the magnitude of HIV spread in the coming five years, and the report will be published elsewhere.

In this paper we will present (1) the epidemiologic prediction regarding the magnitude of HIV spread in Japan, (2) cost-benefit analysis (CBA) of preventive programmes proposed in the spring of 1986 and discuss the limit of CBA in developing a preventive programme.

ESTIMATION AND PREDICTION REGARDING POPULATION OF AIDS PATIENTS AND SEROPOSITIVE SUBJECTS

In the beginning of 1988, estimation was made regarding the population of AIDS patients and HIV seropositives in each risk group classified according to transmission modes of HIV (Soda et al, 1988). It is conspicuous that no case of seropositivity has been identified among prostitutes, drug abusers and convicts. So far AIDS patients and seropositive persons are mostly confined to haemophiliacs, homosexual males and repatriates from countries where the AIDS epidemic is occurring in much greater magnitude. Thus only these three groups will be presented here for the description of estimation method. Figure 1 shows chronological incidence of AIDS patients so far reported in Japan.

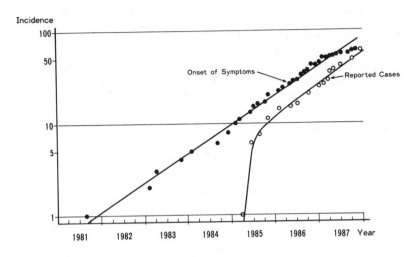

Figure 1. Chronological incidence of AIDS patients.

(a) Homosexual Males

It is at present not feasible to make scientific estimation on the population of homosexual males in Japan, which is far more proscriptive of homosexuality than Western countries. The editor of a gay magazine which has the largest circulation of its kind, estimates that up to 300,000 males practise homosexuality and about 30,000 are probably promiscuous (Ohi et al, 1987c). Since exact prevalence of seropositivity is unknown, the population of seropositive homosexuals and AIDS patients as well as their annual incidence was calculated according to the following mathematical model :-

$$X_t = r\ Y_t - a$$

where Y_t is the incidence of seroconversion in year t, X_t is the incidence of patients in year t, r is probability for a seropositive male homosexual to eventually develop AIDS (30%) and a is the period of latency (5 years).

When t is the present juncture of time, Y for the year
t - a + 1 onwards is calculated based on an assumption that
transmission occurs following the pattern observed in US
homosexual population (1.4 fold average annual increase 1985
through 1987). Though the behavioural pattern of male
homosexuals in Japan is unclear, a study conducted in Nagoya
suggests that the frequency of anal contact is about one half
(37%) of that in the USA and the rate of promiscuity defined as
having more than 10 sexual partners is also about one half
(Isomura: Personal communication). Thus, 50% of actively
practising homosexual males in Japan was calculated to follow
the American pattern in terms of transmitting HIV.

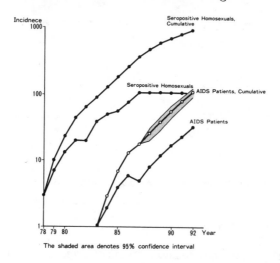

**Figure 2. Predicted incidence of AIDS patients and seropositive
subjects among homosexuals.**

The incidence of homosexual males who seroconverted
during 1987 is 108, with the cumulative number of seropositive
homosexuals being 370 at the end of 1987 and 910 at the end of
1992. (Fig. 2) This estimation (370) is approximately 9 times
greater than the cumulative cases of 43 (18 patients, 25
seropositive subjects so far known).

Assuming that 50% of estimated 30,000 homosexually active
males live in Tokyo metropolitan region, this estimation gives
prevalence rate of 2.5%, in close accordance with 2.8% reported

by Matsumoto et al (1987) who studied 352 homosexual males in Tokyo.

(b) Haemophiliacs

There are approximately 5,000 haemophiliacs in Japan, 40% of whom is estimated to be HIV seropositive (2,000). No seroconversion has occurred since the end of 1985 when thermal disinfection of the blood products was implemented.

The number of patients can be predicted according to the following model:-

$$X_k = r \sum_{j=1}^{k} n_{k+1-j} \; P_j$$

where X_k is the incidence of patients in year k, n_{k+1-j} is the incidence of seropositive haemophiliacs in year k+1-j, P_j is the probability of developing AIDS, j years after the seroconversion, r is the eventual (cumulative) probability of developing AIDS for a seropositive haemophiliac. Assuming that P has Weibull distribution with median of 5 or 7 years, (γ = 2.286 given by Lui (1986) is used as a pattern parameter) and HIV transmission due to contaminated blood products occurred 1979 through 1985, X and n were obtained following the method proposed by Brookmeyer and Gail (1986). We used for calculation the 32 cases reported before July, 1987. The incidence of AIDS patients from this group will reach the maximum of 18.4 in 1989, when the median of latent period is 5 years, and 24.8 in 1990 when it is 7 years (Fig. 3). The final cumulative numbers of AIDS patients among haemophiliacs are 130 and 232 respectively. The rate of developing AIDS for seropositive haemophiliacs is 6.5% in the former setting and 11.6% in the latter.

(c) Repatriates and Entrants from Epidemic Areas

Eleven cases of seropositive repatriates had been reported in Japan as of the end of 1987, with 9 being those from Africa. Some 30,000 persons repatriated from Africa in the preceding year making the seroprevalence rate of 0.03% in this group which is 150 times greater than that of Japanese blood donors (0.0002%).

Assuming the seropositive rate of blood donors in a country to be equal to the seroprevalence of entrants from the country, estimated number of seropositive entrants is given in Table 1.

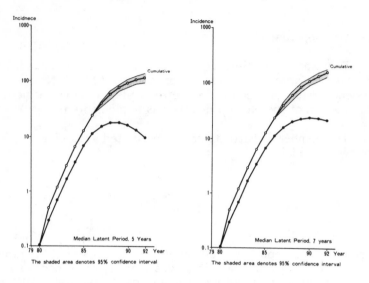

Figure 3. Predicted incidence of AIDS patients amongst haemophiliacs.

From the foregoing data, we can summarize the predicted number of AIDS patients and seropositive subjects. At the end of 1992, roughly 3,000 people will be HIV seropositive and the cumulative number of AIDS patients will be still between 260 and 300 (Table 2).

COST-BENEFIT ASPECT OF CONTROL PROGRAMMES

Benefits

Net benefits expected from a public health programme are the difference between total benefits expected and total costs incurred. Total benefits are equal to direct, indirect and intangible costs that are to be incurred as the consequences of the disease and its complications if they are not prevented. Estimation of intangible costs presents a special problem since there is no rational way of evaluating human emotions such as fear and anxiety. Thus we eschewed this estimation in the analysis. Saving of medical costs for the diagnosis and treatment of the patients with AIDS represents the most direct benefit. Indirect benefits represent the value of productivity loss which would have been saved by the implementation of the programme.

TABLE 1. Expected Number of Seropositive Entrants *

Region	Seropositivity Rate (%)	Entrants (1986)	Seropositive Entrants
Africa	1.0	10,000	100
North America	0.036	550,000	200
South America	0.077	26,000	20
Europe	0.014	358,000	50
Pacific	0.0054	56,000	3
Asia	0.0002	1,015,000	0.2
Total		2,021,000	373

* Soda et al. 1988

TABLE 2. Estimated Population of AIDS Patients and Seropositive Subjects in Japan (1987, 1992)*

Year	Risk Groups	Seropositive Subjects (cumulative)	Patients (cumulative)
1987	Haemophiliacs	2,000	34
(December)	Homosexual males	370	18
	Others	31	7
	Total	2,400	59**
1992	Haemophiliacs	2,000	116-157
(December)	Homosexual males	910	110
	Others	90***	30***
	Total	3,000	260-300

*   Soda et al. 1988
**   Reported cases
*** Less reliable compared with other high risk groups

Benefits related to haemophiliacs. 40% of 5,000 haemophiliacs are estimated to be seropositive. Physicians in charge of their treatment unanimously maintain that they are well educated about the nature of AIDS and have been practising discretion to minimize sexual transmission of the disease (Ohi et al, 1987a). As is the case in the USA, the haemophiliacs are monogamous and there is no evidence suggesting seropositive haemophiliacs constitute a serious source for horizontal transmission of HIV to the heterosexual group. Thus the benefits of surveillance and education of the haemophiliacs can be treated as a constant, null in this case, for the sake of parsimony.

Benefits related to homosexual men. (a) Direct benefits - US $40,000/person (US 1$ = Y130). The Japan Public Health Association recently reported that therapeutic costs of 13 AIDS patients were US $40,000/person with average admission period of 95 days. (b) Indirect benefits - US $440,000/person. Reports from the US and other countries indicate that 90% of adult AIDS patients were males ranging in age from 20 to 49 years. We adopted an economic value of a 40 year old man to calculate the economic loss incurred from the premature termination of a life (based on the value of 1979). Since no reliable figure is available in Japan as regards labour loss, we have omitted this benefit.

Thus without counting intangible benefits, the total benefits (B) are expressed as:-

$$B = Np \times (40,000 + 440,000) = rNs \times 480,000$$

where Np is reduced incidence of AIDS patient, Ns is averted incidence of HIV transmission and r is probability for seropositive homosexuals to develop AIDS (30% in 5 years).

Costs of public health programmes

Control programmes can be subsumed into (1) education and surveillance (Programmes A, B, C, D) and (2) provision of safe blood supply - blood donor screening (Programmes E, F).

A. Serological examination of haemophiliacs. The entire population (5,000) of haemophiliacs will be serologically screened and confirmed (US $15.4 per person, total cost US $77,000).

B. Counselling clinics for homosexual men. Since no strict confidentiality is guaranteed under the current system, we propose to start two counselling clinics (one in Tokyo, one in Osaka) where homosexual clients will be assured of confidentiality. The clinic will be staffed with a physician and two trained counsellors (cost $460,000). Actually, the Ministry of Health and Welfare (MHW) has recently appropriated the budget to implement the counselling clinics for the fiscal year of 1988.

C. Alerting physicians and other health personnel. Physicians (110,000 members of Japanese Medical Association and staff of 8,500 general hospitals) should be kept informed of the current status of the infection and encouraged to educate other health personnel. The Ministry of Health and Welfare (MHW) has asked some 600 hospitals throughout Japan to cooperate in the detection of AIDS (US $400,000).

D. Travellers to high risk countries. A hand-out alerting the risk of HIV transmission should be delivered at passport issuing government offices to applicants travelling to high risk countries. The annual number of overseas travellers was about 5 million in 1985 (US $380,000).

In February 1986, blood screening was implemented for HIV in Tokyo and other metropolitan areas and subsequently expanded in the end of the same year to cover entire Japan. At the end of 1987, 22 out of 11,200,000 donated blood samples were found to be seropositive.

E. Total screening programme. The costs for serological screening which covers entire Japan (8,200,000 donations in 1986) are expected to be US $132,000,000.

F. Partial screening programmes. Aside from haemophiliacs and their spouses, the seropositive blood samples have been found exclusively among men. Thus, screening limited on blood samples from reproductive men (20 - 49 years old) is theoretically expected to be more cost-effective (US $61,000,000).

The total costs may be expressed as either the sum of Programmes A, B, C, D (no donor screening, NDS) or A, B, C, D, E (total donor screening, TDS) or A, B, C, D, F (partial donor screening, PDS).

Figure 4 shows break-even points for the 3 programmes (TDS, PDS, NDS). It is noteworthy that the preventive programme without donor screening will become cost-beneficial when only 3 cases of AIDS are prevented. When the total screening of blood donors is conducted, 290 cases of AIDS will have to be prevented for the the programme to pay-off.

COST-BENEFIT APPRECIATION IN THE SELECTION OF HEALTH PROGRAMME

Our epidemiologic prediction implies that AIDS epidemic in Japan for the coming few years will be relatively small (cumulative incidence of seropositive subjects being 3,000, that of AIDS patients up to 300 in 1992) and still largely confined to haemophiliacs and male homosexuals. However, there is a possibility that the incidence of heterosexual transmission will grow at an increasing rate, especially among entrants and repatriates from African countries. In view of the fact that the two major high risk groups in Japan, haemophiliacs and homosexuals, have only negligible potential to cause AIDS transmission into the public, blood test for those heterosexual high risk groups may be warranted in case their stay is expected to be long.

With the seroprevalence of 2/1,000,000 among blood donors, it is obvious that the current blood screening programme is far from cost-beneficial. However, it does not necessarily mean that the blood screening programme is economically unwarranted. It rather suggests the limitation of CBA which does not permit evaluation of intangible benefits expected from averting such a dreadful disease as AIDS. Our preliminary study using willingness to pay approach demonstrated that potential recipients of blood are ready, without exception, to pay the costs of the screening even if the chance of HIV transmission is as small as 1 out of a half million (unpublished data). People tend to be most fearful in situations where the consequences can be devastating, uncontrollable, involuntary and irreversible, even if the chances of an incident are very small (Fischoff et al, 1981).

Risk perception may be influenced by a variety of factors, making evaluation of intangible costs more difficult. For instance, the plight of AIDS patients and the fatality of the disease has been well publicized, but few know that the seroprevalence of human T cell leukemia virus type I in many areas of Japan is as high as 5%, and 1 out of 2,000 in the seropositive subjects develops adult T cell leukemia (ATL), which is also fatal. As a consequence of receiving unscreened blood transfusion, a probability of dying from ATL is 25/1,000,000 while that from AIDS is 2/1,000,000 (even if we assume that

100% would eventually develop the disease). Certainly no one has made a fuss about ATL and blood screening. CBA underestimates

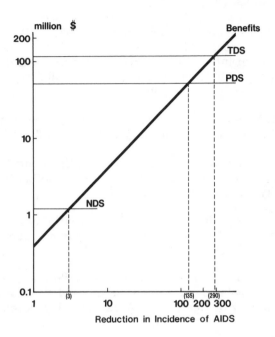

Figure 4. Costs and benefits of donor screening programmes.

the intangible costs related to the emotion of individual human beings or panic of the society. Formulation of a health policy which utilizes CBA must recognize this aspect.

REFERENCES

Brookmeyer R, Gail M (1986). Minimum size of the acquired immunodeficiency syndrome (AIDS) epidemic in the United States. Lancet ii: 1320-1322.

Fischoff B, Lichtenstein S, Slovic P (1981). "Acceptable Risk". New York: Cambridge University Press.

Lui K J, Lawrence D N, Morgan W M et al (1986). A model-based approach for estimating the mean incubation period of transfusion-associated acquired immunodeficiency syndrome. Proc Nat Acad Sci USA 83: 3051-3055.

Matsumoto T, Takahashi H, Yanagisawa U (1987). HIV seroprevalence among male homosexuals. In "Study Report on the mechanism of infection and development of clinical manifestations in AIDS, under the auspices of Ministry of Health and Welfare". pp 63-68 (in Japanese).

Ohi G, Kai I, Kobayashi Y et al (1987a). AIDS prevention in Japan and its cost-benefit aspects. Health Policy 8: 17-27.

Ohi G, Kai I, Terao H, Yoshimura T (1987b). Epidemic potential of AIDS through heterosexual transmission. Jap J Pub Health 34: 211-214 (in Japanese).

Ohi G, Kai I, Kobayashi Y et al (1987c). Potential of AIDS (acquired immunodeficiency syndrome) epidemic in Japan and public health. ibid. 34: 49-54 (in Japanese).

Soda K, Kitamura T, Shimada K et al (1988). "Study Report on the predicted population of AIDS patients and HIV seropositive subjects". Ministry of Health and Welfare, (in Japanese).

The Global Impact of AIDS, pages 263-269
© 1988 Alan R. Liss, Inc.

34. A THIRD FORCE : NGOs in AIDS CONTROL

R N Grose

Global Programme on AIDS, World Health
Organization, Geneva, Switzerland

INTRODUCTION

Most of the massive response to AIDS and HIV infection to date has been in the phase of defining the problem and planning national programmes. This is not to deny, of course, that pioneering roles have been played by organisations, governments and individuals who have established first-rate care and prevention programmes in the worst-hit cities of the developed and underdeveloped world. But at the global scale, it is clear that implementation of comprehensive national projects and programmes of the scope that is required is still in its earliest stages. In this presentation I will look at the potential role for non-governmental organisations (NGOs) in implementation in developing countries. This will involve answering three questions.

1. WHAT IS THE PROBLEM?

In the context of implementation, the problem consists of the difficulties we are all going to face in putting plans into practice: that is, problems we will face in preventing the spread of HIV and in caring for those affected by HIV-related diseases. This, in turn, means successfully encouraging people to change from high-risk to low-risk behaviour, and making sure that facilities are in place to provide care for those who need it, directly or indirectly, as a result of infection. I am going to focus on prevention rather than care.

To succeed in convincing people to change their behaviour, two things, among others, are essential :

* **access :**   channels of communication, either in the information giving sense, or preferably in the information sharing sense, as so succinctly put by Sue Laver (pp 264-270).

* **confidence :**   listeners must be confident that the message is (a) right, and, (b) fundamentally important to them.

This access and this confidence are both critical resources. We all know that in many places one or other or both do not exist, at least not in sufficient quantities for people to change their behaviour. There are a number of reasons for this. Firstly, in relation to communication and access, many states lack the comprehensive institutional development that would enable them to be in close and sensitive contact with all their people - often because of political or economic factors beyond their control.

Secondly, in relation to the confidence of people that the AIDS messages are both right and important, constraints lie in the deep and ancient cultural roots that underlie sexual behaviour, in the enduring beliefs in medical practices that are ineffective against this virus, and in the human response that says, the more our children die, the more children we must bear. The result of these economic and cultural factors is that, for many, government remains a distant irrelevancy.

Having broadly outlined some of the problems underlying implementation, the next question is, what do we do about them - what do we want to achieve?

2.   WHAT DO WE WANT TO ACHIEVE?

What I have just formulated is a potential problem in attaining prevention. The problem is two-fold: lack of access for communication - what we might call institutional distance - and cultural bias against changing behaviour. In this context, what we want to achieve can then be very simply stated: to shorten the institutional distance, that is, narrow the communication gap, and to adapt the message to the cultural context.

Simply stated, but less easily done. How can we achieve it? To answer that question, we need to look at some of the resources we have available.

3. HOW CAN WE ACHIEVE THIS OBJECTIVE?

Apart from the informal, dynamic and effective contribution of individuals, families and friends who are involved throughout the world in the fight against AIDS, we can identify three very broad groups of institutions that are also key participants: governments, intergovernmental agencies (such as WHO, UNDP, World Bank), and, thirdly, non governmental-organisations.

3.1 Governments

In national programmes, it is the government that has the most formal authority. This institutional authority reaches from cabinet to community. Its natural constituency is the entire population of the country. But these strengths are undermined by lack of human and material resources as well as by extraneous economic or civil problems such as debt, disadvantageous terms of trade, and, in some places, armed uprisings or foreign interventions. The result is that although the national structures do exist, communication between government and people is often not effective. The institutional gap remains just partly bridged, and communicating persuasive health messages is hard.

3.2 Intergovernmental Organizations

UN bodies and other intergovernmental organizations can provide some of the missing resources. Resources contributed by this group of agencies include technical assistance, policy advice, and finance. They have accumulated a vast knowledge bank from their worldwide experiences. But these strengths, too, are still not enough, as these agencies provide support mainly at governmental level and they do not usually directly involve communities. Communicating convincing messages is still hard, and community participation is likely to remain at the level of rhetoric rather than reality.

3.3 Non-governmental Organizations

Individual NGOs lack national authority, huge constituencies and the amounts of finance available to governments and intergovernmental agencies. However, their constituencies include many communities that are not well served by national programmes. NGOs include not only international development agencies, but also the small, single-interest organisations made up only of members of the communities they serve. Because

AIDS requires the involvement of sectors beyond health, the NGO group, as a resource, includes labour unions, teachers' groups, women's associations, drama groups, human rights organisations, and more.

Despite their enormous diversity, we can generalise about their strengths. They bring specialised skills; they have local knowledge; they are close to the communities in which they work; over the last few decades they have accumulated considerable project experience; they are flexible, mobile and able to innovate.

A key characteristic of NGOs is their ability to work in networks (Fig.1). Among themselves this may occur at three levels: they may share membership or constituencies, they may belong to umbrella organisations or federations, and even those federations may belong to broad international coordinating bodies. These overlapping networks provide a great opportunity for working cooperatively on AIDS control.

In working with governments, NGOs can operate simultaneously with central ministries, regional offices, and

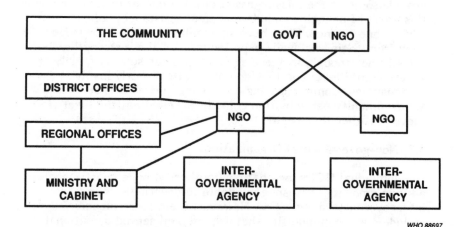

WHO 88697

Figure 1. Networks: NGOs' Strength

local officials. They can liaise between vertical government programmes, for example in health and agriculture. Outside the government sector, they can deal directly with intergovernmental organisations and with other NGOs. Some operate free from official structures for at least part of the time, and some deal only with the communities from which they spring.

If we look back at the problem we are addressing, the institutional gap between national programmes and the people, it becomes clear the NGOs have a vital role to play. Governments and intergovernmental organisations have strengths in authority, institutional frameworks, and technical and financial resources. To some extent they do reach the people, of course. But it is NGOs' ability to work simultaneously in peripheral, isolated communities and with central bureaucracies, and to assist communities themselves to generate the resources they need, that gives them the potential to facilitate communication. Their closeness to the community, and for some their roots within the community, provide at least the potential for incorporating local beliefs and practices in health and sexuality into credible, forceful, and acceptable messages on AIDS.

While on the topic of proximity to the community, it is worth raising, in passing, another facet of AIDS prevention. By looking at known locations of HIV epidemics, patterns of movement of people to and from those areas, and patterns of sexual behaviour in the ethnic groups involved, it should be possible to identify, in broad terms, communities or groups for whom becoming aware of risk is a priority. Existing development programmes can be designed or adjusted accordingly. Similarly, organisations might be able to put together popular strategies for alternative, local, income-earning opportunities. This would reduce the economic need for rural-urban migration and for the family separation and social fragmentation that go with it. This kind of "preventive development" would strengthen rural development policies that have, for years, struggled to counter rural emigration and rural economic decline.

Of course, NGOs have problems too, and not least is the great range of competence among them. But we should also recognise that their very diversity is a strength: the world is a diverse and dynamic place, and monolithic programmes sometimes lack the agility to adjust to changing needs and circumstances. Large projects are usually slow to start, and once started they have so much momentum they can find it hard to stop or to change direction. Diversity allows for innovation: the testing of new ideas and the promotion of the ones that work.

Having clarified that there is a vital role for NGOs in prevention of HIV infection and AIDS, as in other forms of development, we should look at what NGOs need to help them in implementation.

NGOs' IDENTIFIED NEEDS

In recent discussions at WHO, a small group of reasonably representative international NGOs listed difficulties or new requirements arising out of their growing involvement in AIDS programmes. The needs that they identified included new and effective approaches to health education; information on AIDS in general and specifically by country; extra resources in personnel and funds; improved coordination among themselves, in order to learn from each other's experiences; assistance with such universal problems as insurance; assistance in improving coordination with national AIDS committees; and the formulation of positive, developmental ways to work - that is, not merely filling resource gaps but helping build sustainable structures.

WHO needs to strengthen its working relationship with NGOs in order to further its support for national programmes and in pursuit of its global objectives of prevention, care and the reduction of negative impact. One way it can do this is by meeting some of the needs identified by NGOs. At the recent meeting, WHO committed itself to doing just that.

SUMMING-UP

To recapitulate briefly, global AIDS prevention can maximise its chances of success if it draws on the complementary strengths of governments, intergovernmental agencies, and NGOs. Perhaps the most important strengths of NGOs in this context are their abilities to form networks, to close the distance between communities and national programmes, and to amplify the voices of those communities. Helping the people be heard will help problems be better defined and give a better chance for solutions to be found. NGOs have a vital role in strengthening those two resources of access and confidence building: that is, communication to and within communities, and people's confidence that the AIDS message is right and important enough to act upon.

At the same time, NGOs have a role in identifying and providing support for those who are ill and for their families, as well as for the young and the elderly whom AIDS makes destitute.

Finally, giving due respect to the independence and autonomy of NGOs, it is important to point out that we are not talking about organisational domination and control, but about management - specifically, about management by coordination. It is not a matter of asking "what do we have in common, and how can we work together", but "what do we have that is different, and how can we work together".

The Global Impact of AIDS, pages 271-276
© 1988 Alan R. Liss, Inc.

35. NON-GOVERNMENTAL ORGANISATIONS, AIDS AND THE INSTITUTIONAL MEMORY : EXPERIENCES FROM THE LEAGUE OF RED CROSS AND RED CRESCENT SOCIETIES

Bruce Dick

Head, Community Health Department and AIDS Coordinator (ad interim), League of Red Cross and Red Crescent Societies, P O Box 372, 1211 Geneva 19, Switzerland

INTRODUCTION

During the past twenty years there has been a large increase in the number of international and indigenous non-governmental organisations (NGOs) concerned with "health". They have demonstrated that they have flexibility, potential for innovation, effective contact with vulnerable communities and a capacity to respond rapidly to changing circumstances in a way that enables then to **do** what others can often merely talk about. Major donors are increasingly appreciating that NGOs are important and responsible components of the health sector, for relief and development programmes: the AIDS pandemic poses us with elements of both.

NGOs have **already** played an essential part in the prevention and control of AIDS: by highlighting the problem of AIDS and the urgent need for action, carrying out information activities, providing counselling services and counteracting the discrimination that is bubbling to the surface in the wake of this pandemic. The importance of NGOs was clearly recognised and reinforced both by Dr Jonathan Mann in his presentation (pp 203-205) and by the Declaration from the recent World Summit of Ministers of Health on AIDS Prevention Programmes. This is important because not only do NGOs themselves need a long-term commitment to become involved with AIDS but they need the commitment of others to facilitate and support such involvement.

Despite their great potential, many NGOs were rather slow off the mark. Like most other organisations it took us a fair amount of time to move from denial to commitment, from passivity to action. However, now that we are "on the bus", the challenge for us will be to ensure that an involvement with AIDS strengthens our existing programmes and, at the same time, that the lessons learnt from these on-going activities (our institutional memory) strengthen and direct our involvement with the AIDS pandemic.

AIDS AND THE INSTITUTIONAL MEMORY

The initial dilemma that has confronted most NGOs is a hardy perennial and relates to the dialectics of primary health care, what I call the PHC purist - selectivist debate: should we develop integrated or vertical programmes in response to AIDS? "Integration" is encouragingly a key word of most NGO policy documents, although with donor pressures, the high visibility nature of the problem, inappropriate requests for assistance, and many organisations taking on extra staff to deal with AIDS, this is not always going to be easy.

Many of us have already had to deal with this integration/vertical programme issue as we became involved with supporting national Diarrhoeal Disease and Expanded Immunisation Programmes. Based on these past experiences we need to ensure that an involvement with the AIDS pandemic supports, rather than detracts from our on-going activities and commitments.

An involvement with the AIDS pandemic places a magnifying glass on many difficult issues that already face NGOs, in one way or another: how to "move something up the agenda" without allowing it to take over; how to develop general policies and strategies, and ensure consistency of our messages, while at the same time being sensitive to local needs and conditions; how to "coordinate" without being seduced by the aphorism that "to coordinate is good but to control is best"; how to find a balance between being proactive and reactive, between being too pushy and doing things too-little-and-too-late; how to be realistic about what one's own organisation is in a special position to contribute, despite all the donor pressures and the enormity of the problem. How to add substance to our commitment to use existing structures and systems whilst at the same time ensuring that we avoid all the "business-as-usual" type of delays which they so often cause.

AIDS has additionally posed some problems that most of us

have not had to confront with other health programmes: the importance of being sensitive about language both for the people affected and also because the words which we use have an impact on our own attitudes and actions; the importance not only of ensuring that "the community" participates, but that we specifically involve people with high risk behaviours and people who are HIV positive or have AIDS; the importance of trying to **do** something despite the ostrich position which, for a variety of reasons, some governments have chosen to adopt; the importance not only of taking a stand against discriminatory practices that affect people's health but also of counteracting the discrimination that is released by this disease.

THE LEAGUE OF RED CROSS AND RED CRESCENT SOCIETIES RESPONSE TO THE AIDS PANDEMIC

Within the League of Red Cross and Red Crescent Societies we were determined to use our institutional memory as we responded to the AIDS pandemic. We wanted to ensure that our actions reflected the lessons learned from the successes and mistakes of our previous relief operations and development programmes (including the "selective" ones, such as our CHILD ALIVE programme). In particular we wanted to avoid the Atlas fantasy (thinking that a single organisation should, or more importantly could take all the problems of the world on its shoulders) and the Icarus syndrome (getting carried away by high-visibility unsustainable activities) !

As a start, we harnessed the enthusiasm of a number of donor National Societies "to get involved". With their support we organised workshops for Red Cross and Red Crescent Societies in Europe and Africa with the aim of informing and motivating them, generating commitment, exchanging experiences and ideas, and developing general policies and strategies. We also sent an information pack to all National Societies which contained basic information about AIDS, provided some ideas about what could be done and gave some examples of what National Societies were already doing.

Using the information gained from these workshops we drafted a Resolution on AIDS which was adopted at our General Assembly held at the end of last year. This was a unique opportunity for highlighting the important issues, generating commitment and endorsing the broad policies and strategies. It was also an opportunity to begin to ensure that National Societies take a strong stand against discrimination - something which they are mandated to do by the Fundamental Principles of the Movement.

At the same time, we developed effective formal and informal communication and coordination both within the Federation and outside, with WHO's Global Programme on AIDS, other NGOs and relevant individuals and organisations. In general this has been very rewarding and is another positive spin-off to the AIDS pandemic.

Finally during this initial phase we developed basic information and advice for our delegates. This was primarily intended to allay their ungrounded fears that AIDS had suddenly made it "dangerous" to work in developing countries. This of course is far from the case provided that the simple rules are adhered to (as they would also need to be adhered to in Europe or North America) .... condoms are much more important than plasma expanders in a delegate's health kit!

Throughout, we have decided not to set up an "AIDS Unit", but to carry out activities through the relevant operational and technical Departments such as Community Health, Information and the Blood Programmes. The initial difficulties of this approach were relatively easily overcome by setting up an AIDS Working Group with representation from all the Departments concerned, and we are convinced that the long-term benefits will far out-weigh any initial hiccoughs.

During 1988 we will run workshops for the Caribbean and Latin American National Societies, assist National Societies organise and carry out national workshops and develop their short and mid term plans, help to coordinate the funding for the projects which are developed and provide technical assistance as required.

Many National Societies have of course already been actively involved with the AIDS pandemic for some time, exemplifying the many potential roles for NGOs: catalytic, innovative and supportive. The Kenya Red Cross carried out its famous "help crush AIDS" Health Education campaign; the Swedish Red Cross has collaborated with an NGO with less credibility but more expertise in the field of AIDS and developed innovative approaches to counselling and providing support for people who are HIV positive or who have AIDS; the American Red Cross have been responsible for implementing nationwide AIDS information programmes, both general and targeted (for example, AIDS in the work place); the British Red Cross has both disseminated general information in support of the government's programme and also provided specialist services based on their traditional on-going activities; the Norwegian Red Cross Society has played a major role in mobilising and funding advocacy and information activities which counteract discrimination; and many other Red Cross Societies, in both developed and developing countries, have provided support for their governments' national AIDS Control Programmes through their on-going training, information and community health activities, and blood transfusion services.

The activities of National Societies have varied a great deal depending on their existing programmes, resources and commitments, although all efforts have been guided by the need to comply with their government's policies and strategies. The Rwanda Red Cross Society, for example, which is responsible for the country's blood transfusion services, has been very active with screening donated blood as well as implementing an important national Health Education campaign. Across the border in Uganda and in Kenya, the National Societies are not involved with blood transfusion services (except for donor recruitment) and have therefore limited their activities to health education/information (although because of their ability to respond rapidly, with the support of sister Societies they were able to provide a channel for the initial purchasing of HIV screening equipment, reagents, protective clothing, etc., at a time when their governments were still in the process of developing and obtaining funds for their short and medium term plans).

CONCLUSIONS

Red Cross and Red Crescent Societies have a long tradition of responding to disasters and I have often heard it said that AIDS is a "disaster". Certainly AIDS is a disaster. However, if ever there was a disaster that needed to be seen within a context of development or that had serious repercussions for other development programmes; if ever there was a disaster that needed to be seen within a long-term perspective and needed a long-term commitment for its solution; if ever there was a disaster that was going to require the involvement of many different professional skills and expertise; if ever there was a disaster that was going to test our Federation's institutional memory, that was going to test whether we have moved with the times, in terms of our approaches to solving health problems

.... AIDS is it.

There are many questions about AIDS that remain unanswered: some because we still have a great deal to learn about this disease, despite our understanding of the simplicity of the basic messages for preventing its spread; some because they are quite simply difficult and complex questions. What are the long-term implications going to be on development projects; how are we going to ensure that AIDS is not just the latest high-visibility activity which will inevitably suffer from "donor fatigue"; how are we going to develop methods of really encouraging people to alter their behaviour (we haven't always been brilliant at this); how are we going to monitor and evaluate the impact of our programmes (it's much more difficult than with immunisation of diarrhoeal diseases - at least you can see whether a mother is giving a child ORS and has mixed it properly!); how are we going to stay positive and optimistic as we watch AIDS affect our friends and co-workers, and undo the advances in health status indicators that have been achieved during the past twenty years; how are we going to integrate AIDS activities with existing programmes,and cooperate with other organisations, while retaining the "profile" that is as important for NGOs as it is for everyone else?

I don't think that any of these problems are insurmountable, and I remain optimistic and convinced that we have a lot to gain from the AIDS pandemic. Like non-stick frying pans and the space race, I am sure that there will continue to be many positive spin-offs, and I have no doubt that AIDS will provide us with many opportunities to turn past rhetoric into present reality.

The Global Programme on AIDS has generated enormous political commitment, and, for a change, financial resources appear to be much less of a problem than identifying relevant and sustainable ways of spending them. Whilst accepting that NGOs will have a special role to play in confronting AIDS, we will obviously need to avoid the situation whereby they become the organisational equivalent of the Village Health Worker - being off-loaded with all the problems that governments and other organisations either don't want to deal with or don't really know how to tackle ! We will need to identify our own specific contributions and be clear about our objectives and strategies .... to which end, we will need to remember Rudyard Kipling's "six serving men" (what, how, when, why, where and who) and hope that we don't get Alzheimer's disease of the institutional memory!

The Global Impact of AIDS, pages 277–279
© 1988 Alan R. Liss, Inc.

36. THE COMMUNITY AS A RESOURCE

Grace Smallwood

P O Box 771, Hermit Park, Townsville, Queensland
4810, Australia.

I want to discuss an approach to developing AIDS Media and
educational materials, by using the Community as a resource.

Although Australia is not a developing country, my people,
black Australians, have a health status similar to that of Third
World countries. This includes a high prevalence of substance
abuse, widespread malnutrition, poor living environments,
inadequate essential services, low educational achievement and
high unemployment.

The approach of using the Community as the main resource
is applicable to any Society which has limited technical
professional and monetary resources: this is our only strength.
Citizenship was granted to my people 20 years ago, but we have
only one graduate medical doctor and very few registered nurses.
It is therefore essential that black health workers are the key
element in the teaching of all health education. Reasons being:-

* the workers have a practical knowledge of our culture;
* A commitment to raising the health status of our
   Community;
* A knowledge of local health issues;
* An understanding of the restrictions, facing any problems
   in our Community;
and * A degree of credibility in our Community, that visiting
   experts cannot quickly achieve.

Although AIDS is not a major problem yet amongst black
Australians, poor sanitation and nutrition leading to a poor
health status, with a high incidence of hepatitis B and

Chlamydia, lays the Community open to the spread of this virus.

The Western health system has much to learn from the approach taken in the mobilisation of black communities by our own health workers. In the past Western health educators have tried to educate our people, but with little understanding of our culture, and by using their own methods of health education, they have understandably failed. The approach taken has three main components :-

* **Consultation** - to work with black communities with local people.
* **Networking** - to use established black health worker networks.

and * **Pretesting of communication materials,** which involves black health workers in developing, pretesting and running public health campaigns.

It is essential the workshop happens in black environments so that the contributors feel comfortable. The workshop team consists of a doctor, a nurse, a health educator, a communication consultant and graphic artist. The workshop begins with short introductions, and information sessions about AIDS. This is followed by sessions on basic rules of communication - how to develop media materials and plan a health education campaign. Deciding aims and objectives, selecting target audiences, and developing messages conveyed, are key elements of this process. The ideas of the workshop participants are recorded, and the graphic artist and communication consultant develop several concepts based on these ideas. The following day these concepts are presented in rough visual form to the workshop. The participants are enthusiastic in their response when they see their ideas expressed in the communication materials. Once again, note is taken of the workshop reactions, to the various concepts. Particularly what people say, how they physically react - with laughter, puzzlement, seriousness and most importantly, their ideas for changes. These changes are then incorporated into further versions of the materials.

Community members are then invited to review and comment on the materials to gain a wider target audience response, and to refine the materials to a final acceptable stage. The workshop then votes on which posters, slogans or advertisements it thinks are the strongest and most effective. The next session of the workshop, develops action plans related to specific activities, that can be undertaken in the campaign.

These action plans bring together networking, research, planning and evaluation. These elements are then developed into specific activities, related to the networks used by the health workers. In many of the slides, I have used the colours red, black and yellow. These colours are colours of the Black Australian flag and are instantly recognisable to my people. This is an example of being culturally specific in your communications. When my people see these colours, we know the communication is for us, and we usually trust the message.

The most important aspect of the training workshop is that it produces materials, posters, radio ads, action plans on the spot and pretests these materials in local communities. This approach reinforces the importance of black health workers and develops strategies that fit into existing structures and networks. It also trains health workers in the essential ingredients of conceiving, planning and implementing a media campaign concerned with health issues. Most importantly, the health education programme that is developed, is relevant to that particular community and is "owned" by that community.

This programme would not have been a success without community involvement which has been a part of our cultural heritage, spanning over 40,000 years.

The Global Impact of AIDS, pages 281–287
© 1988 Alan R. Liss, Inc.

37. AFRICAN COMMUNITIES IN THE STRUGGLE AGAINST AIDS : THE NEED FOR A NEW APPROACH

Susan M L Laver

Department of Community Medicine, University of
Zimbabwe, Box A173, Avondale, Harare, Zimbabwe.

INTRODUCTION

The saying goes that when you're up to your neck in mud
fighting crocodiles in a swamp, take time to stand back and
remember that you came to drain the swamp in the first place.
Most of us working in the field of AIDS Awareness would
certainly admit that we have often found ourselves to be up to
our necks in conceptual mud, fighting all sorts of conceptual
crocodiles. The problem of AIDS in Africa lies not only in the
dimensions of its transmission. It is fraught with political and
cultural sensitivity, and compounded further by economic and
social problems which already impede progress in many spheres
of development. Misperceptions about the transmission of the
disease are common and diverse, ranging from exogenous and
endogenous theories to the retributionist theories alluded to by
many workers elsewhere (Homans et al, 1987). Given these
problems and the scarcity of available resources for health in
developing countries, any discussion about AIDS where attempts
at control fail to incorporate the fundamental principles of
mobilisation for development through the active involvement of
people at every level, would seem futile. So while it is important
to note that education has been wisely accepted as an
appropriate weapon in the AIDS drama, health professionals
should not discard historical evidence of the successes achieved
in health care programmes, where participation by communities
in the information sharing process, has been accorded equal
weighting as a tool in the struggle against ignorance and
misunderstanding.

THE INFORMATION-SHARING SCENARIO

If we examine information-sharing scenarios for AIDS in
Africa, we find ample evidence of attempts to spread
information in most countries. Faded posters, now the subject of
graffiti, and sometimes reversed and used for other propaganda,
such as football matches, hang apologetically from their stands.
AIDS leaflets, read and unread, understood and misunderstood,
lie idly in any number of public venues - and valid questions
remain unanswered in the minds of many. Despite the cost and
effort behind many of these print media efforts, research into
popular understanding about AIDS demonstrates clearly that
although levels of consciousness about the epidemic have been
raised, misunderstanding still exists. It has also been shown that
shifts of attitude in some countries have been slight after initial
campaigns (Wilson, 1987), and in many cases opposite to that
desired (Spicer, 1987). An analysis of media used in health
education campaigns also clearly reveals that message-content
has often been characterised by incomprehensible language, and
a lack of sensitivity to culture, lay beliefs, traditional values and
emotional needs of the people. Paradoxically, we have almost
reached the situation where target audiences have been disabled
by the mass media.

It is not surprising therefore, to note the growing body of
workers who warn against the indiscriminate use of mass media
as a means of educating the people and stress rather the need to
use interpersonal channels of communication for reaching
selective groups and influencing sensitive behaviours within the
community (Hubley, 1987). Other workers stress that meaningful
and enduring changes in behaviour can only be achieved
individually or collectively if increased opportunities are created
(and subsequently provided) for communities to enter more
actively into the broader issues of the AIDS debate, i.e. its
detrimental effect upon society and development (Homans et al,
1987).

These trends would indicate the need to shift away from
prescriptive traditions of information giving, which seem to
characterise AIDS campaigns, and move more rapidly towards
information sharing. It is therefore essential that we wean
Health Workers, and indeed the public, from a dependency on
mass media as the panacea for AIDS education, and encourage
instead, the adoption of educational approaches which activate
dialogue, generate information exchange and permit greater
participation by lay people and all levels of Health Worker.

A genuinely participatory approach must therefore start from what people already know and allow them to determine what further information and/or skills are required. This requires that Health and Health related Workers stand back and LISTEN to what is being said, what needs are being expressed, rather than imposing set ideas of what is needed.

But how does this work in reality; there are two issues of major concern: **who** participates and **how** do they participate?

WHO SHOULD PARTICIPATE IN SUPPORT ACTIVITIES AGAINST AIDS?

If true participation in support activities against AIDS is to be achieved at every level of the community then this of necessity means that there must be a devolution of educational responsibility from present service providers to men, women and young people in the community to plan, staff and manage that responsibility. This further implies that the outreach network already used in the implementation of PHC is extended beyond governmental and non-governmental organisations to include lay fieldworkers, volunteers and members of the community who practise risky behaviour in AIDS prevention work. In this context we see the Traditional Healer turn from AIDS-Cure Advocate to AIDS-Counsellor, the once stigmatised Downtown Social Lady turn Group Advisor, the Blood Donor turn Donor Motivator, and the previously misinformed Factory Worker turn AIDS educator. Under these circumstances the responsibility for support activities against AIDS devolves from the politician and health professional to include a wider representation of concerned representatives from sub-groups within the community. But are the members of the community ready to assume this front line role? An analysis of abstracts from interviews with a selected range of Zimbabweans would certainly seem to indicate a readiness to become involved.

Downtown Social Lady. How can I fight this problem alone? Others won't believe me, change will be difficult unless it is accepted by my group, I'll be isolated, lose money. I have no insurance, it's hopeless talking about AIDS in these circumstances. We need to be heard as a group, not isolated.

Traditional Healer. They do not believe we have a role to play. We want to help. We could counsel. We are being isolated through newspaper reports, our initiatives are being discouraged. We are being isolated without consultation from an important medical event which affects us all.

Factory Worker. The message which says stick to one partner is unreasonable. It should be stick to one sex unit (i.e., partners within a polygamous marriage), but my voice will not be heard alone.

Young Male Blood Donor. I've been donating blood for a long time now. There are others in my workplace who could join me, but at this time they are uninformed and frightened about the idea of donating blood.

Health Worker. There is not time for teaching about AIDS when the queues are so long. If only there were others in the community to assist us.

THE HOW OF PARTICIPATION IN SUPPORT ACTIVITIES AGAINST AIDS

The HOW dimension of participation adds a somewhat more qualitative aspect to this debate if responsibility for support activities against AIDS is to truly devolve from national levels to representatives within community sub-groupings at every level of society. From the outset a commitment by Governments to the achievement of this objective within an organised plan of action is essential.

In this context forums that respect the confidentiality of sub-groups in the community should be convened and an appropriate participatory methodology evolved to inform and mobilise towards the adoption of a positive intention to participate in support activities against the disease. Participatory activities at one level could include, for example, AIDS Awareness Workshop for Traditional Healers, regular discussion groups for Downtown Social Ladies, Donor Promoter Courses for Blood Donors, and Writers' Workshops such as the one held in Zimbabwe (Laver, 1987), which promote the compilation of culturally specific print media for different target groups within communities.

For this process to be effective however, it is recommended that these activities are carefully guided and that opportunities for participation are sequentially explored by groups, so that the outcome is fruitful. This would basically involve four main steps :-

(1) **Participation** by sub-group volunteers in **exploring** and **identifying** the problems and dimensions of AIDS in terms of its social, economic and environmental contexts, i.e.:-

* What is HIV and AIDS?
* What are the factors which contribute to the transmission of HIV in our group?
* How does present behaviour in my sub-group break with tradition and contribute to the problem?
* How will this problem effect the people in our group?
* What are the long term prospects if we do not act now?
* What are the blocks to attitude/behaviour change?
* What are the risky behaviours practised by our group?
* In what way can we assist in the modification of these behaviours/assist in support activities against AIDS?
* How can we support those already affected?

(2) **Participation** by sub-group volunteers in the **identification** of **selective messages** for information sharing :-

* What do members of our group understand about HIV and AIDS?
* What are the barriers to learning about HIV and AIDS in our group?
* What are the learning problems in our group?
* Which messages will be appropriate for our group?
* What information exists already that is appropriate for our group?
* Where can we get this information?

(3) **Participation** by sub-group volunteers in the **identification** of **strategies** for information sharing and support activities :-

* What are the available opportunities for communication in our group (a) on an individual basis, (b) in groups and (c) in communities?
* What local initiatives can we use for communicating information in our group, (a) artists, (b) singers, and (c) writers?
* What participatory strategies can we use in communication, (a) role play, (b) drama, (c) focus group discussions and (d) meetings?
* What other local initiatives can we use to mobilise information and support (a) political meetings and (b) rallies?

* How can we learn about and practise new communication skills?

(4) **Participation** by sub-group volunteers in **identifying** appropriate methods of feedback :-

* How can we establish a report-back system to the local authority?
* What methods could we use to assess failure, successes?
* How can we generate new ideas, local initiatives?

This list is not exhaustive. It merely alludes to the concept of direct involvement of sub-groups in developing strategies for AIDS communication which should, by the nature in which they evolved, bear messages of relevance for their situation.

CONCLUSION

It is natural for health professionals to want to assume responsibility for the dissemination of AIDS information. However, given the very nature of the virus and the proportions of the epidemic, it is essential that the responsibility devolves from this level to be shared with those, who, given necessary support, will undoubtedly show the willingness and diligence in imparting information that we have come to experience in the broad discipline of Primary Health Care. There are positive indications in many countries which would suggest that a participatory approach to AIDS prevention work has been initiated within existing forums. Local initiatives must be encouraged if efforts to contain the epidemic are to be successful.

REFERENCES

AIDS Awareness Writers Workshop. Harare, Zimbabwe, 7-11 September 1987. Unpublished proceedings.

Homans H, Appleton P (1987). "Learning About Aids. Participatory Health Strategies for Health Educators with a responsibility for Adult education about Aids". Health Education Authority in association with AVERT.

Homans H, Appleton P (1987). "Educating about AIDS". A discussion document for Health Education Officers, community Physicians and others with a responsibility for effective education about AIDS. NHS Training Authority.

Hubley J (1987). "AIDS in Africa. A challenge to Health Education". Leeds Polytechnic.

Laver S. "Participation in Education for AIDS". Paper presented at the First Zimbabwe Psychiatric Conference, Harare, Zimbabwe, 15-16 January 1988.

Spicer E. "Overview of 19 Focus Group Discussions with various groups in Zimbabwe". Unpublished paper, December 1987.

Wilson D. "Areas of Ignorance about AIDS". Paper presented to AIDS Awareness Writers Workshop, Harare, Zimbabwe, 7-11 September 1987.

The Global Impact of AIDS, pages 289-300
© 1988 Alan R. Liss, Inc.

38. PARTICIPATORY APPROACHES TO THE PRODUCTION AND USE OF THE MASS MEDIA

G Gordon[1], J Riber[2], E Spicer[3], S Smith[4].

International Planned Parenthood Federation[1]; Development through Self Reliance, Harare, Zimbabwe[2]; Edwina Spicer Productions (PVT) Ltd, Harare, Zimbabwe[3]; Development through Self Reliance Inc., Columbia, USA[4].

INTRODUCTION

The paper describes the use of participatory approaches, including aspects of focus group methodology, in the generation of content and scenarios for a mini-feature film on AIDS for African audiences. The paper describes the group's perceptions of the problem of AIDS and how these indicate the need for a film which personally involves the audience at an experiential level. The authors suggest how mass media can be used within the context of primary health care programmes which include counselling, follow-up discussions and support for change.

PARTICIPATORY APPROACHES TO THE PRODUCTION AND USE OF THE MASS MEDIA

Education that motivates people to adopt safer sexual practices is the only strategy we have for preventing the spread of HIV at the present time. As a contribution to this strategy, the IPFF AIDS Unit is supporting the production of a mini-feature film on AIDS for African audiences.

African nations contain a rich diversity of cultures and sexual mores, modified by education, travel, changing family structures and economic realities. Many people in every country are aware now of the disease called AIDS, but their knowledge and perceptions will depend on exposure to educational programmes and to people with HIV infection.

How could the film makers find common themes which would meet the needs of as many groups as possible with information on HIV, which would help people to examine their own behaviour and options and motivate them to adopt safer practices, if necessary?

How could the film makers adopt, in Sue Laver's words, (pp 281-287) "a genuinely participatory approach which starts from what people already know, feel and do, and allows them to determine what further information, skills and motivation are required. This requires that we sit back and LISTEN to what is being said, what needs are being expresses, rather than imposing set ideas of what is needed?" How could the film makers produce and use the mass media in a way that is "enabling" rather than "disabling"?

FOCUS GROUP METHODOLOGY - an approach to exploring problems and their causes and identifying solutions

Communicators typically find out about the knowledge, attitudes and practices of the "target" group in order to generate appropriate "messages", which are then disseminated as posters, leaflets or films. In this process, the communicators are placed in an active role and the target group in a passive role. Communicators do Knowledge, Attitude and Practice (KAP) studies or focus group discussions, carry away the data, process them and feed them back to the group.

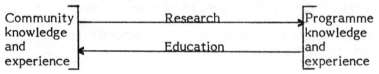

Community knowledge and experience — Research → Programme knowledge and experience ← Education

A more participatory approach would have the social group and communicator as equal participants in an exchange of knowledge and experience, based on an understanding that AIDS is a problem for both parties.

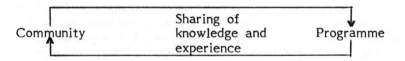

Community — Sharing of knowledge and experience → Programme

Focus Group Methodology is a qualitative research method borrowed by health educators from the world of commercial marketing. Ideally, a focus group consists of six to ten people of similar backgrounds and a representative sample of focus groups is selected to cover each socioeconomic group. In practice a focus group may become larger as members of the community notice and join in the discussion. The facilitator introduces the topic and asks a few key open-ended questions to begin the discussion.

People are encouraged to hold an open-ended conversation together, asking and answering each others questions, commenting on what is said, and interacting with each other rather than the facilitator. Thus the facilitator is not acting as a group leader. The facilitator must create an atmosphere of safety where everyone can talk freely without fear of censure, pressure or gossip. There are both right and wrong answers and no judgements. In commercial Focus Groups this is achieved by getting together a group of strangers. In some Focus Groups the facilitator introduces the topic and then leaves the group to continue the discussion, recorded by tape or a silent notetaker. Any misinterpretations are cleared up **only** after the group has run out of steam.

As used by commercial marketing, Focus Groups are not participatory because the researchers take away and control the information generated. There is no ongoing discussion with the group as an action group.

However, health educators can learn from focus group methodology how to allow people the time and safety to talk freely and share their experience and knowledge without the health educator interrupting the dialogue prematurely with imposed facts and advice.

Focus Group discussions used as a qualitative research method have several advantages over conventional quantitative KAP surveys.

* They enable respondents to explore feelings as well as knowledge, attitude and practice.

* Respondents discuss the topics using their own framework of thinking, not a framework imposed by the researcher. This generates a set of issues of priority concern to the respondents which may never have been identified if a questionnaire was used. "You don't know what you don't know unless they tell you".

* Focus Groups are an empowering method of research because members of the group share their knowledge, define problems and reasons for them, and examine options for solving them. They are in control of the discussion and its outcome. They also learn from the contributions of the facilitator.

* Programme workers trained in the methodology can use this approach in all their communication-activities. The discovery that the target group has much of the necessary knowledge and experience to solve problems and requires only specific pieces of information and material support from the programme can be a powerful way to create a more participatory work-style generally.

* Focus group discussions are quicker and cheaper than large scale quantitative surveys.

However, focus group discussions do not produce quantitative data that can be analysed statistically and the analysis of the discussions is time consuming and can be subject to researcher bias.

Making Focus Groups Participatory

The facilitator's approach to the questions is important. One question, such as "We have a new disease called AIDS in our country, what can we do about this problem?" treats the group as equal participants in exploring the dimensions of the problem and possible solutions.

On the other hand, a long list of questions designed by the facilitator usually results in people merely answering the facilitator's questions as in a group interview, rather than taking over the discussion themselves.

Obviously, Focus Groups must be held with each social group in their own language. A Focus Group carried out by an outsider in the official language with easy to reach, educated urban groups is unlikely to have any meaning for rural groups who have not been to school.

Groups may be made up of people of the same gender or mixed. Same gender groups can usually talk more freely, particularly about sexuality, but they may get locked into one perspective of the situation, for example, that women are powerless and should fear men. A discussion with men and women can bring out areas of conflict and potential solidarity in a very constructive way, as long as men are not allowed to dominate the conversation. The mixed gender Focus Groups described here resulted in helpful interactions between men and women, and people were not shy to discuss matters of sexuality and lifestyle in the group.

Similarly, with age, young people often find it difficult to talk about sex with their elders present and vice-versa, but some groups containing three generations have brought up useful ideas about reasons for changing sexual behaviour, and which traditional values and practices could give meaning to the safer sexual practices being advocated.

Facilitators need training in the methodology, because asking open-ended, non-judgemental questions and listening to others without interfering requires a major change in habits for many of us trained to teach. Practice is needed to develop the skill of being sensitive to the needs of the groups so that members participate freely and the conversation moves on. Note-taking skills also require practice.

Through the discussion, the facilitator helps the groups to:-

* build a good relationship;
* explore the perceptions of the group and the meaning of AIDS in their own situations;
* understand the problem, and options and constraints to solving it more clearly; and
* develop new perspectives and a plan of action.

Focus Groups are powerful tools for evaluating programmes. Focus Groups with service users or social groups reveal the participants' perceptions of the programme - what is helpful and what is less helpful; reasons for utilisation and non-utilisation; what information has been relevant to their own lives and what is still needed. Focus Groups with workers reveal their perceptions of the problem, the groups they work with, and their role in tackling the problem. Analysis of these two sides of the coin indicates what is needed to match the needs of the two groups more closely.

WHAT DO PEOPLE KNOW, FEEL AND DO ABOUT AIDS?
WHAT DO THEY THINK CAN BE DONE TO PREVENT AIDS?

The Focus Groups were held with groups of men, women and young people in urban and rural areas of two African countries. Groups were held in two regions in one of the countries. The discussions were essentially an evaluation of earlier campaigns organised in these countries.

During the discussions it became clear that people need more that a set of facts to enable them to take action against HIV infection. Certainly there was some misunderstanding of the facts, but even when people remembered them correctly, they did not necessarily believe them or act on them.

In this section, some of the main ideas that came up are described. The questions are not those used in the focus group.

Does AIDS exist? Is it a problem in your community?

People found it difficult to believe that AIDS was a problem in their community or region, because they had never seen or heard of a person with AIDS, and they had no idea how many around them might be HIV positive. People felt that they were being asked to make difficult changes in their behaviour and fight against a disease without being given proof of its existence.

"In a war, you are fighting and you are told that so and so has died. He was a victim. Where and who are the AIDS victims? We want to know how they are feeling. We are told that a baby can get AIDS if its parents have it, but we have never seen or heard of a baby born with the disease."

People had many suggestions on how to convince people that the disease was really among them, including display of the number of people with AIDS and HIV positives on a board outside the district hospital; payment to families to release the details of their dead relatives' diagnoses, and allowing the public to meet people with AIDS or see them on film.

Many people thought that AIDS was a disease of cities, and that their rural community was safe from infection as long as outsiders could be kept out or tested. "Outsiders" were defined as foreign nationals from the West or neighbouring countries, or people who have worked or studied in these countries.

Reflection on actual rural behaviour patterns in and out of the village is needed.

What are the signs and symptoms of AIDS?

All groups could mention one or more symptoms of AIDS. The worry was that these symptoms are common with other illnesses and how was one to know when a person has AIDS? Lack of knowledge had resulted in people with a common disease, such as diarrhoea, being made extremely anxious and they and their families being ostracised.

Few people brought up the idea that one can be infected for a long time without knowing it, but when the discussion turned to testing, it was clear that they understood this concept and found it difficult to live with such uncertainty. Many people thought that the test could solve the problem for individuals and communities. If everyone was tested and those positive segregated in some way, the rest of the community could get on with their lives in safety with peace of mind.

People need help to understand that mass testing is neither feasible, logistically and economically, nor advisable because it results in rejection and makes it more difficult for those with HIV infection to act responsibly.

How can a person become infected with AIDS?

Casual sex with many partners was seen by all groups as being the main problem. The details of sexual practices, including condom-use, were rarely talked about spontaneously. Men tended to say that the fault lay with women, while women blamed men. However, women were blamed three times more frequently than men and prostitutes were described as both the source and the transmitters of the virus.

Few people were really convinced that HIV is only transmitted through sexual intercourse, by blood and from mother to child. Many people believed that the disease could be caught "like leprosy" in every possible way that they had heard about for other infections.

This idea is likely to arise not only from misinformation, but also from local theories of disease causation and denial, with people preferring to contemplate every conceivable way that they might catch HIV rather than confront the need to change their sexual behaviour.

This belief leads people to two conclusions:-

* "How can it be worth the trouble to use a condom when you can still catch the disease through the air in so many ways?"

* "AIDS is a contagious disease like leprosy, so infected people must be isolated as they do with lepers. They must test the whole country and isolate those with AIDS in special camps. When everyone is identified and isolated, we will be safe."

How can we prevent AIDS? Are people changing their behaviour? What are the barriers to change? What should be done?

There was consensus that staying with one partner was the best option, with condoms as a poor second if one really could not manage this.

However, both men and women thought that staying with one partner might not be a realistic option.

The women felt that they stayed at home while men went with other women. Men found it impossible to control themselves. It was natural for them to need more than one woman for variety, "like one eats groundnut soup one day and palmnut soup the next". Men needed sex to stay healthy, so if they were away from home, or their wives were pregnant or abstaining, they must find another woman. "So now women must fear men. They won't change and they refuse to use condoms. So the women must just wait to die."

The men felt that any woman will go with another man if thereby she gains materially. "If you are a poor farmer and your wife meets a richer man, she will flirt with him and keep going to the city 'to buy something'. One day you will fall sick and have AIDS. In fact, men now fear women."

One woman then made a powerful statement that "Men and women will have to learn to understand each other better now, otherwise all our children will be orphans".

Condoms were unpopular in all the groups. One woman said that people would only accept condoms if they saw people dying of AIDS in their communities.

The three major problems raised were :-

*   Condoms break frequently, either because the user is "too manly", or the condom too small, or because the user is too impatient to put it on correctly. Deterioration is likely to be a major cause of this problem. Recent studies suggest that in typical storage conditions in the tropics, condoms can only be relied on for one year, and if displayed in sunlight in transparent packages, deterioration is very rapid (1).

*   Condoms reduce sensation. "It's like eating a sweet with the wrapper on or having a shower with a raincoat on." "It's like masturbation." "We have heard of this new protective way of using condoms, but some say that it is quite soundless and tasteless to have sex with Durex on."

*   Men and women foresaw grave difficulties in asking a partner to use condoms. "They spoil a relationship because it means you don't trust your partner or she doesn't trust you."

One wife given condoms at the clinic felt, "so ashamed and depressed to give them to my husband. I fear that he will insult me and say that I have had sex with other men, because condoms can protect against so many things such as diseases and pregnancy." Several women thought that they could avoid this problem by saying that they are using condoms to space births.

Some women wanted methods that they could use independently to protect themselves from AIDS. They were very interested in spermicides containing nonoxynol 9. Even if they are not totally effective they are better than doing nothing, "sitting at home waiting to die".

One woman said, "the people most likely to spread AIDS are those least likely to use condoms. For example, truck drivers would be in too much of a hurry to put a condom on, and drunks won't think of it".

Young people were thought to be the group who were using condoms more frequently and correctly.

Many of the groups thought that prostitution should be abolished, but all acknowledged the difficulty in achieving this.

As one boy eloquently stated, "starvation challenges education and therefore the government must first make sure that everyone has enough to eat so that they don't have to fall into prostitution."

A prostitute warned about the danger of her occupation allegedly shouted, "Never be ashamed of the job you do provided you get enough to support your family. Suffering is nothing as long as there is life."

What should be done with people with HIV or AIDS?

All groups thought that those with HIV or AIDS should be identified and isolated in a more or less caring or coercive way. Asked to imagine how they would react if they themselves had HIV infection, many people thought that they would commit suicide. Some would be sexually responsible, while others thought it "would not be worth sacrificing sexual pleasure when the country is riddled with AIDS", or "I would infect others if they reject me so I take some people with me."

Two people said that they would share their experience with others so that they could avoid the same suffering - "the loss of one, the saving of a million".

THE SCENARIO FOR A FEATURE FILM

The discussions showed clearly that people need a medium that enables them to experience at a personal level the reality and meaning of AIDS for people like themselves. They need to live through the life of a family touched by AIDS, to experience how its members are feeling, how they cope and the consequences of the infection. They need to examine the fear that leads to a desire to isolate, and how people can get through this fear and live with and care for people with AIDS safely. They need to have reinforcement of their own belief that men and women can learn to communicate about sexuality and support each other, and that their own social groups have the power to tackle the problem of AIDS.

Story-telling has been a medium of education in Africa for generations. The ideas expressed in the Focus Groups could easily be woven into short stories for telling at small group meetings. The stories could be presented through local drama groups and puppeteers.

MEDIA IN THE CONTEXT OF PRIMARY HEALTH CARE

A film of the story is a powerful way of moving people motivating them to take action. But because a film can have such a powerful effect on people's emotions, it is best to use the film in the context of a primary health care programme. Optimally, after watching the film, people will be able to discuss their concerns and develop plans of action in small group discussions or counselling sessions.

Existing primary health care networks can provide this follow-up. Health and family planning workers, teachers and community members who already "counsel" others could meet with groups and counsel individuals. This does not imply long training and specialists. The skills of counselling are essentially those of listening and helping the client to look at options and make decisions. Many people already have these skills and only need a short training to use them for HIV counselling.

It is planned to end the film with a sequence which suggests how people watching the film could get together to decide what to do or seek out local counsellors to talk over their concerns. Even if the film is shown alone, for example in a city video theatre, the story aims to defuse the fear that has been generated by past campaigns, and show people coping with HIV and AIDS in a positive way. The film suggests that everyone, whatever their HIV status, still has the opportunity to avoid further infection in themselves and their families.

CONCLUSIONS

Communities can become actively involved in the development of mass media through small group discussions, which enable members to express freely their perceptions of a problem. The feelings and ideas of the group are used to develop scenarios, which accurately meet their needs both for information and personal involvement at an experiential level.

The small group discussions showed that people need more than facts about AIDS to enable them to change their lifestyles. They need to experience at a personal level the reality and meaning of AIDS for their own lives. Drama, stories and films provide this experience, albeit at second hand.

Mass media can be developed and used in the context of existing primary health care programmes if communities are actively involved in expressing their educational needs and developing media, and existing networks are involved in follow-up support.

REFERENCE

1. Monitoring condom quality. Outlook (PIACT) 5, (3), September 1987.

The Global Impact of AIDS, pages 301–306
© 1988 Alan R. Liss, Inc.

39. THE FAMILY AS A RESOURCE

Philista Onyango and Pervin Walji

Department of Sociology, University of Nairobi, Box
30 197, Nairobi, Kenya

The family, whatever its form and functioning, remains the
basic social institution to which all human beings belong, and
nothing affects an individual without touching the individual's
family. However, when it comes to issues regarding disease,
often the family is considered as a last resort to which health
providers turn, mainly to ease their burden. The family is turned
to, for example, because the hospitals have no empty beds, or
the disease is terminal and the beds should be left to the
"deserving patients". This relationship alienates the family from
the process of preventing the spread of diseases and ill-equips it
to manage its sick ones. The health authorities or providers may
not perceive the family as a resource, although at times the
family may be the only meaningful resource available. The
family members, on the other hand, may not perceive themselves
as a resource for disease intervention. We are familiar with
situations where families abandon their sick members in
hospitals and decline to fulfil their responsibilities simply
because they are used to situations where formal institutions are
doing what the family is supposed to do. The family may even
request external resources to look after their sick ones. For
example, a nurse is requested for visits to a family with an
invalid, or the family sends its sick one to live in a hostel. All
this illustrates that the modern set up under-utilizes the family
when it comes to the control, prevention and management of
diseases. The family is only called upon to sort out hospital bills,
collect their recovered relatives, and be advised on how to
manage their ill ones at home.

The family seems to be the most valuable and dependable
resource the society has to control, prevent and manage

infection by HIV and AIDS. A review of the limited information reveals :-

- there is no known cure yet
- the treatment, even if discovered, will not reach the majority of the sufferers in the near future; the estimated cost to treat 10 AIDS patients greatly exceeds the budget of the largest hospital in Africa
- those at the greatest risk of being infected by the virus are those closest to the victim, that is the spouse and newborn children
- a social stigma is attached to this disease, more so than the traditionally dreaded diseases such as leprosy or mental illness
- the spread of the deadly virus can only be stopped through behavioural change.

On the other hand, significant observations about the family include :-

- the family is the basic institution where members learn socially approved as well as disapproved behaviours
- the role behaviour learned in the family becomes the mode and prototype for the role behaviour required in other situations
- the individual's behaviour is easily visible to the family, the family can evaluate with accuracy that behaviour and act as a source of pressure on the individual either to adjust or change
- it is through the family that the society is able to elicit from the individual his necessary contribution to the society
- one of the tasks the family still proudly performs for its members is the maintenance of the health of the members through the provision of food, shelter and clothing, and the family is a primary source of care for ailing persons.

The family has been observed to have made considerable contributions in the care of AIDS patients. Although shocked and stunned at the revelation of the disease, family members have rallied behind their sick and dying relatives. The family members have opened the doors of their houses to the AIDS victims and lived with them until the victims died. Often, they washed, fed and changed the clothes of the victims without asking for or expecting compensations. In the process they have provided the psychological and emotional support the victims needed and actually in some instances prepared the victims and allowed them to die with dignity.

In situations where the external institutions have failed to protect the AIDS victims, the family has gone to great pains to protect them as well as itself, by safeguarding the information about the patient's disease. Thus families say that their relatives are suffering from cancer, or those diseases that are perceived by the society to be respectable, mainly to ensure that its members and the victims are not ostracised. Some family members have restricted their social contacts only to professionals and relatives of AIDS patients, to avoid any form of external threats to their existence. This arrangement, although it may be deemed unfortunate since it isolates the family, is perhaps the most realistic response that may enable an AIDS victim to go through the traumatic experience in a more peaceful manner when other systems have declared their inability to do anything.

The family may look for resources to enable it to send its AIDS victims for second medical opinions at renowned international medical centres or from the traditional healers. What better way of providing hope and support?

The family at its worst denies the presence of AIDS among its members or attributes it to either witchcraft or to God's will. This attitude may be due to lack of proper information, leading to obvious negative implications for the control and prevention of the spread of the infection. However, in other situations, the denial becomes a useful defence mechanism and acts to maintain the family's homeostasis in a state of crisis. For the family, life has to continue with or without AIDS.

Where the AIDS victims are parents who eventually die, the other family members have been taking care of the victims' children and supporting other dependent relatives.

What does the family need to perform effectively its tasks regarding AIDS? Medical facilities are indeed limited, while hostels, isolation wards and the like are too expensive for most families. The need to empower families to keep their AIDS victims in their homes becomes crucial. This requires involvement of the family in the initial stages, when the discovery of AIDS or HIV is made, through open discussion restricted to family members and the victim regarding plans of action, as well as providing material assistance according to the identified needs.

Most familes are still ill-informed about the disease and how its virus is transmitted. This calls for targetted education, such as workshops or seminars for AIDS patients and their immediate families (those the victims consider significant), run and conducted by skilled professionals.

Because of stigma attached to this disease, the family members of AIDS victims tend to opt for isolation to protect themselves from shame and gossip. Often the family members suffer silently from rage, anger, guilt and even shame until their member quits the stage. Even after death, the burial arrangements and mourning processes may be cumbersome to family members. The concealment of the disease obviously puts one in a conflicting state. The family needs to have access to some proper counselling services, either as groups or individuals, where the feelings of fear and guilt can be expressed. There is the need to promote networking among the families of AIDS and HIV victims. The network could lead to a powerful force of informing others about the disease as well as designing strategies to stop the spread of the infection.

Family members need not only to be equipped with knowledge regarding AIDS and HIV, but also need essential services, such as provision of condoms. The family members can have advice through a dialogue with health professionals how they would like the service to be provided.

Efforts have been made and are being made to elicit the participation of most formal institutions to combat the spread of AIDS. The only institution that is still to be involved is the family. For the family to be effective it will have to be involved in designing and even implementing some of the programmes aimed at combating the spread of the deadly disease.

AIDS has been received with mixed feelings in Africa. In some parts of Africa (only few countries) the presence of AIDS has been acknowledged and health education programmes to combat the disease developed. However, in other parts (unfortunately most countries in Africa) the presence of this deadly disease has not been recognized and accepted and therefore hardly any meaningful programmes exist to combat the spread of the infection. These reactions influence the way the family members, health workers and decision makers respond to the disease and its victims. The medical facilities and the information with regards to AIDS are extremely inadequate in the continent and most institutions (health, education, religion, political etc.) are ill prepared and unable to adequately handle the disease! Under such circumstances, the only institution (although it may be ill prepared too) that is constantly available and dependable for AIDS victims in the continent is the family.

The family has always taken care of its sick ones in Africa, using other alternative sources whenever the recognized sources become ineffective or not accessible. In most parts of Africa, families are aware that there are diseases that are "African" and can only respond to African forms of treatment. AIDS unfortunately fits into the African concept of disease, simply because it is terminal. The AIDS victim is automatically granted the support and understanding often given to the individuals suffering from the so-called "difficult African disease". As such the victim is regarded as any member of the family who is suffering from a disease brought by God or some jealous relatives.

This situation is made worse in Africa because of the way the disease presents itself. Most AIDS sufferers in Africa have been observed to be in their prime and are heterosexual men and women living legitimate marital relationships. In situations where AIDS programmes are done with caution (everything has to be approved) and services on AIDS provided through "hide and seek" methods leading to inadequate information to the public, it is extremely hard for family members to associate AIDS with sexual behaviour since, in normal circumstance, most human beings are extremely discreet about their sexual behaviour. As such most AIDS victims are actually treated with sympathy by their families. Even in situations where the disease and the virus have been diagnosed by modern medicine, the victims may actually decline to tell their relatives the type of diseases they have. The medical profession may also opt not to inform the relatives, not only to observe the patient's privileged confidentiality, but also to avoid creating sensation.

In most parts of Africa when one dies, especially when one is young, the practice is that the widowed person remarries. Therefore, for the most part, when AIDS patients die, it is automatic for the remaining spouses to remarry through whatever available method (e.g. inheritance of wives by relatives of the deceased). Although the practice has both psychological and economic functions for the family members of AIDS victims, it has major implications for the control and prevention of the spread of the infection.

Thus, considering that there are mixed feelings regarding the disease, inadequate resources to combat it, cultural practices that actually may escalate the spread of the infection, and the experience that families have in taking care of their sick members, the involvement of the families in AIDS programmes becomes paramount in the continent.

In conclusion, it seems that the family has been playing a leading role in providing material and emotional support to AIDS victims with little or no recognition of its contribution. Among all the institutions dealing with AIDS, the family seems to be the most dependable, available and natural resource.

This calls for research to determine the contribution the family is making and what the family is capable of doing, as well as providing support to the family in terms of knowledge and material. Finally, the family will be involved in the entire process of AIDS control, prevention and management.

REFERENCES

Goffman E (1963). "Stigma Notes on the Management of Spoiled Identity". Englewood Cliffs, N J Prentice Hall.

Goode W J (1964). "The Family". Englewood Cliffs, N J Prentice Hall.

Kayongo-Male D, Onyango P (1984). "The Sociology of the African Family". London, Longman.

IPPF. People : Aids and the Family 4, 1987, pp. 3-24.

Leslie G R (1979). "The Family in Social Context" (4th Ed.) New York, Oxford University Press.

Odetola T O, Oloruntimehin O, Aweda D A (1983). "Man and Society in Africa". London, Longman.

Onyango P (1976). "The Views of African Mental Patients Towards Mental Illness and Its Treatment". Unpublished M.A. Thesis, Nairobi, University of Nairobi.

Orley J H (1970). "Culture and Mental Illness". Nairobi, E. African Publishing House.

Shelp E E, Sunderland R H, Mansell P W A (1987). "Aids: Personal Stories in Pastoral Perspective". New York, The Pilgrim Press.

The Panos Institute; Panos Dossier 1. "Aids and the Third World", (2nd Ed.), 1987.

UNICEF. State of the World's Children, 1987.

The Global Impact of AIDS, pages 307-311
© 1988 Alan R. Liss, Inc.

40.   INDIVIDUAL FREEDOM AND THE PUBLIC INTEREST

C Everett Koop

Surgeon General, U.S. Public Health Services, Room
18/67, 5600 Fisher Lane, Rockville, Maryland 20852,
USA.

We have had three days to look at the myriad ramifications
of AIDS upon the health of individuals and of societies. I have
been asked to address one of the non-medical issues: that is, how
does the AIDS epidemic affect the balance between individual
freedom and the public interest? One of the extraordinary
aspects of this epidemic, is the very fact such an issue can be
raised at all, and it does not seem out of place.

We talk of individual freedom, of professional responsibility,
of civil rights and wrongs, and of many other issues which seem
to be appropriate in the context of the AIDS epidemic, but which
would be of marginal interest, or of no interest at all, in the
context of almost any other infectious disease, with the possible
exception of leprosy.

In any event, I would like to explore this issue of individual
freedom and the public interest. One way would be to do it in an
abstract philosophical fashion. For example, people in our
society, once given the facts, are able to make a free choice on
the basis of those facts, and they individually and collectively
will benefit. That's the theory. Conversely, the person in our
society who does **not** know the facts of life and health, facts that
are known by most of his or her neighbours, is not a free
individual, able to make a choice: that's not a theory, it is
reality.

Such a person, in the real world of our inner cities, for
example, may lack information about nutrition, about personal
and environmental safety, about a great many other aspects of
daily life that shape his or her day-to-day existence. And we,

who now feel a compelling need to relay information about AIDS
to hundreds and thousands of such individuals at risk of infection,
we must face the possibility that our messages today about AIDS
may be as unsuccessful as our messages yesterday about diet,
family planning, smoking, fire prevention, syphilis and alcohol
abuse. We've tried to deliver the facts about those and many
other public health matters in order to help our citizens freely
make their own choices of behaviour based on good information.
In other words, to help them act as free people **should** act, for
their own benefit as well as for the benefit of their community
or society. But, for whatever reasons, they have not been able to
use the information and, therefore, I would submit that they are
not free.

But I think you would prefer that I speak to the specific
issue of how we serve the public interest and permit individual
freedom which is the hallmark of our society in the global sense.
Before addressing the problem, I must remind you that, at least
in the United States, everything that is thought, said and done
about AIDS is coloured by three facts.

(1) In spite of all we know about AIDS, it is still somewhat
of a mystery, especially to non-medical people, (2) the disease is
virtually 100% fatal, (3) people get AIDS by doing things most
people do not do and of which most people do not approve.

The rejection of such individuals, coupled with the fear and
the mystery of AIDS, inevitably means that the diagnosis of
AIDS will bear a stigma. This stigma, at least in the U.S., has
been known to deprive one man of his rented housing, keep a
family from going to the barber, shopping at the supermarket, or
attending school or church. Such ostracism has led to a
heightened suicide rate among persons with AIDS and, in at least
one instance, the arson of the home of three HIV positive
children with hemophilia.

Such unfair and unjust treatment of a family points out the
widely held public health position of the need for confidentiality
with test results, and with the diagnosis of persons with AIDS.
Confidentiality is not in conflict with the pursuit of the public's
interest in the long term. Indeed it augments it by not driving
the AIDS patient underground, by permitting his/her treatment
of other STDs, by winning confidence, thus enabling counselling
of the individual and his/her sexual contacts or drug sharing
partners.

In the matter of testing, I have argued against any kind of universal compulsory test for AIDS. Even the most generous estimate of the number of people walking around with the virus today, and it's currently 1.5 million at the outside, even that estimate is an extremely small fraction of the total U.S. population of 240 million. And, in any case, we already know that **90 percent** of all persons with AIDS thus far have either been IV drug abusers or homosexual or bisexual men, and these two groups are themselves, not large. In addition, the overwhelming majority of homosexuals and bisexual men have been untouched by the epidemic. Apparently, only a minority of these individuals have engaged in the kind of specific high-risk behaviour that spreads the virus. And we gather from surveys done here and there that this community of men has undergone a very serious and positive change in behaviour. We might even expect a decline in the rate of AIDS reporting from this group in a year or so. If it seemed unlikely **before** the public education programs that all homosexuals would be stricken with AIDS, it seems even less so today.

The IV drug abuser presents us with a different problem. The people of the United States see the **drug habit itself** as the issue. The appearance of AIDS within the drug culture is just another potential catastrophe for the drug addict, along with hepatitis, tuberculosis, dementia, starvation, suicide and so on. It's true that many drug addicts have voluntarily presented themselves for AIDS testing, but we suspect that the majority of them have not, and will not. Over the years, we've been singularly unsuccessful in penetrating the drug-addicted culture with every other public health message we've ever had, including the one that says "Stop!" In addition, the sheer volume of non-AIDS drug-induced violence, is still very high, about 5,000 according to the F.B.I. and our own National Institute of Drug Abuse. Hence, the heart of the problem, and the urgent need for a solution, is the **addiction itself** and **not** the specific act of needle-sharing among addicts.

Testing for HIV antibodies will not in itself contain the epidemic. Nor will any of the measures some advocates of mandatory testing support, such as : (i) quarantine, (ii) use of identity cards, (iii) compulsory contact tracing and (iv) public recording of the identity of HIV positives, none of which I support.

Mandatory testing has a place with some groups, but not for the majority. Let me give an example of one group where it makes sense and another group where it does not: the armed forces and those applying for marriage licences. The U.S. armed forces mandate testing of all recruits and active duty personnel, for two reasons. First, they are immunized against every disease for which there is a vaccine: a live virus vaccination could be lethal to HIV positive personnel. Secondly, the armed forces are their own walking blood bank: the latter reason is also why our foreign service personnel are tested.

Pre-marital testing on the other hand, is expensive and would not contain the epidemic. There was a day when a negative pre-marital test for syphilis was required for a marriage licence. However, there was not only a cure for the syphilis, but living together outside the bonds of marriage was frowned upon. Today, that is not the case. Not only is there no such cure for AIDS, but the majority of those getting married have already been living together. Unfortunately, those who practise high risk behaviour, in general, are not applying for marriage licences. The combination of the possibility of false positives and the stigma accompanying HIV positivity is a risk many young people do not wish to take. And finally, the cost benefit ratio is very high, because only a very small number of those tested would be true positives in most communities. In some states it would take approximately $100,000 to find a single case.

Another area which needs mentioning is the freedom of the physician, nurse, dentist or other health care worker to refuse to treat patients with AIDS or those they may think might be HIV positive. This freedom is certainly not in the public interest. Never before have health providers in the U.S. turned down a class of patients because of their diagnoses. We never did it for leprosy, yellow fever, smallpox, influenza or polio. And we must not do it for AIDS. There are in the U.S. more than seven million health care workers. Fewer than a dozen have seroconverted because of job related activity, and eight or nine of them would not have done so if they had followed the simple guidelines set down by the Centers for Disease Control several years ago.

The issue of testing patients in hospitals for HIV antibodies is being managed in many places on a voluntary basis, which threatens no one's individual freedom, yet does seem in the public interest. Voluntary testing with confidentiality is being urged in many circumstances, one major target group being couples who contemplate a pregnancy.

One can hope that as we become more familiar with the disease of AIDS and as we drop the myths and misinformation, the stigma associated with the diagnosis will diminish and that information and education will ultimately change behaviour to bring about the containment of the epidemic. The economic, legal and ethical implications of AIDS are enormous and threaten the social cohesion of whole societies. The challenge to maintain the balance between individual freedom and the public interest is also enormous. If we can manage it in fairness and with understanding, we may give the world something as precious as the scientific breakthrough we all seek in prevention and treatment.

The Global Impact of AIDS, pages 313–316
© 1988 Alan R. Liss, Inc.

41.   AIDS-RELATED HEALTH LEGISLATION

D C Jayasuriya

Attorney-at-Law, Institute of Comparative Health
Policy and Law, 40-12 Swarnadisi Place, Koswatte
Road, Nawala, Sri Lanka

The year 1983 was a watershed in the annals of health
legislation. In a matter of two years after the first AIDS cases
were detected, several countries around the world recognized
the role of health legislation in minimizing the spread of the
virus. By March 1988, over 50 countries have taken steps to
introduce new legal measures which specifically address AIDS
(Jayasuriya, 1988; Fluss, 1988; WHO, 1987). Several others have
extended to AIDS cases provisions in existing laws such as public
health codes and communicable disease statutes. Over 3,000
million people live in the countries which have AIDS-specific
legislation.

In its evolutionary process, health law responds to medical
developments, realities and expectations in different ways. At
the outset, laws of many countries addressed only AIDS or AIDS
patients, though now it is not uncommon to find references to
"HIV", "ARC" and "high-risk groups". Laws which first began
with blood donors as the target group now address other groups
such as prostitutes, intravenous drug users and even
homosexuals. As the medical community became sensitized to
the incidence of "false-negative" and "false-positive" blood test
results, legislatures in some countries responded by requiring
"confirmatory" testing such as by way of the Western blot. The
strength of health law lies in its dynamic nature, adapting to
changing medical realities.

AIDS-related laws can be broadly classified into three
categories, namely (a) product-related laws, (b) behaviour- and
attitude-oriented laws, and (c) institution-oriented laws.

Product-related laws are those which seek to protect supplies of blood, semen, tissue, organs, and from more recent times even breast-milk. Many developed countries lost no time in subjecting donations, transfusions and transplants involving these products to stringent controls. However, most developing countries are yet to move in this direction. Another product which has been the subject of legislation is condoms. Countries are beginning to appreciate the need to relax restrictive laws and policies affecting the importation, exportation, distribution, taxation and advertising of condoms. Like in many other areas of health law, the goals of law reform can be achieved only with appropriate behavioural and attitudinal changes. Indeed, one writer recently suggested that every maypole erected today ought to be covered with a condom (Goldsmith, 1987).

Behaviour- and attitude-oriented laws which seek to reduce the incidence of high-risk behaviour by making it an offence to engage in sex whilst being infected, by requiring compulsory screening, quarantine and contact tracing, by providing for deportation and for the refusal of visas, etc., always bring into sharp focus the rights of individuals within the broader social framework. Screening has been by far the most controversial approach. It is a public health measure which brings in is wake numerous ethical and constitutional issues. Countries such as the United States, USSR, Austria, the Federal Republic of Germany, Iraq and Hungary have introduced legislation for this purpose. Over 40 countries now require AIDS cases to be notified, though it is only about one-third of them that require HIV seropositive cases to be reported as well. International travel restrictions have been introduced in a few countries and the time seems to be opportune now for the existing International Health Regulations to be reviewed in the light of our current knowledge of communicable disease control. A few countries have amended their drug laws to provide syringes and needles to intravenous drug abusers. At least one country now permits the termination of pregnancies of AIDS infected women. Some countries where prostitutes have to be licensed now provide for such licences to be cancelled in the event of seropositivity. Writing on safe sex, a researcher recently remarked that "sex with a prostitute may be riskier than sex with a neighbour, but if neither has been tested for HIV then neither can be truly safe" (Goedert, 1987).

Institution-oriented laws seek to promote not only research but even the education, counselling and care of AIDS patients. National AIDS committees have been established in over 130 countries, though only a few have a legal basis. Some countries have specially designated research institutes as well as reference laboratories. Measures to promote the development of drugs, vaccines and test kits include financial support and relaxation of regulatory controls on clinical trials. With a view to preventing discrimination against AIDS patients and HIV infected persons, some countries have amended the laws and practices relating to insurance, social security, education, housing, and labour.

What has been the impact of the AIDS pandemic on health legislation in particular and on national legal systems in general? First, the pandemic has been an emotive stimulus for countries to re-examine their health laws, and health-related concepts. In some countries this has meant a review of several 19th century legal enactments. Secondly, concern with blood supplies has led to new controls and better internal management systems. Thirdly, safety guidelines issued by agencies and organizations such as the US Centers for Disease Control, the DHSS in the UK and by WHO have led to a better appreciation of the dynamics of contagious diseases and risk prevention. Fourthly, the relationship between regulation and drug innovation is being investigated in some countries with a view to relaxing existing controls in respect of drugs for special diseases such as AIDS. Fifthly, some countries are responding to the problem of drug abuse by providing for compulsory treatment, which is one of the most desirable long-term goals of any drug abuse policy. And, sixthly, the movement to promote human rights, to protect the confidentiality of medical records, and eliminate discrimination against patients and infected persons has now assumed an entirely new dimension. We are witnessing the articulation of new health-related human rights concepts and proposals for the establishment of monitoring mechanisms.

Taking a closer look at the crystal ball, what do I see for the near future? As a consequence of some countries having rushed in with legislations which have encroached into the rights of individuals, there has been a challenge to the legitimacy as well as the credibility of public health law. Fortunately, other countries seem to be adopting a more cautious approach, observing at close hand what countries with restrictive legislation may or may not be able to achieve over the next few years. Comprehensive AIDS-related legislation is essentially a developed country phenomenon and there are tremendous pressures on countries with limited resources to emulate countries with highly evolved health-care and legal systems. An example in point is the pressure to screen students being sent abroad for higher education. In the nature of things, it is likely

that we will see more AIDS-related legislative activity from the
Third World but in order to avoid having to follow a path studded
with pitfalls, any contemplated AIDS-related measure must be
carefully evaluated in terms of (a) medical, scientific and
technological readiness and validity, (b) constitutional, ethical,
cultural and social acceptability; (c) political expediency and (d)
economic feasibility. Health law now faces its greatest
challenge, and it is only through a truly multidisciplinary effort
with carefully evaluated control measures that health law can
continue to command the influence, the respect and the sanctity
it has had to its credit over the centuries.

REFERENCES

Fluss S (1988). The AIDS pandemic: some global legislative and
legal aspects. In Schinazi RF, Nahmias AJ (eds): "AIDS in
Children, Adolescents and Heterosexual Adults", New York:
Elsevier, pp 58-66.

Goedert J J (1987). What is safe sex? N Eng J Med 316: 1339.

Goldsmith M F (1987). Sex in the age of AIDS calls for
commonsense and "condom sense". JAMA 257: 2266.

Jayasuriya D C (1988). "AIDS: Legal and Public Health
Dimensions". The Hague: Martinus Nijhoff.

WHO (1987). "Tabular Information on Legal Instruments Dealing
with AIDS and HIV Infection". Geneva: WHO.

The Global Impact of AIDS, pages 317–322

42.   AIDS - RETURN TO SACHSENHAUSEN?

The Hon. Justice Michael Kirby CMG

President, Court of Appeal, Supreme Court, Sydney, Australia.

Recently, I was in Bangalore, India, attending a conference of judges called to review the remarkable growth of international human rights law. I clutched a few spare hours to visit the fading remnants of British rule to be seen at every turn in that temperate cantonment town. Here, the statue of Queen Victoria, Empress of India. There, the masonic lodge. Nearby, the great parade ground, now overgrown with bougainvillea. I wandered into Holy Trinity Church - once the bastion of Anglican Christianity -now fallen on harder times. In this crumbling pile I sat in the front pew marked "The Hon'ble The Resident". All about me were the symbols of yet another foreign empire which India had finally absorbed. Yet this was my empire. And it had passed away in my lifetime.

I looked at the wall of plaques which commemorated the servants of Empire. One by one they told the tale of earlier epidemics. A sapper dead at 21 from cholera. Twin brothers dead, within one month of each other, from plague. And so the list went on. The priest dead in two years of service for his flock. Smallpox, dysentery - many forgotten deaths. The encounter of the foreigners with unfamiliar viruses challenged their resistance. And I asked myself, in that quiet place, is AIDS just another infection? Is it simply part of the inescapable cycle of life and death on this planet?

The slightest acquaintance with the history of humankind now shows the importance for human events of these cyclical infections (1). It demonstrates the frightful havoc and toll of death and suffering of the millions whom disease carries off. Few of the dead are memorialised in the ruined churches of lost empires. They are just more human souls who die in pain and despair. I asked myself if we mortals were so insignificant that epidemics of this kind have no meaning - just something inevitable, to be endured in waves.

As I left the church my eye caught one plaque with a text from the Letter of James (2). "Blessed is the man that endures temptation: for when he is tried, he shall receive the crown of life". We are certainly being tried. But shall we, in the end, receive the crown of life? The trial of AIDS has only just begun. Our scientists and technologists are being tested. International cooperation and world bodies will be extended. Our democratic institutions will be put to a test by public alarm and fear. Respect for human rights will be tested - for they matter most when they are hardest to accord. Patients, and their families, in every land will be tested by human suffering, pain and grief. Above all, it will be a test of human ethics. The history of previous encounters with infection has not always been an uplifting one. People panic. Out of panic come irrational and ineffective policies and, worse, harsh and oppressive laws. We must be on guard against the risk of adding to the mounting toll of suffering a burden of ill targeted, ineffective laws.

Sachsenhausen Revisited

How can we do this? This century has been so full of misery, destruction and cruelty that, near the close of it, we can surely learn some lessons from our earlier mistakes. One of the lessons to be derived from the Nazi holocaust against unpopular minorities - especially the Jews - is the danger of depersonalising human suffering. This is, I am afraid, a growing danger with AIDS. When the problem becomes a matter of statistics, graphs, bar charts, trend lines and the other necessary paraphernalia of modern communication, there is a danger of acceptance of the unacceptable. This, after all, is how civilised and even pious and religious people accepted the horrors of participation, or acquiescence, in Belsen, Buchenwald and Sachsenhausen.

A few weeks ago I read an item in a Netherlands journal. It must be false I thought. At least I hoped so. A journalist, Suzanne Schneider, presented herself as a representative of "Midinvest", an organisation specialising in the building of clinics for incurable diseases. She went, according to the report (3), to a number of mayors in the district of Sachsenhausen. She asked these worthy civic fathers whether they would be interested in the establishment of a closed institution for AIDS patients. She used the old plans of Sachsenhausen concentration camp. Even the watch-towers of the former camp were not deleted. According to the report, eight of the ten mayors interviewed immediately said that they were interested. The idea of a multimillion mark project within the boundaries of their municipalities was too good to resist. One of them said :"It is about time something was done about this. The health of the general community is more important than 300 AIDS patients". Another mayor was even recorded as saying: "Once the clinic is in operation we will say that a medicine has been found there". The prospect of ordinary labouring jobs for the local population attracted others. Only two of the ten would have nothing to do with it.

We should not be surprised at such a report. We have seen it all before. It is there in earlier living memory (4). Anyone who doubts the stigmatisation of patients during epidemics should read of the way, in Australia in the 19th Century, that the small Chinese populations were rounded up and put in shocking conditions in hulks off the coast (5). And if you think that we have now become more civilised - with a heightened international conscience about human rights - remember Sachsenhausen, then and now.

The Human Dimension

In the big cities of the developed world as in the villages of central Africa, the day is not far off (if it has not already arrived) when every person will know someone who has died from AIDS -or be the friend of someone who has died. A problem with these large international gatherings is that the human dimension may be insufficiently focused. Yet that dimension is vital, both to mobilise our energies, whatever our respective expertise, and to toll loudly the bell of ethics. Good ethics in the global fight against AIDS will be derived from good data and from never forgetting that this is a problem of fellow human beings - people like ourselves with families, and with the joys and disappointments of living.

At a conference in Paris, last October, I announced my isolation of three new mutants of the AIDS virus. To distinguish them from HIV, I called them "HIL" - highly inefficient laws (6). HIL I represents laws for mandatory testing of the entire population for the presence of HIV. HIL II is mandatory testing of particular groups deemed specially at risk to exposure to the virus. HIL III is mandatory certificates at the frontier. My thesis was that these were ineffective, inefficient and potentially even harmful approaches to the social regulation of AIDS - at least at this time. Until there is a vaccine and a cure, the whole thrust of effective social policy and lawmaking must be to promote the spread of information and of measures for prevention of infection. Difficult though it will be for some societies to accept a number of the measures of prevention necessary to contain the epidemic, those measures will eventually have to be taken. If we are serious about the protection of life, the sooner this is done, the better.

I suggested in Paris that no AIDS conference should convene without the voice being heard of those who have acquired the virus. True, it will not be the only voice. But it is a voice that should not be silenced.

Mark was at school a few years behind me. He was a good athlete. He showed talent in languages. He went to the university and marked out a career in what seemed to me to be a number of esoteric aspects of foreign literature. I kept contact with him over the years after school days.

Six months ago he asked to see me. He told me that he had been diagnosed as antibody positive to HIV. He was frightened. Would I speak at his funeral, if the worst came to the worst? Of course I would. I laughed, telling him not to worry. The statistics were against his progression to "full blown" AIDS. The scientists would find a cure. Jonas Salk even talked of a vaccine for the already infected. Mark smiled with relief and we ate our dinner. But I noticed that he took no wine and chose the simplest of food. Mark was scared.

I returned to Australia from Europe in late January to the news that he had been admitted to hospital. It had all happened very suddenly. He was without symptoms until mid-January. He had been meditating and dieting. Then suddenly he was too weak to work. He was losing weight rapidly. A mass was discovered in his stomach. He was admitted to hospital for tests. I went to see him at once after my return. Down the long hospital corridor I walked. Throwing a glance to right and left, the scene was the same. Rows of beds. Young men emaciated. Tearful families clustered in the corridors. Retching and coughing were the only sounds to break the silence. The epidemic was certainly here.

Mark's concern was how he could tell his colleagues that he

would not return next week to work. He had already braved that journey once and told his parents. To the fear of death was added, for him, the hurt of embarrassment and stigmatisation - even of loathing amongst some at the mention of the fearful acronym. I composed a letter for him. It just said, accurately, that he had been diagnosed with cancer and would need chemotherapy. He would probably not be back this semester. It was a great relief for him when he signed the letter. He wanted to act professionally and honourably.

They diagnosed a lymphoma. He was going to have chemotherapy. But he told me:- "I must face the fact that I probably have only eighteen months to live. My life has telescoped". I looked at him - his grey face and frightened eyes. I shared his fear. I tried to encourage him. But it was hard. We both knew that he was on a short journey from which there would be no return.

Mark seemed just a little bitter. "The rules changed", he said, "But they didn't tell us quickly enough". The words kept recurring. The "rules" for "safe sex" for Mark had taken too long to save him. He was the kind of person who would have obeyed the rules - if only he had known them.

I saw Mark a few days later. He had undergone surgery. He was trembling and shaking uncontrollably. I grasped his hand. "Hang on", I told him. He could not talk. He could not stop shaking. But he nodded to me. It was the last time I saw him. I had to leave Sydney and travel to Bangalore. In Bombay I received word of his death. I never spoke at his funeral, as I had promised him I would. But I speak for him now and I dare to speak for all those like him. I speak for their familes; for their doctors and nurses; for their loved ones and for their fellow citizens who care.

If we see the problem of AIDS as a problem of statistics then we may face the dangers of the new Sachsenhausens. If we continue to deny its existence and call it by other names we will prolong grieving and diminish our resolve to act. If we content ourselves with treating the ill and refuse to face the necessities of education and counselling we will have the deaths of many on our collective conscience. But if we see this calamity as the problem of Mark and of men, women and children in every land, we will surely redouble our efforts to find a cure and to develop a vaccine. And meanwhile we will guard ourselves against the danger of laws and policies that are ineffective and yet damaging to human rights. There is, of course, no human right to spread infection - AIDS or otherwise. The central human right is the right to life. Close behind is the right to the pursuit of happiness which subsumes most other rights. As we bring to a close a century of so many mistakes and of unprecedented suffering and destruction, we should seek to redeem ourselves by at least tackling this problem efficiently and ethically.

That means a global approach - for no hidden corner of the world exists that will be immune from AIDS. It also, at the moment, means prevention. Unless we learn from the errors of the past we will repeat its mistakes. The surest way to guard against that danger is to keep steadily in mind the human dimension of AIDS. First and always it is an illness. People are suffering and dying. Their families and friends are grieving. No law and no policy, no rule and no judgment that concerns this topic should, even for an instant, forget those central facts. To the burden of illness, fear and even despair, we must certainly not add the burdens of stigmatisation, shame and discrimination. To do so would not only be immoral. It would be seriously counterproductive (7). At least at this time, the effective global attack on AIDS requires urgent behaviour modification of those specially at risk. No other strategy holds out hope of containment to protect the uninfected. Spreading urgently and clearly the word of the changed rules to the Marks of this world - not their confinement in new Sachsenhausens - is the way of the moment.

The views stated are personal views only.

REFERENCES

1. W H McNeill (1976). "Plagues and Peoples". New York: Anchor.
2. The General Epistle of James, I, 12.
3. "Sachsenhausen herleeft", reported in "The Gay Krant", Amsterdam, Netherlands, October 1987, No.10, p9.
4. Plant R (1986). "The Pink Triangle." New York: Henry Holt.
5. Curson P H (1985). "Times of Crisis." Sydney: University of Sydney.
6. Kirby M D, "The New AIDS Virus - Ineffective and Unjust Laws", unpublished paper delivered at the Symposium International de Reflexion sur le SIDA, Paris, France, 23 October 1987, reprinted, The Washington Post, 2 February, 1988, p12.
7. Mangold T. "The Plague mentality makes victims of us all", The Listener, 2 July, 1987, 546.

The Global Impact of AIDS, pages 323-327
© 1988 Alan R. Liss, Inc.

43.   AIDS IN PRISONS IN ENGLAND AND WALES

John L Kilgour

Director of Prison Medical Services for England and
Wales, H M Prison Services, Headquarters, Cleland
House, Page Street, London SW1P 4LN

General

This paper is necessarily over-abbreviated. The nature of
the spread of HIV has focused epidemiological attention on the
high risk behaviour groups which are disproportionately largely
represented in the prison population. The injecting drug misusers,
and the sexually promiscuous are present in numbers related to
the rising proportion of drug-related crime and the numbers of
prisoners who exhibit anti-social behaviour. The potentially, and
often actually, dangerous nature of the prison environment,
influenced by the prison sub-culture and by irrational and
irresponsible reactions of prisoners (and sometimes staff),
presents particularly acute problems requiring intelligent,
sensitive, and specific management responses.

The spread of HIV in the UK has broadly followed the US
pattern in the community at large, but following some three and
a half years behind. However, the development in the prison
system has shown significant differences from the US experience
and from that in mainland Europe, the numbers in all cases being
significantly lower.

Numerically, there has been only one case of the full-blown
syndrome reported in the prison population since formal
recording started in 1985 in England and Wales. There have also
been 4 cases of AIDS Related Complex (ARC) and 164 cases of
HIV antibody positivity. There were 51 known cases of HIV
antibody positive prison inmates in England and Wales on 4th
March 1988. No mandatory testing takes place and there is
probably the same proportion of under-identification as in the

general community.

These numbers occur against a background of an average daily prison population of 49,000, or 160,000 prison receptions per year, which include selectively higher than average numbers of those most exposed to the risk of infection. If the prison population were a genuine undistorted reflection of the community at large, which they are most arguably not, one would have expected so far 3 cases of AIDS and (assuming a total of 50,000 HIV antibody positives in the community at large) 480 HIV antibody positives in the prison population as a cumulative total since 1985.

Principles

The prison medical service in England and Wales has found it salutary to maintain its AIDS policy in the handling of prison inmates on the following principles :-

*   First, a prisoner is punished by being deprived of his liberty. He is sent to prison as punishment and not for punishment. He retains all other human rights including access to medical, nursing and pharmaceutical care of the same standard and accessibility as is available in the community at large.

*   Secondly, it follows that no medical procedure may be undertaken without the informed consent of the prisoner/patient.

*   Thirdly, he should receive all the advice and health education available to the general community relating to health promotion and the control of infectious disease, including AIDS, and this should be enhanced as necessary if special hazardous factors relating to the prison environment obtain.

Health Examination

All prisoners undergo a health screening on reception by hospital staff and a medical officer, which includes the use of a questionnaire specifically directed to elicit the possibility of high risk HIV-related behaviour, among other enquiry.

Each prison establishment has medical and nursing staff who hold daily clinics. Cases of AIDS or ARC are extremely unlikely to be missed. However, it is known that members of high risk behaviour groups (drug dependent prisoners, homosexual and bisexual men) are advised by those organisations who protect their interests not to disclose their HIV antibody status if known, or to seek a test to establish it, for fear of discrimination in their prison life either by the staff or other prison inmates.

HIV Antibody Testing

HIV antibody testing has been available on demand by prisoner patients on the same conditions as it has been available to the general community and from the same date. Specialist counselling facilities are available throughout the system which must be used by medical officers before any such test is carried out, and post-test counselling is also given for any patient with a positive result. No testing without positive informed consent is undertaken. Such testing may obviously be recommended by an individual doctor who may regard it as part of the diagnostic process, but before it is carried out it will still be subject to the same conditions of informed consent described above.

Management

A clear policy statement devised by the Prison Medical Service with the prior consultation and agreement of the Prison Administration and the industrial organisations representing the staff involved is maintained and updated. The need for confidentiality is firmly stressed (this is a particularly difficult point in the closed environment of a prison). No restriction on the regime is placed on any HIV antibody positive prisoner except that he will be accommodated either in a single cell or share accommodation with another who is also HIV antibody positive, and will not undertake activities involving sharp instruments or body contact sports. There is no medical requirement for isolation, although the danger of irrational prisoner reaction in some cases and places requires to be taken into account to protect the individual. Where opportunistic infection develops, the patient will be transferred to National Health Service specialist facilities where this is considered necessary on clinical grounds on the independent clinical judgement of the doctor in charge.

Control and Education

Without a vaccine or effective drug therapy, great effort is put into a programme of education and training. Specifically different programmes have been devised for staff training, where clearly knowledge and competence have led to the sharp diminution and near-disappearance of irrational over-reaction by staff towards inmates who are, or are thought to be, infected. A comprehensive training programme has been devised and will be maintained. It includes what has been widely regarded as an excellent staff training video, a video-based leaflet for all members of staff, a training manual which is very detailed yet easy to understand, and a series of more locally based initiatives involving local specialist staff.

A parallel but separate educational programme exists for prisoners who have received all the material produced by the UK government on the subject, together with a leaflet specifically devised by the Prison Medical Directorate and a voluntary organisation for prisoners, and a prisoner-targeted video has been distributed for viewing throughout the system. This video will be reinforced by a second more sensitively directed video later this year.

Other Problems

Condoms. It has been argued that in the light of the spread of HIV by anal intercourse, and because male prisoners are deprived of heterosexual intercourse in prisons in the UK, homosexual acts must occur and therefore condoms (currently prohibited for security reasons) should be made available. The legal situation in the UK is that homosexual acts are legal between consenting adults in private. In the prison system there is nowhere for a prisoner to be where he is not capable of being under surveillance for security considerations. The provision of condoms could therefore be perceived as condoning an illegal act, or an act against prison rules. Condoms are also widely regarded as a means of smuggling other contraband material such as illicit drugs into prison establishments. While the issue remains under review, condoms remain contraband in prison.

Sterile needle supply. On a similar basis, it has been suggested that clean sterile needles should be supplied to injecting drug misusers in order to minimise the spread of HIV. The prison administration makes strenuous and largely successful efforts to prevent the entry of illicit drugs of all kinds into prisons. The provision of needles would certainly condone an illegal act (possession of illicit drugs) and security reasons would completely rule out the provision of a potential weapon, possibly contaminated, for prisoners. There is therefore no intention of agreeing to such a measure.

General Points

Provided the ethical stance adopted in the UK is maintained, the situation seems to present only the foreseeable problems related to increasing numbers. The ready collaborative support available from the National Health Service is of enormous help. The difficulty remains in maintaining the effectiveness of the educational campaign both for staff and inmates, but the resources devoted to this are very well justified, and are proving very effective. It is to be hoped that one of the positive aspects of a prison transit will be to improve the chances of minimising spread by irresponsible behaviour in a potentially irresponsible little educated group, and to prevent the ignorant acquisition of the disease among those members of the community most likely to be at risk.

Work and policy guidance provided by the Council of Europe and the recent Consensus statement from the World Health Organization special programme on AIDS, as one constructive result of the expert consultation held in Geneva from 16th to 18th November 1987 for which I had the privilege of being consultant and rapporteur, are regarded as an excellent basis for developing prison policy on the management and control of HIV among prison inmates in all countries whether developed or under-developed, East or West.

The Global Impact of AIDS, pages 329-334
© 1988 Alan R. Liss, Inc.

44. REACHING THE PUBLIC : GENERATING INSTITUTIONAL SUPPORT FOR BEHAVIOUR CHANGE

Anthony J Meyer

Global Programme on AIDS, World Health
Organization, Geneva, Switzerland

The World Summit of Health Ministers in January 1988
affirmed the conviction of public health experts around the
world by recognizing that:-

"........ in the absence at present of a vaccine or cure for
AIDS, the single most important component of national
AIDS programmes is information and education because HIV
transmission can be prevented through informed and
responsible behaviour. In this respect, individuals,
governments, the media and other sectors all have major
roles to play in preventing the spread of HIV infection".
(London Declaration on AIDS Prevention)

In recognizing the importance of prevention through
informed and responsible individual behaviour, the London
Summit recognized equally the role of institutions across sectors
in establishing and supporting that behaviour. The individual and
his social institutions are seen in a cooperative relationship in
the battle against AIDS.

These affirmations are warranted by what we know about
introducing behaviour change in the face of other public health
initiatives, such as the prevention of heart disease, the reduction
of tobacco use, family planning and child survival programmes.
People learn when they are motivated to do so; when people
learn, they can use the new information and integrate it into
their lives; during this learning process, individuals are
influenced in their behaviour by others - their families, their
peers and their institutions.

AIDS prevention and control programmes must influence knowledge and attitudes in entire populations, as well as influence behaviour among target audiences in diverse circumstances of risk. To achieve these twin objectives of developing public knowledge and discouraging risk behaviour, these programmes will need to engage actively a broad range of individuals at risk and institutions capable of working with them.

The following study of 30 national AIDS programmes and control plans indicates an auspicious beginning in mobilizing an array of organizations for this shared agenda.

STUDY DESCRIPTION

The Global Programme on AIDS (GPA) of the World Health Organization is collaborating with its Member States to implement a global AIDS prevention and control strategy. As part of this strategy, multisectoral National AIDS Committees are established under the leadership of the national health authority. These committees develop national AIDS prevention and control plans to guide and coordinate activities across sectors.

The Global Programme on AIDS has assisted National AIDS Committees in over 100 countries to develop short-term plans (covering six to eighteen months) or long-term plans (covering three to five years) for AIDS prevention and control. Information and education programmes represent an important element of each plan.

As part of its support to these programmes, the Global Programme on AIDS is maintaining a worldwide profile of the scope and impact of information and education programmes to combat AIDS. To prepare an analytical frame of reference for this profile, 30 national AIDS Prevention and Control plans were studied to identify recurring target audiences and collaborating institutions. The 18 short-term and 12 mid-term plans selected for study represent a diversity of countries where the Global Programme on AIDS has assisted in preparing plans. Ten plans were included from countries in Sub-Saharan Africa (five Anglophone, four Francophone and one Luzaphone); five plans are from the Americas; five from the Middle and Near-East; five from Asia; and five from the Pacific Region. Of these 30 plans, 21 describe their countries as having a low prevalence of AIDS and HIV infection.

RESULTS

Concerning the objective of influencing public knowledge and attitudes, all plans include explicit efforts to inform the public about AIDS, how HIV infection is transmitted and how HIV infection is not transmitted. Correct knowledge about AIDS is seen to:-

*   reduce fearful and stigmatizing public reaction;

*   decrease the spread of HIV infection through ignorance; and

*   promote cooperation with AIDS control programmes.

Some plans specifically call for information, testing and counselling services and the marketing of the services to encourage their use.

Even countries with a low level of HIV infection are planning public information campaigns, although of varying magnitude and urgency. One plan states that "the success of any control programme requires the cooperation and responsible action of every individual in the community". The justification for these campaigns is not necessarily that the public at large needs to change risk behaviour, but rather that prevention of the spread of HIV infection requires informed public support.

All plans recognize the media as important channels for information. Some plans call for the systematic use of the press as an educational instrument, taking advantage of the high level of public interest in AIDS.

Against this background of an informed public, other programmes can be tailored to mobilize organizations and to support behaviour change in specific audiences.

All plans give the highest priority to the AIDS-related education of health sector personnel including physicians, medical technicians and health care workers, including midwives, traditional birth attendants and injectionists.

The focus of additional specific audiences within the plans appropriately corresponds with the dominant modes of transmission within the respective country.

Table 1 presents the most frequently mentioned target audiences for specific behaviour change interventions.

TABLE 1. Target Audiences

Audiences	No. of Plans
Most Frequent	
Prostitutes and clients	25
STD patients	19
Gay and bisexual men	18
Selected Countries	
Travellers	12
IV drug users	11
Military	11
Seropositive mothers	8
Prisoners	8
Low HIV Countries	
Sea/airline personnel	9
Tourists	5

Prostitutes and their clients and attendees of Sexually Transmitted Disease (STD) clinics are important throughout plans, in all areas of the world. Gay and bisexual men are included in virtually all plans where heterosexual transmission is not verified as the dominant mode of transmission. This inclusion of these audiences may not be surprising, since HIV infection is spread primarily through sexual activity and the risk of transmission is increased through unprotected sex with multiple partners, all the more so if they are unknown partners. Nevertheless, the plans are very forthright in identifying these audiences and in candidly discussing approaches to working with them. Considering the sensitivity often associated with discussing sexual behaviour, this forthrightness is itself an encouraging sign for the development of successful AIDS education programmes.

Travellers are identified as an important target audience where HIV prevalence is low and where travelling across national boundaries for work or pleasure is common. In countries where HIV infection is perceived to have spread more extensively, plans may additionally include seropositive mothers, military personnel and prisoners. In addition, IV drug users are included in plans where HIV transmission through the sharing of needles is a problem.

Countries with a low prevalence of HIV infection focus on points of entry for HIV infection to their country. Educational plans for these countries include maritime workers, airline personnel and tourists, in addition to prostitutes and travellers other than tourists, as target audiences.

These education programmes for specific audiences depend upon diverse public and private institutions to inform and educate. Considering provider groups and organizations, all plans give the highest priority to engaging all elements of the health care system. Twenty-three plans expressly seek to involve the Ministry of Education in programmes to train teachers and to introduce AIDS education in school systems. Collaboration between national health and education authorities constitutes the most extensive cross-sectoral planning revealed by the study.

TABLE 2. Channels of Influence Emphasized in Addition to Health and Formal Educational Systems

Channel	No. of Plans
Community/Political leaders	13
Religious leaders	12
Family Planning Associations	10
Red Cross	9
Employer/Employee groups	7
Women's groups	6
Youth leagues	6

Table 2 presents the channels of institutional influence most frequently included in plans, in addition to health and formal educational systems. These include national and local political organizations, church organizations, family planning associations, employer and employee groups and leading public and private agencies associated with particular constituencies such as the Red Cross, women's groups and youth leagues. Table 2 includes only clearly identified organizations appearing in five or more plans. A great variety of other country-specific organizations, including NGOs, are mentioned in the plans overall. Additionally, 22 plans include the provision of condoms and discuss a variety of institutional mechanisms for their distribution.

DISCUSSION

It is possible to criticize or minimize the importance of this planned response to AIDS. Sime individual plans have omitted mention of institutions of likely importance to them. Overall, the plans pursue only the simple epidemiological logic of the disease. From a public health perspective, the plans follow the expected rules for containing an infectious disease. There is nothing surprising that they should plan in this way. Yet, the range and magnitude of planned institutional response remains humanly impressive. The Member States of the World Health Organization are remarkable in this respect in the plans studied: that they are attempting to do what the epidemiological evidence indicates they ought to do; that their ambition to implement what the rules of good public health practices suggest they implement; that they are planning in fact to engage every institutional channel of communication that appears reasonable to inform and educate their public. It is possible that when history places the global impact of AIDS in perspective one of the most significant impacts of AIDS will be seen to have been the positive institutional response it engendered.

The Global Impact of AIDS, pages 335–340
© 1988 Alan R. Liss, Inc.

45. INTERVENTION POLICIES

Lars O Kallings

Professor, Director, National Bacteriological
Laboratory, Stockholm, Sweden and WHO
Collaborating Centre for AIDS

INTRODUCTION

This paper may serve as a summary of currently existing
intervention methods, but not of vaccination or of curative
treatment, which are powerful tools for intervention in other
infectious diseases.

INFORMATION

The current intervention policies are all based on the
knowledge of the mode of spread of HIV. That knowledge is the
most important tool and it may turn out to remain the only tool
available to control the HIV epidemic. Therefore, it is a
challenge to mankind - to *Homo sapiens sapiens* - to prove its
wisdom and ability to use the simple fact that HIV is only spread
by blood, from mother to offspring, and by sexual intercourse.
Furthermore, HIV seems to be transmitted only slowly through
ordinary heterosexual intercourse in healthy adults.

The most important preventive measure is to inform people
about the cause of AIDS and the mode of transmission of HIV.
The information has three objectives :-

*   to teach the general public about the cause of AIDS and the
    modes of transmission of HIV
*   to teach the individual about risk behaviour and how to
    prevent infection
*   to counteract anxiety among the population and ostracism
    of HIV infected people.

Evaluation of nationwide information campaigns in several countries shows that the first goal may be attainable. Evaluation attempts have been performed in e.g. Rwanda, Australia, Sweden and the United Kingdom. What can we learn from these evaluations? The exposure to information was high and improvement in the general knowledge of HIV/AIDS and how to protect oneself was evident. On the other hand, there was no evidence of changed behaviour in the general population. After all, the goal of the information is to influence the individual to refrain from risk behaviour. Obviously, we cannot expect short term effects on practices for the general population. The information needs to be repeated and targeted, particularly to persons that are at risk. There are studies showing self-reported changes of practices among homosexuals and drug addicts.

SEX EDUCATION

Many countries now teach about HIV infection and other sexually transmitted diseases in the **schools.** I think that it is important to incorporate that information into sex education and to teach about the biological, social and emotional aspects, suitably adapted according to the ages of the children. In countries where sex education in schools is not practised due to religious or cultural reasons, the essential information may be a natural part of the family education.

Boys can be reached for further education also during **military service** when most of them start sexual activity. Military service often coincides with the age when sexually transmitted diseases are most prevalent in men.

Another possibility to reach people for education is at the **work-place.** Particularly for young people that have left their families, the work-place is a central point in the daily, social life. The opinions expressed there probably play an important role in influencing behaviour. Therefore, in our country, for instance, we are emphasizing information at the work-place in close cooperation with the employers and the trade unions.

Other important channels for information and discussion are **political parties, religious organizations, sport clubs** and **women's organizations.** Naturally, other voluntary organizations like the **Red Cross/Red Crescent, Save the Children** and, not least, the **associations for homosexuals, hemophiliacs** and against **drug addiction** are playing a very important and pioneering role for information. In short, in many countries, the whole society is now being mobilized in the struggle against HIV/AIDS in an impressive and unprecedented way. I think that the grass-roots approach involving face-to-face contact is the most important factor for the long term effect in the attempts to influence behaviour and to counteract discrimination against the HIV infected.

CONTROL OF BLOOD PRODUCTS AND BLOOD TRANSFUSION

Further spread of HIV by blood transfusion is now effectively prevented in many countries and preventive measures are being instituted in others. The blood products for clotting disorders are treated to free them of infectious HIV. In many countries, efficient sterilization of skin-piercing medical equipment has been the rule for a long time, but in many developing countries there is still a lack of sterile supplies or sterilization equipment. This is a problem and an area for further intervention.

VOLUNTARY TESTING OF PREGNANT WOMEN TO COUNSEL THE HIV INFECTED

In some countries, it is legal and feasible to test pregnant women for HIV antibodies, and so break vertical transmission through counselling those who are HIV-infected about abortion and the prevention of further pregnancies. In Sweden, for instance, HIV testing is now offered to all pregnant women. The acceptance rate is high. The test results are kept confidential.

IMPROVEMENT OF PRIMARY HEALTH CARE FOR MOTHERS AND CHILDREN, FAMILY PLANNING

I would like to stress the importance of strengthening primary health care, particularly for mothers and children, as an intervention measure to prevent HIV infection. For instance, if the health of pregnant women is well monitored, then there could be less demand for blood transfusions in developing countries in connection with delivery. As so well described by Dr Fleming (pp 357-367) in developing countries, one of the big groups receiving life-saving blood transfusions is women anemic already before delivery and then brought to hospital exsanguinated after complicated delivery or in conjunction with caesarian section.

Another big group in need of blood transfusion is young children anemic due to malaria and other parasitic diseases.

Today many women and children are infected by HIV through transfusions with unscreened blood. Prevention of anemia could make a significant contribution to diminishing the spread of HIV. These are only examples of the importance of maintaining and strengthening primary health care. Do **not** remove the scarce resources for family health care to the hospitals for the treatment of the many AIDS cases. It should be the responsibility of governments to reallocate resources to the health area and for rich industrial countries to give the necessary support so that the preventive measures for the health of mothers and children do not need to compete with the humanitarian need to diminish the pain and agony of the fatally ill!

CONDOM CAMPAIGNS

It is also important to pursue the family planning programmes and to use that network for information on HIV/AIDS and for promoting the use and supply of condoms and other barriers.

CONTROLLING DRUG ADDICTION

The prevention of HIV transmission caused by exchanging blood through syringes used by intravenous drug abusers can be divided into short term tactic interventions and long term strategic interventions. The short term measures necessitate emergency activities, such as the supply of clean syringes, disinfection practices and methadone-programmes. The long term interventions are attempts to stop the abuse of intravenous drugs. As the HIV infections will be with us for decades or centuries, the long term actions are important. To control drug addiction is extremely difficult, as we all know, as there are strong economical and political forces promoting the international drug trading and as there is a deficient commitment to fight against the addiction in many affected countries. The international custom council has estimated the cash flow of illicit drugs in the world to 200 billion dollars a year. The national custom and police authorities, Interpol, United Nation Agencies, and the bank authorities are now stepping up their efforts to control the production of drugs, the distribution over the borders and the transfer of large amounts of currency. The primary prevention by social and medical activities to trace, support, treat and rehabilitate the drug addicts is laborious, time consuming and expensive. These activities need now to be pursued in a more energetic and determined way. There is a need to allocate considerably more public resources for crash programmes. Let us sincerely hope that the unique commitment by the politicians to fight against AIDS will include also improved actions against drug addiction, particularly to stop recruitment of young people to become drug addicts.

CONTROLLING SEXUALLY TRANSMITTED DISEASES

There are direct intervention policies trying to reach people with high risk sexual behaviour through clinics for sexually transmitted diseases or gay health centres. All should be counselled, and by HIV testing programmes, HIV positive individuals may be instructed to inform their previous and present sexual partners in attempts to break transmission chains. All testing programmes should be based on informed consent and confidentiality. Intervention measures directed against HIV infections will at the same time be directed against all other sexually transmitted diseases and vice versa. Therefore, the measures need to be integrated. In some countries syphilis, gonorrhoea and chancroid are frequent, in others chlamydia, herpes and papillomavirus, causing condyloma, are the currently most commonly observed STDs. It has also been shown by multivariate analysis that several of the common STDs, particularly those causing ulceration, will increase the risk of transmitting or contracting HIV infection. Therefore, controlling other STDs, e.g. by condom-campaigns and treatment, will help diminish the spread of HIV.

In addition, I would like to mention the increasing interest in the risks of young women contracting STDs, including HIV, associated with the more vulnerable mucous membranes on the cervix of the uterus. In young women, the outer part of the cervix, mechanically exposed in the vagina during intercourse, is covered by the same type of delicate epithelium as inside the cervix. In the adult woman, that vulnerable epithelium is replaced by a robust vaginal membrane. The vulnerable cells are sensitive to infection by papillomavirus, gonococci and chlamydia and to abrasions causing bleedings. In young women, the hormones used for contraception tend to increase the ectopia. The increase of cervical cancer in young women reported from many countries has been associated with a frequently occurring infection with certain types of papillomavirus. It seems reasonable to advocate delaying the first sexual experience and the use of condoms or diaphragms to protect the vulnerable portion of the cervix in young women against abrasions and exposure to infections. However, the direct importance in the prevention of HIV infection needs to be further studied. I have allowed myself this diversion to more specific aspects to emphasize the importance of incorporating new knowledge of other infections into the intervention against HIV infection.

I will finish this overview of intervention policies by emphasizing the prerequisite to achieve results by the intervention efforts; that is to get the confident cooperation of the individuals by voluntary measures, confidential handling of test results, warranty against discrimination and by offering psycho-social and medical support. That means that the resources for counselling and social support need to be available before other measures are taken. The security of the individual through the active support by the society and actions to prevent discrimination are indispensible parts of the policy to prevent further spread of HIV.

The Global Impact of AIDS, pages 341–345
© 1988 Alan R. Liss, Inc.

46.   THE IMMUNE SYSTEM APPROACH IN TEACHING AIDS
TO YOUNGSTERS : TWO UNIQUE PROGRAMS FOR
SCHOOLS

Inon Schenker

AIDS Project, School of Public Health and
Community Medicine, Faculty of Medicine, Hebrew
University, Jerusalem, Israel

The first case of AIDS in childhood was traced back to 1979.
Since then, the number of children affected by the disease has
been steadily increasing.

Two risk factors are primarily associated with infection by
the AIDS retrovirus in the child population :- (a) children
receiving blood transfusions or blood products for various
medical conditions; (b) newborns infected in-utero, at birth or
(possibly) by breast-feeding by mothers who are carriers of the
HIV.

Today, AIDS in children is no longer an American and
African phenomenon. Throughout the world, reports of pediatric
cases are rapidly being published. On December 30th 1987, Israel
reported to the WHO Collaborating Center on AIDS about 43
AIDS cases of which 32 had already died. One pediatric case was
reported and that was of a haemophiliac child. In January 1988, 6
more adult cases have been reported and Israel's total is now (1st
May, 1988) 59 AIDS cases (39 having died) in a population of 4
million citizens. The accurate number of reported carriers is 376
but the estimated number is 3,500.

The fatal outcome of the disease, when at present there is
no therapy available, has caused fear, stress and anxiety, not
only in the high risk groups but in the general population as well.

AIDS has become a front-page disease, the lead item on the
evening news and a frequent topic on TV talk shows. All these
are part of children's everyday life, as well as of adults. This
state of anxiety is of special concern in the child population,

especially in societies where children infected by HIV want to go to school, play in parks and meet with friends.

The increasing number of children and adolescents affected by AIDS, and the special psychosocial problems regarding AIDS in the child population introduces two major challenges for the health educator in the school setting :-

(a) Taking part in the prevention of the disease, and

(b) Reducing fears and anxieties about AIDS in the general child population.

It would be a disservice to pupils **not** to provide them with knowledge and opportunity to increase their awareness, and to dispel misperceptions about AIDS.

The main problem remains: What is the proper way to carry out AIDS education into the school?

The purpose of this paper is to introduce two unique health education programs on AIDS for youth in schools.

Taking into account the psychosexual development of children and their sexual identity, I have decided, after consulting with experts in psychiatry and psychology, not to combine the AIDS issue with sex education, but to link it to the immune system.

I look at the acquired immune-deficiency syndrome as a special infectious disease, but do not stress it as a "pure" sexually-transmitted disease, since this is not the case in all high-risk groups. The idea is not only to fight AIDS, but rather to promote healthy behaviours and life styles. For example :-

By combining AIDS education with the immune system approach, we increase awareness of the importance of routine vaccinations and that is a goal by itself.

The goals of the programs are :-

(a) To increase in the target population the knowledge about the immune system in human beings;
(b) To decrease fear of routine immunization;
(c) To increase the knowledge about AIDS, its causes and its prevention;

(d) To decrease the fear of AIDS; and
(e) To provide the tools to cope with the case of a child with AIDS at school
(f) (in high-schools) To increase the awareness of "safer sex".

The programs were designed for students from as low as grade 6 in elementary schools (that is, "kids" at age 11) and up to 12th grade.

Our first program on AIDS consists of 6 units. It is named: **"Explaining AIDS to Children"** and is aimed at 6-9th grades.

The first unit is an introductory game to the subject of AIDS and the immune system. We draw a large circle in the courtyard of the school. The children standing inside the circle act as the lymphocytes protecting the human body from infections. The children outside the circle act as pathogenic agents, who wish to go inside the body, and capture the object in the center of the circle (hat, book, etc.) without being caught by the "lymphocytes". If the "pathogens" are successful, it means that the person will be infected by them.

Along the same principles, two additional games teach the children the role of the T-helper cells and the macrophages in the immune system and what is an immune deficiency.

The second unit explains the immune system through the use of a series of slides demonstrating by cartoons a fight between the "bad guys": pathogenic viruses, bacteria, and the "good guys": lymphocytes, antigens, phagocytes. The characteristics of the immune system, its specificity, its ability to memorize, and its effectivity are explained in the slides as well.

The third unit is devoted to a discussion of the medical achievements in the field of infectious diseases. The pupils are instructed to read special stories from famous books, on the medical victories against bacteria. Through the reading and the discussion, they are shown the great successes of medicine in curing fatal diseases of the past.

The fact that in Jerusalem all girls in the 6th grade receive a German measles vaccination, and all children in the 7th grade receive the BCG immunization is used to teach the **fourth unit** in our program. This unit, requiring the participation of a school nurse and/or a physician, stresses the importance of immunization and gives guidelines for the proper use and care of the immunization card.

The issue of AIDS is introduced to the class only in the **fifth unit.** In this unit, we use a second series of slides which show the origins of the disease, its modes of transmission, the high-risk groups, the outcome and the possible ways of prevention.

The sixth unit is devoted to the problem of a child infected with HIV, in school. Using role-playing, the writing of a composition on the subject, and an open discussion, we try to make the class and the individuals analyze carefully the situation of a child with AIDS, discovered at school, and the ways to cope with it. The unit stresses the fact that the child with AIDS causes no special danger to his teachers and classmates.

Stressing the importance of the pupil's responsibility in spreading the true facts about AIDS and not relying only on the popular media concludes this program's message.

The second program: **"The Immune System and AIDS"** is for 9-12th grades. In this program we delete the first unit of the first program, and while incorporating materials from the first program, we place here more emphasis on AIDS and its prevention. The 6th and last unit in this program deals with "safer sex" and with drug abuse. In this unit, we discuss the spread of AIDS in the world, the students calculate their individual risk of acquiring AIDS and are taught about the importance of condom-use and reducing the number of sex partners. The risks of drug abuse are explained as well.

Going step by step, using cartoons as a non-threatening tool, we explain fully and scientifically, the acquired immune-deficiency syndrome and its consequences. The programs include a teacher's manual and students' work-sheets in addition to the slides, together with other explanatory material.

Combining the issue of AIDS with the immune system allows us to be brief when discussing the delicate subjects of sexuality and specifically homosexuality in that age group. By starting off with the neutral issue of the immune system, we **don't** have to focus on the sexual transmission of HIV, although this way of transmission is fully explained in the later stages pf the programs. This approach is better accepted by conservative parents, teachers and officials.

Given the sensitive nature of the subject, we felt that it was vital to solicit feedback from experts in fields related to AIDS education prior to testing the program in the field. 26 Israeli experts from the fields of medicine, psychology, education, public health and others, were asked to comment in detail about the written program sent to them. They have all approved the program in principle. Some argued we should begin at grade 8, not 6, and others insisted that we should combine AIDS solicitously with sex education.

The WHO Special Program on AIDS has included examples of the programs in its special folio on AIDS education materials distributed officially at the London Summit of Health Ministers on AIDS (January 1988).

The WHO Euro-expert Committee on AIDS recommends the use of the programs in different countries after "minor modifications" are made.

"Explaining AIDS to Children" and "The Immune System and AIDS" are now under review in Germany, Switzerland, the UK, Spain, Denmark, the Netherlands, Hungary and the USA.

In Israel, the Minister of Education, Mr. Navon, and a team of his experts has examined the programs from the scientific and pedagogic aspects and after consulting with the Israeli National AIDS Committee, has decided to recommend their nationwide use to Israeli primary and secondary schools. The implementation, which started on 1st September 1987, is followed by a program trial.

As modular programs, carefully prepared for youth in schools and suitable for different curriculums, the two programs can be provided in the school setting by teachers, nurses, doctors, health educators and other trained personnel.

It is my belief that these programs can serve as an excellent base for modification to suit other cultures in developed and in developing countries.

The Global Impact of AIDS, pages 347–355
© 1988 Alan R. Liss, Inc.

47. GALLUP INTERNATIONAL SURVEY ON ATTITUDES
TOWARDS AIDS

Norman L Webb

Gallup International, London, UK

SUMMARY AND CONCLUSIONS

Gallup International has performed an international survey
on attitudes and opinions about AIDS. The survey is the first of
other voluntary projects launched at its own expense by Gallup
International as a memorial to Dr George H Gallup, the founder
of our group and a pioneer in opinion polling research. This
survey was conducted in 36 nations, and preliminary results for
33 of them are given here.

In most countries AIDS is regarded as the most urgent
medical problem, and for some Third World countries it was not.
Nevertheless, 90% of the populations of many countries were
aware of the condition, but a few countries, notably in Africa
and Asia were less aware than would have been thought. Concern
about contracting the disease in the general population was
relatively low, but the exceptions were in the Americas and
some Asian countries. As far as becoming an epidemic was
concerned, throughout the world there was a clear realisation
that this was likely to occur in the case of homosexuals,
haemophiliacs, intravenous drug users, and promiscuous people.
At the same time there was widespread concern about the risk of
becoming HIV positive amongst those who receive blood and
occasional experimenters with partners other than their own.
Relatively few people thought that they should change their
behaviour or had already changed in their sexual activities.

In terms of the risk of catching the disease, most of the
peoples of the world were aware of the clear situations in which
it could be caught. However above and beyond that there was

much concern about other ways in which it might be caught, which can only be counter-productive. Substantial minorities in many parts of the world, for instance would refuse to work together with a person carrying the AIDS virus, though minorities around the world have a sympathetic view towards AIDS victims.

Our conclusions are the following. For the most part, populations of peoples of the world are now informed about the risks of AIDS. There remain some areas where this is not true. However, it can be said that the fears expressed by many people are a problem in themselves. Firstly, there is a problem of receiving blood, which may be dangerous in some areas but not in others. Secondly, there is a fear that one can get AIDS by means which are not supported by scientific practice, for instance sharing a drinking glass or via insect bites. Lastly, there is the cumulative effect of these fears upon the behaviour of people's of the world, in particular in respect of being close to people who have the condition, which may have some important social effects, and in terms of their willingness to make sacrifices in respect of a proportion of the population that are on their way to dying from the condition.

Clearly there is a substantial need for a somewhat differently directed programme of information and of avoiding some misinformation in respect of this challenge.

METHODOLOGY OF THE SURVEY

At Gallup's International conference in Japan in 1987 it was agreed that the member countries should cooperate in carrying out a study of attitudes towards AIDS as a first manifestation of their respect towards the late Dr Gallup, who was in his lifetime keenly interested in international cooperation and particularly interested in the contribution that the Group might make towards health and towards peace. Accordingly, after some months spent in preparation of a questionnaire to be addressed to the populations of a number of countries, this questionnaire was despatched to our member affiliates with instructions to pose the questions to the populations of their own countries. In addition an example of the format of the results was included, since the British had carried out the survey in advance of other countries, and had provided this particular format. To date 33 countries have cooperated, and more will produce results within a relatively short time, so that results are available for most parts of the world. It must be confessed that some countries, after looking at the questionnaire, adopted slightly different practices in the way that they administered the questions to the population, in particular by slightly changing the form of the question and using show cards, so that technically speaking there are a number of countries whose results are not so comparable with others as would be desired. Nevertheless the data are here given for the value they may contain. Samples in each country were, with few exceptions, national and carried out in the period August 1987 to February 1988.

The Dutch, who carried out the survey in the Autumn of 1987 for the first time, and who deviated from the required method of interviewing, have repeated their survey in March 1988 strictly in accord with other countries. The nature of these results are given here, and while it is remarkable that these make the Dutch results more comparable with other western European countries in most respects, a marked lack of sympathy for AIDS sufferers is expressed. Whether this is due to specific national attitude of the Dutch or to a hardening of attitudes over the last six months cannot be decided. It is known that a number of events have occurred in the Netherlands which could change the situation. This leaves open the question of whether attitudes to AIDS have also changed in other countries between the last part of 1987 and now.

The highlights of the data are given in five tables in the appendix. The first page of these covers urgent health problems and awareness of AIDS. Naturally, it was only worthwhile to put further questions to those people who were aware of AIDS. Consequently the base for the third question on Table 1 (the degree of concern about AIDS) and for all questions on subsequent pages, was that proportion of the original sample who were aware of AIDS. In most cases this was well over 90%, but in a few cases, in particular Nigeria and blacks in South Africa, the proportion was distinctly lower.

THE RESULTS AND SOME OBSERVATIONS

The results have been despatched both to London and Princeton, USA in the form of tabulations. In these analyses by age, sex, marital status and other demographic criteria were provided. In addition, tapes or diskettes of the survey material are being accumulated. Some time will elapse before a master tape of all data becomes available.

The results presented here give no demographic analysis at

all, and are given as national totals in percentage form in Tables
1-5 of the appendix. Although there is a wealth of information
contained in the data, the present paper deals only with their
main results, and, it can be stated that although there are
differences within countries according to different sectors of the
population, they do not invalidate the broad conclusions drawn
here.

From two questions posed in the survey, the first about the
likelihood of AIDS becoming an epidemic amongst different
sections of the population, and the second addressing itself to
ways in which the virus can be caught, two broad conclusion can
be drawn. The first is that there is very considerable, though not
complete, public awareness of what has happened with
haemophiliacs and intravenous drug abusers who share needles.
The dangers of homosexual practices and general promiscuity are
clearly well known. However in some parts of the world there
appear to be disturbingly large numbers of people not aware of
these risks.

Turning to the reverse side, the awareness of what has
happened to haemophiliacs seems to have spilled over to all
forms of receiving blood. In some societies this may be a real
risk still, but I believe this is conquered in the West. However,
other perceived risks, such as sharing a drinking glass, coughs
and sneezes, friendly kissing etc appear to be identified. Further,
working alongside someone known to have AIDS is perceived by
some as a definite risk.

The social consequences of such fears could be great.
Clearly many more people suffering from AIDS are bound to
emerge in our midst, according to the known epidemiological
facts. With such greater acquaintance and contact with the
existence of the disease the effects upon people's behavior at
work, at school, in all forms of social gathering, and in terms of
willingness to undergo necessary medical treatment could be
dramatic.

This points out a duty to the responsible authorities to
redouble their efforts in terms of public education in two
directions. The first is education and persuasion in respect of the
real risks, and the second, and possibly far more difficult, is the
question of putting into perspective overdramatic and unrealistic
fears, both counter-productive and dangerous in their social
effects. It is reassuring that the Gallup International survey
showed that majorities of the population, though misinformed on
some things, still feel that AIDS sufferers should be treated with
compassion.

TABLE 1.

Sample Size		AIDS	Cancer	Heart Disease	Stroke	Senility	Alcoholism	Drug Abuse	Mental Illness	Pollution/ Radioactivity	Other	Don't Know	Yes	No	Very Concerned	A Little Concerned	Not Very Concerned	Not At All Concerned	Don't Know
		Perceived Most Urgent Health Problems — What would you say is most urgent health problem facing this country at present time?											**Awareness of AIDS** — Have you heard of AIDS?		**Degree of Concern about AIDS** — How concerned are you that you will get AIDS?				
1569	USA	68	14	7	–	–	1	3	–	1	14	3	99	1	20	22	21	37	–
1041	Canada	57	24	6	–	–	1	1	–	–	6	4	100	0	12	18	19	50	1
	Mexico																		
1163	El Salvador	10	17	1	–	1	32	25	1	2	10	5	76	24	9	7	12	46	26
1014	Colombia	44	8	–	–	–	3	14	2	2	14	3	99	1	18	27	21	34	–
1204	Ecuador	9	19	19	–	–	2	6	1	1	43	2	70	30	22	24	35	17	2
1252	Brazil	79	7	1	–	1	1	–	1	1	8	4	100	0	35	20	8	37	–
1028	Argentina	24	14	8	–	1	2	10	4	–	26	2	91	9	16	21	17	45	1
1041	Chile	35	24	10	1	–	10	6	1	–	10	2	95	5	11	14	31	37	8
800	Uruguay	26	44	10	–	–	1	3	2	–	12	2	97	3	17	18	12	50	3
969	Great Britain	48	19	13	–	1	5	2	–	1	9	7	99	1	6	16	14	62	2
1001	France	39	4	4	–	1	5	2	3	1	5	7	97	3	5	16	31	51	2
1012	Germany	39	29	13	3	1	2	9	1	–	–	2	92	8	6	14	27	42	11
707	Switzerland	62	13	4	1	1	6	6	3	–	6	4	98	2	2	8	25	61	4
1000	Austria	44	56	29	11	–	19	22	3	1	1	5	99	1	6	19	23	50	2
968	Belgium	33	40	8	1	1	6	4	1	–	5	6	97	3	2	6	24	64	4
1090	Netherlands	34	26	27	–	–	7	6	–	–	1	–	97	3	1	6	16	76	2
1005	Luxembourg	28	40	9	2	1	5	6	2	–	7	12	96	4	4	13	21	57	4
1081	Denmark	44	39	11	1	1	7	4	1	–	1	4	98	2	12	14	17	55	3
995	Norway	63	25	23	1	1	7	9	2	–	8	1	99	1	7	16	28	47	2
1110	Sweden	51	34	15	–	–	5	7	1	1	2	4	99	1	2	8	34	50	6
959	Finland	33	24	18	–	5	4	2	3	–	12	6	99	1	6	13	25	54	1
716	Iceland	32	20	11	5	1	8	4	1	–	5	9	97	3	–	3	32	63	–
1398	Ireland	27	30	16	1	1	2	6	–	1	4	5	93	7	8	13	17	57	5
1020	Spain	31	37	8	1	–	3	10	1	–	2	9	86	14	11	22	15	50	2
803	Portugal	31	38	8	1	1	–	4	–	–	2	14	95	5	11	25	20	39	5
1000	Greece	25	38	17	1	–	–	9	1	–	–	7	95	5	25	20	12	42	0
1113	Australia	52	16	12	–	–	2	4	–	–	9	5	99	1	10	18	22	50	–
1493	Korea	22	42	5	1	1	3	–	4	–	12	12	84	16	6	17	22	55	1
1387	Japan	13	25	5	1	9	–	1	–	–	47	12	95	5	3	12	40	44	1
2000	Phillipines	23	11	3	1	–	2	15	1	–	38	36	78	22	38	18	12	31	–
1500	India	13	36	14	–	1	5	9	1	–	11	8	78	22	13	23	22	36	6
1400	Turkey	28	31	8	–	1	5	5	1	–	13	8	87	13	27	26	28	13	6
4039	Nigeria	10	8	11	7	2	12	17	11	4	19	–	46	54	40	11	5	39	5
	South Africa																		
1300	Blacks												72	28	46	14	14	21	5
1000	Whites												99	1	18	16	16	48	2

TABLE 2. Likelihood of AIDS developing into Epidemic for Certain Groups. Do you think it likely or is it not likely AIDS will eventually become an epidemic for the following groups in society?

% answers "it is LIKELY in the following groups"

	Population at large?	IVDAs?	Haemophiliacs?	People who need blood transfusions?	Married people who have affairs?	Homosexuals?	Couples who are faithful?	People who have several sexual partners?	Doctors/nurses and other hospital staff?	Men?	Women?
USA	51	93	67	59	59	96	9	87	34	53	43
Canada	47	87	64	53	65	94	4	90	32	36	28
Mexico											
El Salvador	52	72	64	71	67	71	21	57	45	61	59
Colombia	69	93	88	90	85	98	11	94	55	77	63
Ecuador	56	100	83	83	55	100	2	71	31	90	48
Brazil	67	92	84	95	88	97	15	96	54	79	69
Argentina	27	92	78	72	72	95	11	95	46	56	46
Chile	51	82	67	75		93	13	81			
Uruguay	45	86	71	80	82	94	8	86	53	72	64
Great Britain	34	95	55	37	49	90	5	84	23	42	29
France	23	83	58	54	67	84	7	74	33	42	36
Germany	13	92	64	52	59	93	3	86	21	36	32
Switzerland	23	91		38	76	91	3	83	13	45	39
Austria	14	88	56	45		87	4	76			
Belgium	12	84	41	47		88	5	78			
Netherlands	14	83	37	24	43	75	2	79	12		
Luxembourg										10	9
Denmark	20	86	53	38	46	85	2	78	16	78	21
Norway	17	90	52	36	49	83	4	82	24	30	24
Sweden	23	94	48	42	50	88	5	87	34	32	27
Finland	17	82	36	38	60	85	3	80	16	28	21
Iceland	14	89	37	33	59	78	2	87	15	16	11
Ireland	29	95	67	48	63	90	5	89	21	30	23
Spain	37	92	72	71		87	11	82	36	40	35
Portugal	26	81	72	73	72	84	8	83	37	69	59
Greece	46	93	72	76	75	94	11	88	34	50	46
Australia	10	67	15	22	15	79	2	56	7	4	3
Korea	18	50	49	75	68	83	6	87	29	51	20
Japan	28	76	79	60	78	89	10	87	42	56	37
Phillipines	62	80	50	81	89	89	12	92	33	78	73
India	6	38	8	42	16	53	3	52	5	7	6
Turkey	34	69	65	78	73	88	12	70	36	56	38
Nigeria	50	46	37	74	70	72	11	90	48	76	76
South Africa Blacks	47	66	44	53	71	75	11	92	29	65	62
Whites	45	85	56	55	63	96	4	90	28	62	44

TABLE 3. Overall Change in Behaviour Because of the Risk of AIDS

Which one of these statements applies to you?

	Because of the risk of AIDS I have changed my behaviour	Because of the risk of AIDS I am seriously thinking of changing my behaviour	Despite the risk of AIDS I have not changed my behaviour	I do not need to change my behaviour	Don't know
USA	11	3	15	68	3
Canada	4	3	9	84	1
Mexico					
El Salvador	4	5	12	51	28
Columbia	7	7	7	79	–
Ecuador	20	23	28	29	–
Brazil	14	8	10	67	1
Argentina	4	5	9	82	–
Chile	9	4	6	80	–
Uruguay	5	3	3	86	7
Great Britain	4	3	4	89	–
France	4	4	13	78	1
Germany	4	3	13	80	0
Switzerland	4	7	9	77	3
Austria	5	5	7	82	2
Belgium	2	2	9	85	2
Netherlands	3	2	4	92	–
Luxembourg					
Denmark	4	2	14	80	0
Norway	3	2	5	90	0
Sweden	5	1	7	85	2
Finland	4	3	9	82	1
Iceland	7	4	2	91	–
Ireland	2	1	4	92	1
Spain	2	2	12	84	–
Portugal	2	3	9	85	2
Greece	10	9	20	61	0
Australia	5	2	7	83	2
Korea	5	15	28	51	1
Japan	1	4	4	87	4
Phillipines	19	15	11	49	6
India	14	6	8	60	12
Turkey	8	10	18	64	–
Nigeria	31	14	5	50	–
South Africa					
Blacks	12	21	18	49	–
Whites	2	2	5	91	–

TABLE 4. Perceived Ways of Catching AIDS

As I read off each item, one at a time, would you tell me whether you think it is a way for people to catch AIDS from someone who has it?

	Working alongside or in close proximity to someone with AIDS?	Intimate sexual contact with a person of the opposite sex?	Intimate sexual contact with a person of the same sex?	Friendly kissing on the cheek?	Being coughed or sneezed on?	Receiving blood transfusions?	From a drinking glass?	Sharing needles?	Insect bites?
	IS	IS	IS	IS	IS	IS	IS	IS	IS
USA	11	88	95	8	25	86	26	97	30
Canada	8	88	92	8	18	84	26	96	22
Mexico									
El Salvador	48	59	70	30	46	70	42	67	41
Colombia	42	93	96	57	52	97	55	97	51
Ecuador	41	54	98	3	20	96	14	97	11
Brazil	29	84	88	10	31	97	85	97	56
Argentina	24	93	93	17	31	92	34	93	43
Chile	39	62	77	12	31	85	34	88	32
Uruguay	16	85	84	11	23	87	27	87	36
Great Britain	6	87	92	3	9	75	10	97	14
France	13	62	73	4	12	73	19	88	22
Germany	3	88	91	3	6	72	6	92	17
Switzerland	8	81	86	2	6	58	10	95	13
Austria	2	86	88	2	6	58	9	90	15
Belgium	10	75	84	5	12	76	16	90	22
Netherlands	10	58	70	1	7	58	9	97	16
Luxembourg									
Denmark	4	79	82	2	8	70	7	94	20
Norway	7	88	87	8	15	84	21	96	23
Sweden	5	83	89	2	10	84	12	97	21
Finland	14	79	86	6	13	82	16	91	29
Iceland	11	93	92	7	24	89	27	97	44
Ireland	11	74	87	6	12	69	14	90	19
Spain	19	72	77	12	23	84	27	81	36
Portugal	20	75	73	13	27	79	28	83	38
Greece	19	86	92	11	20	86	19	92	27
Australia	6	67	75	7	49	63	3	81	5
Korea	51	94	92	62	26	94	61	92	75
Japan	20	61	78	15	54	79	25	78	18
Phillipines	56	88	84	33	7	89	56	77	57
India	25	41	52	22	38	51	12	33	10
Turkey	45	70	77	35		83	37	82	53
Nigeria	34	89		48	56	85	55	85	67
South Africa									
Blacks									
Whites									

TABLE 5. Attitudes Concerning AIDS Victims

I am now going to read some statements about AIDS.

As I read off each statement, one at a time, tell me whether you agree or disagree with it.

	I would refuse to work alongside someone who has AIDS.	In the main, its the peoples own fault if they get AIDS.	Everyone should have a blood test to see if they have AIDS.	AIDS sufferers should be treated with compassion.
	AGREE	AGREE	AGREE	AGREE
USA	25	51	47	87
Canada	23	45	60	90
Mexico				
El Salvador	50	29	68	57
Colombia	53	61	86	69
Ecuador	89	67	69	47
Brazil	27	46	83	69
Argentina	34	40	64	66
Chile	46	35	74	52
Uruguay	29	65	80	68
Great Britain	14	61	48	81
France	16	28	74	93
Germany	19	47	48	74
Switzerland	14	52	41	92
Austria				
Belgium	24	50	68	92
Netherlands	6	33	38	14
Luxembourg				
Denmark	8	48	38	70
Norway	10	52	58	63
Sweden	11	32	61	90
Finland	17	57	52	76
Iceland	13	44	74	86
Ireland	23	56	47	84
Spain	20	28	78	57
Portugal	31	43	68	62
Greece	36	61	81	89
Australia	7	24	47	67
Korea	77	63	79	54
Japan	68	45	59	71
Phillipines	62	67	79	72
India	21	35	46	35
Turkey	63	53	56	57
Nigeria	52	61	85	
South Africa				
Blacks				
Whites				

The Global Impact of AIDS, pages 357–367
© 1988 Alan R. Liss, Inc.

48. PREVENTION OF TRANSMISSION OF HIV BY BLOOD TRANSFUSION IN DEVELOPING COUNTRIES

Alan F Fleming

London School of Hygiene and Tropical Medicine

Transmission of HIV by blood transfusion makes a relatively small contribution to the epidemic of AIDS, but is a matter of particular concern as the infection is acquired not through any voluntary action by the individual, and children and pregnant women are especially at risk.

The frequency of transmission will depend on (i) the number of blood transfusions administered, (ii) the prevalence of HIV infection amongst the potential blood donors, and (iii) the efficiency of the Blood Transfusion Service in excluding HIV infected units. The situation in equatorial Africa is grim because of the large numbers of patients requiring blood transfusions, the high frequency of HIV infection amongst potential blood donors, the absence of any easily recognised high-risk groups to be excluded as blood donors, and the inability of most laboratories to screen for anti-HIV antibodies.

BLOOD TRANSFUSION IN THE THIRD WORLD

Practically all the blood transfused in the Third World is either concentrated red cells in the treatment of anaemia, or whole blood to patients who are exsanguinated.

Anaemia

Malnutrition, infection and inherited defects of red blood cells are the commonest causes of anaemia. The commonly eaten staples, including rice, wheat, maize, sorghum and millet, are poor sources of bioavailable iron and folate. At least 500 million people are exposed to malaria. Around 450 million are infected with hookworm, 40 million in Africa and Asia with *Schistosoma haematobium*, 30 million in Africa and America with *S. mansoni* and 46 million in eastern Asia with *S. japonicum*. About 150,000 infants are born annually with sickle-cell disease, of whom 120,000 are Africans. Up to 74,000 newborn each year have beta-thalassaemia major and 60,000 have haemoglobin-H disease, the great majority being Asians.

Anaemia from all these causes is both more prevalent and more severe in pregnancy and early childhood (Fleming, 1987a).

Pregnancy. There is a greater susceptibility to malaria during pregnancy, especially in primigravidae. Raised nutritional demands may lead to depletion of iron, while high physiological requirements and malarial haemolysis are followed commonly by folic acid deficiency. Patients with haemoglobinopathies have already poor immune status and high requirements for folic acid, so that their anaemias are made more severe by the pregnant state. Estimates of frequency of anaemias in pregnancy (haemoglobin (Hb) less than 11g/dl) range from 24% to 88% in different tropical countries. Severe anaemia (Hb less than 7g/dl) is common; for example over 250 patients are seen each year at University College Hospital, Ibadan of whom one third have profound life-threatening anaemia (Hb less than 4g/dl). Maternal malaria and severe anaemia result in about 30% perinatal deaths: surviving infants are of low birth weight, poor nutrition and poor immune status, and have entered already the vicious cycle of infection, malnutrition, anaemia and immune suppression (Fleming, 1987a).

Childhood. From around six months of age, infants suffer from frequent and intense malaria and from many other recurrent infections. They are exposed while crawling to heavy hookworm infection, and later to *Schistosoma*. Weaning foods are often inappropriate and poor sources of energy and essential nutrients, including iron, folic acid and protein. As beta-chain synthesis replaces gamma chains and fetal haemoglobin, the major haemoglobinopathies become manifest. As a result of all these factors, anaemia (Hb less than 11g/dl) occurs in from 30% to 90% of preschool children in the third world (Fleming, 1987a).

Haemorrhage

Heavy demands are made on blood transfusion services for the treatment of haemorrhage arising from obstetric delivery and from trauma; exsanguination may be profound because of the long delays before arrival at the hospital. Obstructed labour, complicated by haemorrhage from the placental site or ruptured uterus, is seen commonly in young girls who have not completed growth, or in women whose pelvises have not developed during a childhood beset by malnutrition and infection (Harrison, 1985).

The rapidly increasing load of traffic, the poor state of many roads, often inadequate maintenance of vehicles and fatigue or lack of skill of many drivers, all contribute to numerous road traffic accidents, frequently multiple, spectacular and involving many victims.

The demand for blood

About six to eight units of blood are required per year for each general hospital bed in the United Kingdom; there are no great differences in the demands made by obstetricians and gynaecologists from those made by physicians, surgeons and paediatricians. Overall, the demand in Africa is about three times greater: 20 units of blood are required per bed per year in a well staffed general hospital. In northern Nigeria, up to 60 units were demanded per bed by the obstetricians and gynaecologists, around ten times the demands made by their British colleagues (unpublished observations).

TRANSMISSION OF HIV BY BLOOD TRANSFUSION

The principle of voluntary blood donation is upheld more-or-less throughout Africa, but smaller blood banks rely on relatives of patients, and the relatives may recruit and pay donors without the knowledge of the donor panel organisers. Obviously, blood donors are drawn from the sexually active age range, and in urban central Africa, this means that they have a high prevalence of infection by HIV. Anti-HIV seropositivity amongst blood donors has been reported as 18% in Kigali (Rwanda), 14% in Bukoba and 4.4% in Dar-Es-Salaam (Tanzania), 10% in Brazzaville (Congo), and 18.4% in Lusaka (Zambia) (Fleming, 1988a).

There have been three major studies in Zaire which assessed the transmission of HIV by blood transfusion in three age groups (Table 1). The most frequent mode of transmission of HIV to infants is vertically from the mother, but of 238 children with seronegative mothers, 16 (7%) were seropositive; of these 5 (2% of all or 31% of seropositive children with seronegative mothers) gave a history of previous blood transfusion (Mann et al, 1986a). Children two to fourteen years of age have the greatest relative

TABLE 1. HIV-1 Seropositivity and Previous Blood Tranfusions in Zaireans of Three Age Groups

Subjects	Seropositive		Seronegative		Ref.
	No	%	No	%	
Patients, 1-24 months with seronegative mothers					
History of blood transfusion	5	31	16	7	Mann et al, 1986 a
No previous transfusion	11	69	206	93	
Patients 2-14 years					
History of blood transfusion	24	60	108	33	Mann et al, 1986 b
No previous transfusion	16	40	220	67	
Adult hospital workers					
History of blood transfusion	14	9	106	5	Mann et al, 1986 c
No previous transfusion	138	91	2126	95	

risk of infection through blood transfusion; out of 368 hospitalized patients, 40 (11%) were seropositive, of whom 24 (7% of all or 60% of seropositive children) had received earlier blood transfusions (Mann et al, 1986b). Another study in the same hospital showed that of children receiving blood transfusions, 69% had malaria and 97% had anaemia (haematocrit less than 0.25) (Greenberg et al, 1988).

The relative contribution to HIV seropositivity is least amongst adults; of 2834 Zairean hospital workers, 152 (6%) were seropositive, of whom 14 (0.6% of all or 9% of seropositives) had a history of receiving blood transfusion (Mann et al, 1986c).

Patients with sickle-cell disease have emerged as a group at high risk of infection by HIV through repeated blood transfusions (Fleming, 1988b). High transfusion regimes are a recommended management of children with thalassaemia major; however, the majority of patients live in Asia, where there is as yet little HIV, and high transfusion regimes are not practicable. Patients with thalassaemia in Europe have been infected by blood (De Martino et al, 1985), and it may be anticipated that this will become common in Asia, even without systematic high transfusion regimes.

PREVENTION OF HIV TRANSMISSION BY BLOOD TRANSFUSION

Blood transfusion services in the western world may congratulate themselves on the virtual elimination of HIV infection through blood and blood products. This has been achieved by encouraging self-exclusion as donors by members of high risk groups (male homosexuals and intravenous drug abusers), the serological testing of all donations and the inactivation of virus during the processing of blood products (Petricciani et al, 1987). This achievement has been relatively easy compared to the problems facing the developing countries, and these need different approaches.

The transmission of HIV by blood transfusion may be reduced by three lines of action: (i) applying stringent indications for transfusion and so reducing the number of units of blood given, (ii) preventing situations where blood transfusions are essential to save life, and (iii) excluding infected blood from the Bank.

Indications for blood transfusion

It is unjustified and unethical to transfuse blood unscreened for HIV, except as a life-saving measure. Such situations include (i) profound anaemia (Hb less than 4g/dl) with incipient cardiac failure, (ii) severe neonatal jaundice (serum bilirubin greater than 300 μmol/l) and (iii) blood loss of more than 25% of total volume, when the blood pressure and oxygen carrying capacity cannot be maintained by plasma expanders. Any decision to transfuse unscreened blood in other situations must be made after extremely careful assessment.

No serological testing is going to detect all infected blood donors, and even after the introduction of HIV screening, clinicians must remain cautious about ordering blood for transfusion, especially in populations with high frequencies of seropositivity.

TABLE 2. Measures to Prevent Anaemia in Pregnancy in Tropical Africa

---

Family Planning

Delay first pregnancy until growth completed

Spacing pregnancies

Antenatal Clinic

Chloroquine at first attendance: if resistant parasitaemia, trials in order of Fansidar, amodiaquine, mefloquine and quinine

Proguanil 100mg daily (200mg if more than 170cm in height)

Ferrous sulphate 200mg x 2 daily (or x 3 for grande multigravidae or proven deficiency)

Folic acid 0.5mg daily (combined with ferrous sulphate)

Prevention of the need to transfuse blood

The three groups at highest risk of being infected with HIV through blood transfusion are pregnant women, children under five years of age and patients with sickle-cell disease.

There should be investment of time and money into strengthening or establishing Antenatal Clinics, Under-Fives' Clinics and Sickle-Cell Clinics: the prevention of anaemia, however, extends beyond these clinics, and involves Primary Health Care at villages and clinics, Family Planning, hospitals and policies of Ministries of Health. The prevention of the need to transfuse blood is an essential part of any AIDS control programme and both are integral to the health policies of a nation.

Pregnancy. The supervision of pregnancy includes as high priority the prevention of malaria and anaemia; the measures summarised (Table 2) have been shown to be safe, highly effective and costing not more than US $2 for antimalarials and US $ 40c for nutritional supplements (Fleming, 1987b). The advantages of good prenatal care and skilled supervision of complicated deliveries are not confined to the mother, but contribute largely to the prevention of neonatal jaundice and anaemia in infancy and childhood (Tables 3, 4) (Harrison, 1985; Fleming, 1987a, 1987b).

Investment in the Antenatal Clinics is crucial to any AIDS control programme, as it would include also the education of all women attending as to the nature of the epidemic, and screening for HIV leading to advice on termination of early pregnancies of HIV-infected women and the avoidance of subsequent pregnancies.

Preschool children. The principles for maintaining health in preschool children are well known and focus on nutrition (breast-feeding, supplements to risk groups and suitable weaning foods) and prevention of infection (extended immunization programmes and hygiene) (Tables 3, 4). The majority of African children requiring blood transfusion have malaria-related anaemia (Greenberg et al, 1988), and Primary Health Care workers could play a major role in reducing the need to transfuse through the early presumptive diagnosis and treatment of malaria.

Sickle-cell disease. With (i) early diagnosis, (ii) explanation of the disease to the family and patients, (iii) the establishment of **Sickle-Cell Clinics,** where health is maintained through (a) prescribing prophylactic antimalarials and (b) folic acid supplements, (c) advice given on avoidance of factors which precipitate crisis (fatigue, cold, dehydration etc), (d) the expanded immunization programme, and (iv) the prompt treatment of infection and crises, the need for emergency blood transfusion is reduced to nearly nil in the population with sickle-cell disease (Fleming, 1988b).

Exclusion of HIV-contaminated blood and blood products

There are two strategies for the exclusion of HIV-contaminated blood (Petricciani et al, 1987). First, donors who belong to groups at high risk of infection by HIV are requested not to donate blood. In the western world, these high risk groups include male homosexuals and intravenous drug abusers, but in tropical Africa, neither of these two groups exist to any noticeable extent. Some blood banks in Africa have stopped recruiting from convicts, as it is believed that prisons are the few places in tropical Africa where male homosexuality is practised commonly, and from the uniformed services, who have generally a higher rate of seropositivity than the civilian population.

The second strategy is to test serologically all blood donations, and discard all infected blood. Screening of blood in the third world presents difficulties of (i) training of staff, (ii) costs and (iii) choice of tests to be applied.

Staff-training. In some countries, the investment in medical laboratory technology is appallingly low and standards of training in blood transfusion have been allowed to slip until workers cannot be relied upon to perform ABO blood grouping consistently correctly. Ministries of Health should give priority to medical laboratory technology training, which would include techniques for identification of HIV contaminated blood, and to raising the prestige of the profession by providing attractive career structures and conditions of work.

Cost. The cost of delivering one unit of blood to a patient's bedside has been estimated variously as being between US $16 and $30 in different African countries. The cost of materials per HIV antibody screening test is approximately US $1, to which must be added the costs of importation, distribution, training, overheads and staff salaries. It may be concluded that anti-HIV testing should add less than 20% to the total cost of blood transfusion, and that these expenses can be met by Blood Transfusion Services, with or without financial support from overseas agencies.

TABLE 3. **Measures to Prevent Neonatal Jaundice and Anaemia in Infancy in Tropical Africa**

Prenatal

Prevention of maternal malaria and anaemia

Avoid triggers to haemolysis in G6PD deficiency (oxidant drugs, infections)

Delivery

Supervised delivery of small women

Avoiding birth trauma and infant haemorrhage

Allowing placental-infant transfusion

Infancy

Breast-feeding for up to two years

When necessary, expressed breast milk

When UNAVOIDABLE, artificial feeding of correct formula, sterile, not boiled excessively, not goats' milk

For premature, iron and folate supplements from week 2

For diarrhoea, continue breast-feeding, ORT, folic supplements

Prevention of sepsis

Treatment of infection

Choice of tests. At the time of writing, of the commercially and readily available kits, I would recommend the Wellcozyme as the first screening test for HIV-1 in Africa, it being simple to perform, specific, sensitive and reasonably priced. Radioimmunoprecipitation and immunofluorescent assay are extremely sensitive and specific confirmatory tests, but are too expensive and complex for general use. Western blotting gives non-specific weak bands with African sera, making interpretation difficult. One of the ELISAs using synthetic antigens, such as Hoffmann-La Roche or Abbott, is suitable as a confirmatory test, being based on a system different to that of Wellcozyme.

TABLE 4. **Measures to Prevent Anaemia in Preschool Children in Tropical Africa**

Prenatal

Prevention of maternal malaria and anaemia

The Home and Under-fives' Clinic

Breast-feeding for up to two years

Weaning foods rich in energy, protein, bioavailable iron and folate

Road-to-health charts

Immunization

Clinical diagnosis of malnutrition

Presumptive diagnosis and treatment of malaria

Early diagnosis of sickle-cell disease

It may be predicted that in the future (i) screening tests will incorporate a mixture of pure synthetic antigens to detect a wide range of antibodies to both HIV-1 and HIV-2 antigens, (ii) that testing for viral antigens will close partially the window of time between infection of the potential donor and seropositivity, and that (iii) further tests will be based on single antigens to give specific diagnosis of the infecting viruses and to identify antibodies whose presence may have prognostic value.

REFERENCES

De Martino M, Quarta G, Melpignano A et al (1985). Antibodies to HTLV-III and lymphadenopathy syndrome in multi-transfused βthalassemia patients. Vox Sang 49: 230-233.

Fleming A F (1987a). Anaemia as a world health problem. In Weatherall D J, Ledingham J G G, Warrell D A (eds): "Oxford Textbook of Medicine" 2nd edition, Oxford: Oxford University Press pp 19.71-19.79.

Fleming A F (1987b). Maternal anaemia in northern Nigeria : causes and solutions. Wld. Hlth. Forum 8: 339-343.

Fleming A F (1988a). AIDS in Africa - an update, AIDS Forschung 3: 116-138.

Fleming A F (1988b). AIDS and AIDS related complex (ARC) in twenty Zambians with sickle-cell anaemia and HIV contamination by blood transfusion. Cent Afr J Med: in press.

Greenberg A E, Nynyem - Dinh P, Mann J M et al (1988). The association between malaria, blood transfusions, and HIV seropositivity in a pediatric population in Kinshasa, Zaire. J Am Med Ass 259: 545-549.

Harrison K A (1985). Child-bearing, health and social priorities: a survey of 22 774 consecutive hospital births in Zaria, northern Nigeria. Brit J Obstet Gynaecol 92: supplement 5.

Mann J M, Francis H, Davachi F et al (1986a). Risk factors for human immunodeficiency virus seropositivity among children 1-24 months old in Kinshasa, Zaire. Lancet 2: 654-657.

Mann J M, Francis H, Davachi F et al (1986b). Human immunodeficiency virus seroprevalence in pediatric patients 2 to 14 years of age at Mama Yemo Hospital, Kinshasa, Zaire. Pediatrics 78: 673-677.

Mann J M, Francis H, Quinn T C et al (1986c). HIV seroprevalence among hospital workers in Kinshasa, Zaire: lack of association with occupational exposure. J Am Med Ass 256: 3099-3102.

Petriccianni J C, Gust I D, Hoppe P A, Krijnen H W (eds) (1987). "AIDS: the Safety of Blood and Blood Products". Chichester: John Wiley & Sons.

The Global Impact of AIDS, pages 369–373
© 1988 Alan R. Liss, Inc.

49. A FIRST EVALUATION OF THE NEEDLE/SYRINGE EXCHANGE IN AMSTERDAM, HOLLAND

E C Buning, C Hartgers, G van Santen, A Verster and R A Coutinho

Public Health Service, Amsterdam, Holland

INTRODUCTION

In this presentation, a controversial issue will be discussed, namely the **needle and syringe exchange** in Amsterdam. In this programme, intravenous drug users can exchange their used syringe/needle for a sterile one.

Before going into this exchange system, we will first discuss the AIDS problem among IV users, and the drug policy of Amsterdam.

AIDS

By January 1st 1988, 420 cases of AIDS were reported in the Netherlands (population 14.5 million). In 21 cases (5%), IV drug use was a risk factor; it concerned 15 heterosexual and 6 homosexual IV drug users. An epidemiological study carried out by van den Hoek and others (1) showed that in a sample of drug users in Amsterdam, 88 (28%) out of 310 drug users were seropositive.

DRUG SITUATION AND POLICY

The number of hard drug users in Amsterdam is estimated at 6,500 to 7,000. Interestingly, only some 38% are injecting whilst the remaining 62% "chase the dragon" (a way of smoking heroin or cocain). We see a different pattern of drug use among different subgroups: 37% of those of Dutch origin inject, only 4% of the ethnic group and 69% of foreigners, primarily from West Germany and Italy.

The drug policy of the city of Amsterdam can be characterised by the words "pragmatic" and "non-moralistic". The helping system is pluriform i.e. facilities are available on a continuum from harm-reduction to drug free treatment. Harm-reduction is a key word in this approach. Our definition of harm-reduction is that if it is not possible, at a particular moment, to cure a drug addict, one should at least try to minimise the harm that the drug addict does to himself and his environment. Harm-reduction is being done through medical and social care, methadone distribution and needle/syringe exchange. An example of harm-reduction programme is the methadone-bus. This programme can be described by :-

* easy accessibility (no waiting list, outreach to drug scene)
* medical/social intake (including central registration)
* fluid methadone on the spot
* no urine checks
* needle/syringe exchange.

NEEDLE/SYRINGE EXCHANGE

The number of needles/syringes that were distributed increased rapidly over time from 25,000 in 1984, to 100,000 in 1985, to 400,000 in 1986 and to 700,000 in 1987.

A First Evaluation of the Needle/Syringe Exchange

In the summer of 1987, a first evaluation of the needle/syringe exchange system was undertaken (2), using the following research design:-

* recruitment at 11 exchange - and 3 "non-exchange" locations;
* 148 addicts were interviewed with a standardised questionnaire (Table 1);
* participation was on a voluntary basis;
* no blood samples were taken.

Two groups were differentiated, "exchangers" and "non-exchangers" (Table 2)."Exchangers" are defined as IV drug users, who make use of the exchange system in 90% to 100% of the occasions when they needed a needle/syringe.

TABLE 1. Characteristics of 148 Intravenous Drug Users

	Male (N=105)	Female (N=43)	Total (N=148)	Significance P
Average age (years)	30.1	28.4	29.6	NS
Average length of drug use(years)	11	9	10	less than 0.05
Average length of IV drug use(years)	9	7	8	less than 0.05
Dutch origin (%)	48	40	46	NS

TABLE 2. Characteristics of Exchangers and Non-Exchangers

	Exchangers (N=73)	Non Exchangers (N=75)	Significance P
Males (%)	66	76	NS
Average age (years)	31.1	28.1	less than 0.001
Average length of drug use (years)	12	9	less than 0.001
Average length of IV drug use (years)	9	7	less than 0.05
Dutch origin (%)	55	37	less than 0.05
No contact with methadone programme in last 5 years (%)	25	50	less than 0.05

Regarding the question of their current drug use compared to six months ago, there was a different pattern between the two groups: exchangers 29% more, 33% same, 38% less; non-exchangers 50% more, 15% same, 35% less.

The interviewed group was also asked how often they found themselves in a "high-risk situation", a situation in which they had had hard drugs in their possession but no clean needle available. Again a different pattern for the two groups was found: exchangers 50% never, 25% at least once a month, 22% at least once a week, 3% daily; non-exchangers 31% never, 21% at least once a month, 20% at least once a week, 28% daily.

Crucial to the issue of the spread of HIV is the question relating to what they did when they had no clean equipment. Did they then actually share needles? In this matter, there were also differences between the two groups: exchangers 34% never, 31% not for last two years, 26% not for last month, 9% still sharing; non-exchangers 22% never, 20% not for last two years, 36% not for last month, 22% still sharing.

If we take a look at the general drug situation in Amsterdam, we can see an increase in the patient-load of drug free treatment, especially the out-patient treatment (data available period 1981-1986). The mean age of drug addicts in Amsterdam increased from 26.5 in 1981 to 30.1 in 1987. At the same time, the percentage of addicts under 22 years decreased (14.4% in 1981, 4.8% in 1987). Since the estimated number of addicts has been stable in that period, it seems to indicate that the absolute number of young addicts is decreasing.

CONCLUSION

On the basis of the data from this first evaluation we can draw the following conclusions :-

* no indications of an increase in drug use among exchangers.
* no reduction in clients of drug free facilities.
* no indication for recruitment of new IV addicts (percentage of young addicts is declining).
* differences among exchangers and non-exchangers
* needle/syringe exchange helps certain groups to use drugs in a safer way.
* effect on the spread of HIV yet unknown.
* the needle/syringe exchange contacts IV users outside the methadone programmes

Although we need to do more research (in particular follow-up studies that look at sero-conversions among IV drug users), to date these data indicate that a needle/syringe exchange was implemented in Amsterdam without considerable negative effects and that it helps a large group of IV drug users to minimize the risk of being infected with the AIDS virus.

REFERENCES

van den Hoek J A R, Coutinho R A et al (1988). Prevalence and risk factors of HIV infections among drug users and drug-using prostitutes in Amsterdam. AIDS 2: 55-60.

Hartgers C, Buning E C et al. Submitted for publication.

Buning E C. "De GG&GD en het drugprobleem in cijfers, deel I en II", December 1986, December 1987.

The Global Impact of AIDS, pages 375-384
© 1988 Alan R. Liss, Inc.

50.   THE ENIGMA OF AIDS VACCINES

Arie J Zuckerman

Professor, Department of Medical Microbiology and
World Health Organization Collaborating Centre for
Refererence and Research on Viral Hepatitis, London
School of Hygiene and Tropical Medicine (University
of London), Keppel Street, London WC1E 7HT, UK.

It has been said that "never in the history of human progress
has a better and cheaper method of preventing illness been
developed than immunisation". This is well illustrated by the
World Health Organization's (WHO) Expanded Programme on
Immunisation (EPI), which in developing countries is preventing
nearly a million deaths annually from measles, pertussis and
neonatal tetanus, and for which there is a commitment by WHO
and the United Nations International Children's Emergency Fund
(UNICEF) to protect all children by immunisation by the end of
the decade. To this ambitious programme must now be added the
urgency and high priority of developing a vaccine against the
human immunodeficiency viruses (HIVs) and which will require
the ingenuity and the application of novel strategies by the
world's biomedical research community. This enormous
undertaking will be facilitated by the rapid advances in
molecular biology and recombinant DNA technology, the
understanding of immunological mechanisms, and the production
and application of monoclonal antibodies so that the structure
and location of important antigenic epitopes can be determined.
Chemical synthesis of oligopeptides by manual or automatic solid
phase techniques has been simplified, and computer programmes,
X-ray crystallography and other methods provide the tools for
determining the three dimensional structure of proteins so that
the structure and location of antigens or epitopes can be
predicted. These techniques have led to the development and
production of novel vaccines against hepatitis B (Zuckerman,
1987a, b; Moss et al, 1984, Delpeynoux et al, 1986) and foot and
mouth disease virus (Clarke et al, 1987) and the application of
such methods to the development of vaccines against AIDS is

discussed briefly below.

The development of AIDS vaccines is beset with difficulties not only because of the nature of the virus, but also because antibodies to the structural components of the virus are present in infected persons often to high titre, although it has been argued that such humoral antibodies before the onset of infection may be protective; the surface lipoprotein envelope of the virus is subject to variation, and because of the lack of suitable small laboratory animals which are susceptible to this infection.

Inactivated virus vaccines

Traditionally vaccines against virus infections are based on inactivated whole virus (e.g. influenza, Salk poliovirus vaccine) or its component (e.g. plasma-derived hepatitis B surface antigen). This approach, however, presents several problems. HIV will have to be grown to high titre under conditions of high and secure containment. Complete inactivation of the virus, without loss of antigenicity and immunogenicity, must be assured – a difficult task in the absence of suitable susceptible and available small laboratory animal models. The use of cell culture systems for this purpose raises the difficulty of insertion of viral nucleic acids into the host cell chromosome and its eventual expression leading to the production of new and infectious virus (Greenaway and Farrar, 1987).

HIV 1 and HIV 2 are classified as lentiviruses; immunisation and post-infection vaccination against two animal lentiviruses have led to severe clinical syndromes on subsequent challenge with live virus. Thus goats inoculated with inactivated preparations of carpine arthritis and encephalitis virus (CAEV) develop a more severe disease when challenged with live virus, and the same effect is observed following post-infection immunisation of sheep with purified, detergent-disrupted visna virus. Caution will therefore be required in the development and testing of such vaccines (Ellrodt and Le Bras, 1987). Furthermore, inactivated HIV vaccines may induce immunosuppression.

Attenuated live virus vaccines

The use of live HIV vaccines is precluded by many of the considerations outlined above. The construction in vitro of non-pathogenic virus by gene deletion appears an attractive option.

This approach suffers, however, from several disadvantages :-

1. Reverse transcription of the viral genome into DNA copies and integration into the cellular genome may occur.

2. There is the possibility of recombination with endogenous retroviral sequences restoring pathogenicity.

3. Recombination with cellular proto onc genes may generate acute tumour virus.

4. Promotion of adjacent cellular onc genes or their activation near the integration site may occur through viral enhancers.

Production of vaccines by recombinant DNA techniques

The identification and analysis of genes coding for biologically active substances, and the application of technique for the transfer of genetic material within and between organisms with expression of proteins under controlled conditions have been applied to vaccine development. In particular recombinant DNA techniques have been used for expressing the gag and env genes of HIV in prokaryotic and eukaryotic cells. This approach has a considerable safety advantage since such preparations do not contain viral nucleic acid. However, it is not known whether such subunit proteins would elicit neutralising or protective antibodies, and the extensive variation and genomic diversity among HIV isolates from different geographical regions and patients pose difficulties although there are conserved as well as variable epitopes for neutralising antibodies. The genomic variability may offer the virus a number of advantages enabling it to escape the immune system of the host, to infect different cell types and to adapt to a different environment.

Hybrid virus vaccines

Live vaccines using recombinant viruses have been constructed for hepatitis B, and for other viruses. Foreign viral DNA is introduced for example into the vaccinia DNA by construction of chimaeric genes. This is accomplished by homologous recombination in cells since the large size of the genome of vaccinia virus (198,000 base pairs) precludes in vitro gene insertion. A chimaeric gene consisting of vaccinia virus promoter sequences ligated to the coding sequence for the desired foreign protein is flanked by vaccinia virus DNA in a plasmid vector. The hepatitis B surface antigen made by vaccinia virus recombinants was similar or identical in its polypeptide composition, buoyant density, sedimentation rate and antigenicity to material obtained from the plasma of hepatitis B carriers. The recloned vaccinia virus containing hepatitis B surface antigen coding sequences was used to vaccinate rabbits with the production of typical vaccinia lesions in the skin and high titres of hepatitis B surface antibody in the circulation. Preliminary studies in chimpanzees indicated the feasibility of using a recombinant vaccinia virus. The vaccinated chimpanzees had a secondary antibody response when challenged intravenously with live hepatitis B virus of a heterologous subtype with a mild inapparent infection characterised by seroconversion to surface antibody and hepatitis B anti-core. Although the chimpanzees had little or no circulating surface antibody after vaccination when the recombinant vaccinia was growing in the skin, they were immunologically "primed". As a result the chimpanzees had a brisk and sustained antibody response, presumably due to newly synthesized surface antigen after challenge with live hepatitis B virus (Moss et al, 1984). Recombinant vaccinia HIV env gene vectors have been constructed and are under evaluation.

However, there are no accepted laboratory markers of attenuation or of virulence of vaccinia virus for man, either in the host directly inoculated with the virus or after several passages in the same species. Alterations in the genome of vaccinia virus and possible changes in the viral envelope which are concomitant with the selection of recombinants may alter the virulence of the virus. Furthermore, the vaccinia vector can generally only be used once since antibody is induced to the vaccinia vector. Little is also known of the ways in which other pox viruses are maintained in nature, and the possibility that recombinant strains may become established in nature requires investigation.

The advantages of vaccinia virus recombinant as a vaccine include low cost, ease of administration by multiple pressure or by the scratch technique, vaccine stability, long shelf-life and the possible use of polyvalent antigens. The known adverse reactions with vaccinia virus vaccines are well documented and their incidence and severity must be carefully weighed. There are also reports of spread of current strains of vaccinia virus to contacts and this may present difficulties, particularly in populations where infection with HIV is common (Zuckerman, 1987a), although this difficulty might be overcome by the inclusion of the gene for IL-2 in a live vaccinia virus vaccine (Ramshaw et al, 1987). Other recombinant viruses as vectors have been constructed including oral adenovirus vaccines, for example adenovirus type 4 or 7 which have been used for many years for the immunisation of military recruits.

Novel vaccines using hybrid hepatitis B particles

The use of the envelope proteins of hepatitis B virus (hepatitis B surface antigen) in a particulate form by expressing the proteins in mammalian cells is an attractive option. In-phase insertions of variable length and sequence of another virus (poliomyelitis virus type I) were made in different regions of the S gene of hepatitis B virus. The envelope proteins carrying the surface antigen and the insert is assembled with cellular lipids in the cultured mammalian cells after transfection. The inserted polio neutralization peptide was found to be exposed on the surface of the hybrid envelope particles and induced neutralizing antibodies against poliovirus in mice immunised experimentally (Delpeynoux et al, 1987). A number of other immunogenic peptides including HIV peptides could be incorporated into the surface of an organised multimolecular complex in secreted hybrid envelope particles by established cell lines licensed for vaccine production.

Another potentially attractive carrier vehicle for vaccines is the use of the core particles of hepatitis B virus. The advantage of the core structure as a particulate carrier vehicle includes its ability to induce antibody with approximately 100 fold greater efficiency than the surface antigen particle, and an ability to augment T-helper cell function. The feasibility of this approach was recently demonstrated with synthetic and biosynthetic peptides of foot and mouth disease virus (FMDV) after fusion to hepatitis B core antigen (Clarke et al, 1987).

Chemically synthesized vaccines

The development of chemically synthesized polypeptide vaccines offers many advantages in attaining the ultimate goal of producing chemically uniform, safe and cheap viral immunogens which could replace many current vaccines which often contain large quantities of irrelevant and sometimes undesirable microbial antigenic determinants, proteins and other material additional to the essential immunogen required for the induction of a protective antibody. The preparation of antibodies against viral proteins using fragments of chemically synthesized peptides mimicking viral amino acid sequences is now a possible alternative approach for immunoprophylaxis. Several amino acid moieties mimicking determinants of viral antigen have been synthesized and, when coupled to a carrier protein, induced the production of neutralizing antibody in experimental animals (Zuckerman, 1987b). Cell receptors and viral antibodies, elicited antibodies by blocking the attachment of virus to the cells. Whether these results can be translated to man remains to be established.

However, designing proteins with the correct tertiary structure and with functional activities is difficult, since it is not possible to predict the tertiary structure of a protein from its amino acid sequence alone. X-ray crystallography and interactive computer graphics are essential and available tools. The first step is to obtain a highly purified protein which can be crystallized to diffraction quality. The electron density of the crystal can then be calculated and since crystallography provides information on the non-hydrogen atoms in proteins it is possible to build a scaffold model for fitting the known amino acid sequence into this structure. The model can then be refined by using sets to test co-ordinates to improve the density map. More recent techniques using synchrotron X-ray sources may allow the collection of structural information from protein in solution. Two-dimensional proton nuclear resonance techniques, which assign peaks to specific protons in the protein are also available now and the results can be converted to a set of coordinates for the molecule.

An alternative approach is to develop comprehensive algorithms to simulate the mechanisms which determine protein structures coupled with establishing libraries of protein data base. Another approach is to design synthetic proteins based on the natural folding patterns of the alpha helix configuration and the beta pleated sheet.

These studies are in agreement with several reports which show that the modification of peptides based on secondary structure predictions and model building is now feasible. Peptides have been synthesized which retain biological function and appropriate secondary structure, even though they have a limited sequence homology with the natural peptide or are much smaller. For example, studies with hormones have shown that it is possible to stabilize a beta-turn by cyclization of the molecule either by introducing a disulphide bond, or by designing a cyclic peptide.

Synthetic HIV peptides may therefore be employed in due

course as vaccines, although mixtures of more than one of the peptides may be required. Of the many questions which remain to be answered, the critical issues are whether antibodies induced by synthetic immunogens will be protective and whether protective immunity will persist. Some of the carrier proteins and some of the adjuvants which had been linked to the synthetic molecules cannot be used in man, and it is therefore essential to find acceptable and safe material for covalent linkage, or alternatively, to synthesize sequences which do not require linkage. One approach is the synthesis of sets of overlapping linear peptides extending the entire range of the *gag* and *env* gene coding sequences. Alternatively, the sequences for the preparation of HIV synthetic peptides may be based on predictions of computer programmes. Promising results have been reported including the induction of neutralising antibodies.

Novel antigen presentation

Protein micelles are aggregates of polypeptides arranged so that the hydrophobic regions are sequestered in the interior of the particles with the hydrophilic residues on the surface so that the resulting particulate forms are water soluble. The extraction of antigenic hepatitis B polypeptides with the non-ionic detergent Triton X-100 followed by detergent removal allowing membrane polypeptides to reassociate into water-soluble protein micelles was a method developed at the London School of Hygiene and Tropical Medicine (Skelly et al, 1981). The immunogenicity per unit weight of the viral surface polypeptide was greatly increased by breaking down the cross-linked lipopolypeptide complex and converting these to monomeric polypeptide units which were then aggregated into the micellar form. This presentation of the antigen was very effective in eliciting neutralizing antibodies against hepatitis B. Safety tests and protective efficacy studies of the micelle vaccine in non-human primates and limited clinical trials have been completed. More recently, polypeptide micelles have also been prepared from hepatitis B surface antigen protein expressed by recombinant DNA technology in yeast and in mammalian cells at several laboratories in the United Kingdom and in the United States.

Immune stimulating complexes (ISCOMS) based on the use of Quil A and consisting of various glycosides have been used successfully for the preparation of several experimental animal vaccines (including a vaccine against feline leukaemia virus). The viral antigens interact with the ISCOMS to form artificial rosettes which are cage-like and composed of both proteins and lipids. These structures appear to present the viral proteins to the immune system as a repetitive array and may therefore circumvent the problem of the relatively poor immunogenicity of the antigens. It is not known yet whether protective immunity is induced by such preparations, but the use of proteins expressed by recombinant DNA techniques may overcome the problems of preparing subunit antigens from whole virus from cultured cells and their purification.

Cell fusion and syncytia

Virus infected cells may serve as an important means of infection given the propensity of HIV to induce cell fusion and the formation of syncytia, so that little free virus remains in the tissue fluids. The activation of T and B cells and the production of antibody would not be sufficient to provide complete immunity nor to eliminate the virus. Secondly, the role of macrophages and the importance of phagocytosis have received little attention in complex process of establishing protective immunity. Indeed, it has been suggested that transient neutralization by antibody will be of little value if the virus-antibody complexes are simply phagocytosed by macrophages particularly as it appears that macrophages are susceptible to infection by HIV and may well be a primary target cell for the virus. Thus if the majority of macrophages can be infected by virus-antibody complexes the prospects for a conventional vaccine are poor (Langley and Spier, 1988).

Anti-idiotype antibodies

In simple terms, an anti-idiotype is an antibody to an antibody. A region of the antibody recognises the shape of a particular antigen, and this variable part of the antibody is the idiotype. The idiotype binds to the part of the antigen referred to as the epitope.

Antibodies can also act as antigens; these on injection into a second host are treated as foreign and the antibodies produced against them are referred to as anti-idiotype antibodies since they recognise the idiotype of the first antibody. The result is therefore an antibody case in the shape of the original antigen.

Anti-idiotype antibodies can neutralise HIV and closely related strains. One experimental approach, therefore, is to produce antibodies against the CD4 receptor so that the binding site on the envelope glycoprotein of the virus, which is believed to be highly conserved, is blocked. The task is to produce human monoclonal antibodies directed against identified epitopes on HIV which are essential for infectivity. These antibodies could then be used as antigens to produce anti-idiotypes. This is technically an attainable goal and offers an important, if unique approach to immunisation against AIDS.

Finally, little attention has been directed hitherto to the importance of cell mediated responses in protective immunity against infection with HIV, but such studies are now underway.

It need hardly be emphasized that any candidate vaccine must be subjected to meticulous evaluation and premature unsubstantiated claims may result in loss of confidence by the public and may have a serious impact on other immunisation programmes. Because of the lengthy incubation period of 5-8 years it is unlikely that an HIV vaccine will be generally available for at least another 5-10 years.

REFERENCES

Clarke B E, Newton S E, Carrol A R, Francis M J, Appleyard G, Syred A D, Highfield P E, Rowlands D J, Brown F (1987). Improved immunogenicity of a peptide epitope after fusion to hepatitis B core protein. Nature 330: 381-384.

Delpeynoux F, Chenciner N, Linn A, Malpiece Y, Blondel B, Crainic R, Werf van der S, Streeck R E (1986). A poliovirus neutralization epitope expressed on hybrid hepatitis B surface particles. Science 233: 472-475.

Ellrodt A, Le Bras P (1987). Hidden dangers of AIDS vaccination. Nature 325: 765.

Greenaway P J, Farrar G H (1987). Prospects for an AIDS vaccine. Microbiology Digest 4: 26-39.

Langley D, Spier R E (1988). Is a vaccine against AIDS possible? Vaccine 6: 3-5.

Moss B, Smith G L, Gerin J L, Purcell R H (1984). Live recombinant vaccinia virus protects chimpanzees against hepatitis B. Nature 311: 67-69.

Skelly J, Howard C R, Zuckerman A J (1981). Hepatitis B
polypeptide vaccine in micelle form. Nature 290: 51-54.

Zuckerman A J (1987a). Tomorrow's hepatitis B vaccines.
Vaccine 5: 165-167.

Zuckerman A J (1987b). The development of novel hepatitis B
vaccines. Bulletin of the World Health Organization
63: 265-275.

The Global Impact of AIDS, pages 385–395
© 1988 Alan R. Liss, Inc.

51. ANTIVIRAL THERAPY IN HIV INFECTION PAST,
PRESENT AND FUTURE

I V D Weller

Wellcome Trust Senior Lecturer in Infectious
Diseases, Academic Department of G U Medicine,
James Pringle House, University College & Middlesex
School of Medicine, London W1N 8AA

INTRODUCTION

Prior to the spring of 1987, the accepted treatment of
human immunodeficiency virus (HIV) infection was largely
limited to the management of its complications, namely the
opportunistic infections and tumours. There have been advances
in the diagnosis of infections, such as induced sputum
examination for *Pneumocystis carinii* pneumonia (PCP) and
modified acid-fast staining of faeces for the identification of
cryptosporidium. There have been advances also in treatment,
such as the recent use of pentamidine in aerosol form for PCP
and the introduction of ganciclovir for cytomegalovirus induced
retinitis. However, most of the opportunistic infections are due
to reactivation of latent organisms in the host or, in some cases,
to ubiquitous organisms to which we are exposed continuously.
Where antimicrobial therapy exists, it suppresses rather than
eradicates infection, so that relapses are common when
treatment is stopped. Furthermore, many of the antimicrobial
agents used have considerable toxicity.

Similarly, therapy for the opportunistic tumours, Kaposi's
sarcoma and non-Hodgkins lymphoma is palliative rather than
curative, has considerable side effects and may further
compromise the immune system. Faced with these problems, we
must look towards specific antiviral therapy. The rationale for
this is based on the hypothesis that continuing viral replication is
involved in the pathogenesis and progression of disease.
Suppression of productive viral replication may lead to recovery
of immune function and a decrease in the incidence of
opportunistic infections and tumour. Again, suppression rather

than eradication of infection is the likely end point of available antiviral compounds, and implicit in this is life long treatment.

As a result, the ideal anti-HIV drug should be specific (that is, be active against the virus and not host cells), have low toxicity, protect uninfected cells and decrease viral production from infected cells. It should also be absorbed orally and penetrate the cerebrospiral fluid (CSF). Specificity and an easy route of administration are essential for long term therapy. Currently most attention is focused on inhibitors of the viral reverse transcriptase enzyme, which makes a DNA copy of the viral RNA.

ANTIVIRAL THERAPY : PAST AND CURRENT

The assessment of an antiviral compound's action against HIV begins with demonstration of an *in vitro* effect on the virus in lymphocyte culture. Its toxicity *in vitro* in cells and *in vivo* in animals is then evaluated. If these assessments are promising and demonstrate low or acceptable toxicity, small trials in humans are conducted (Phase I studies). These provide information about toxicity (side effects), how the drug is metabolised (pharmacokinetics) and some information about its likely antiviral effects. To demonstrate significant efficacy in terms of its antiviral effect and its effect on reducing, delaying or preventing disease expression, large double-blind placebo controlled studies are required (Phase II studies). Currently only a few drugs have completed this pathway of assessment. Our patients, often influenced by the media, extrapolate from promising *in vitro* studies to assume that a given compound will be beneficial *in vivo*. This has led to patients seeking, at considerable personal financial cost, compounds available on the black market with no demonstrated efficacy.

It is convenient to divide past and current therapies into three groups (Table 1).

Group A are drugs which have been shown to have *in vitro* activity against HIV and which have undergone phase I and phase II studies, i.e. have progressed to evaluation in placebo controlled trials to ascertain efficacy.

Group B are drugs which have been tested *in vitro* and have undergone or are undergoing phase I studies, but as yet have not been evaluated in large controlled studies.

TABLE 1. Antiviral Therapy - The State of the Art with Single Agents

	In vitro	Phase I	Phase II
Group A			
Zidovudine	+	+	+
Ribavirin	+	+	+
Alpha interferon	+	±	±
Diethyldithiocarbamate (Imuthiol, DTC)	+	?	+
Group B			
Suramin	+	+	
HPA-23 (Antimoniotungstate)	+	+	
Mismatched ds RNA (Ampligen)	+	+	
Phosphonoformate	+	+	
Gamma interferon	+	±	
Ansamycin (Rifabutin)	+	+	
Fusidic acid	+	+	
Dideoxycytidine	+	+	
Group C			
TNF (Tumor necrosis factor)	+		
Sodium oxychlorosene	+		
Glucosidase inhibitors	+		
Oligonucleotides	+		

+ = stage of evaluation, from published work and abstracts

Group C are drugs whose activity has been demonstrated only *in vitro* so far.

Group A

Zidovudine, being the most promising agent, will be discussed later. Ribavirin is an analogue of guanosine, one of the four nucleosides (Guanosine, Adenosine, Cytosine and Thymidine) which are the building bricks of nucleic acid. It has *in vitro* activity against a wide range of RNA viruses and has been used in respiratory virus infections and Lassa fever. It is believed to act by inhibiting messenger RNA synthesis (the nucleic acid which carries the message for protein synthesis). In a phase I study in 23 patients with lymphadenopathy, it inhibited reverse transcriptase activity measured in lymphocyte cultures in some patients receiving 1200 mg daily or more, suggesting that it had some antiviral activity. However, there are problems in interpreting data on antiviral activity based on virus culture and reverse transcriptase activity. In a phase II study in 163 patients with lymphadenopathy, six patients developed AIDS in a 600 mg daily dose group, ten patients developed AIDS on placebo and no patients developed AIDS on 800 mg daily. Unfortunately, due to a quirk in randomisation, a group of patients with low T helper lymphocyte counts were disproportionately represented in the placebo arm. Therefore the interpretation of efficacy in this trial is difficult. Furthermore, as yet no significant changes in serum levels of HIV core antigen (p24) have been demonstrated in patients treated with Ribavirin. However, patients with AIDS or ARC treated in a recent phase I study have become reverse transcriptase and HIV-1 RNA negative in lymphocyte cultures (Crumpacker et al, 1987). Recently it has been shown that Ribavirin may antagonize the effect of zidovudine *in vitro*, which if confirmed, may herald problems with its use in combination antiviral therapy.

Alpha interferon has activity against HIV *in vitro* and acts synergistically with zidovudine. High doses have been used to treat Kaposi's sarcoma. There is little data on whether it has action against HIV *in vivo*, but logically it might be expected. Because alpha interferon has been used in Kaposi's sarcoma in phase I and phase II studies, it should be possible to determine retrospectively whether alpha interferons have an effect on p24 antigenaemia, if serum is stored. In patients with Kaposi's sarcoma and asymptomatic patients treated with 35 mega units/m^2, Kaposi's sarcoma patients who responded to interferon developed negative HIV cultures, and among asymptomatic patients more became culture negative on treatment than did placebo patients. However, the number of virus isolations carried out in this study was small.

Diethyldithiocarbamate (Imuthiol, DTC) binds metals (chelator) and has been shown *in vitro* to "partially inhibit" HIV and to have some immunomodulatory properties. In a placebo controlled trial, as yet unpublished, of 90 ARC patients using 10 mg/kg weekly, in 72 out of 90 evaluable patients there was an improvement in symptoms, a decrease in serious events and an increase in T4 counts. These results are promising, but further controlled trials are underway in Europe.

Group B

Suramin was one of the earliest drugs to be used in HIV infection. Early small phase I studies showed an apparent antiviral affect in some patients, but not in others. Further studies have shown no clinical or immunological benefit and an unacceptable toxicity, largely on renal function. Similarly, HPA23 was evaluated in small pilot studies and unacceptable bone marrow toxicity occurred.

Mismatched double stranded (ds) RNA polymers (e.g. Ampligen), induce lymphokines such as the interferons and tumour necrosis factor. They also act as cofactors for an enzyme 2-5A oligoadenylate synthetase (and therefore promote cleavage of viral RNA) and protein kinase (which may interrupt protein synthesis), i.e. they have an interferon like effect. Double stranded RNA polymers were used in cancer more than 10 years ago but were given up because of unacceptable toxicity, which included shock, renal failure and coagulopathies. The introduction of mismatched or mispaired regions into double stranded RNA allows for retention of lymphokine induction but loss of toxicity. These agents have been shown to inhibit HIV *in vitro*. In a phase I study, 10 patients with AIDS, ARC or PGL, treated with Ampligen twice a week intravenously 200-250 mg for 18 weeks, revealed no toxicity (Carter et al, 1987). There was symptomatic improvement with a decrease in lymph nodes and splenomegaly. There were antiviral affects demonstrated by a loss of HIV RNA in peripheral blood mononuclear cells, a decrease of viral antigen in the supernatant of lymphocyte cultures at 14 days, a decrease in serum p24 in two out of three patients and an increase in 2-5A synthetase activity. Immunologically, T helper cells were said to increase, but no data were presented. There was an improvement in allergy and an increase in neutralising antibodies, but again no data were presented. These promising results need to be confirmed.

Phosphonoformate is a pyrophosphate analogue which inhibits nucleic acid polymerases and has been shown to have activity against HIV *in vitro*. Two phase I studies have been published. In one, 11 patients with AIDS or ARC were treated intravenously for three weeks. Virus isolation studies suggested an antiviral affect, but there was no improvment in immune function. One patient developed renal failure. In a second study in 15 patients with AIDS treated for 6-21 days, 70-80% of virus cultures remained positive during treatment. However, five out of eight antigen positive patients became negative. There was no clinical or immunological improvement. Nine out of fifteen patients developed renal impairment. Further work continues with phosphonoformate, but a major drawback would seem to be its toxicity and route of administration. It is possible that side effects may be less severe in asymptomatic patients.

Gamma interferon is a lymphokine and, like alpha interferon, has *in vitro* activity against HIV. Trials of gamma interferon in Kaposi's sarcoma have been conducted and it may be possible retrospectively to look at stored sera for an effect on p24 antigenaemia. Prospective trials are underway.

Ansamycin (Rifabutin) is a Rifamycin derivative. The Rifamycin group act as RNA polymerase inhibitors. This group of compounds was shown to inhibit a murine retrovirus reverse transcriptase in 1974. Ansamycin has been used in AIDS for the treatment of atypical mycobacterial infection. Although *in vitro* activity against these organisms has been demonstrated, *in vivo* results have been disappointing. However, it would seem to have fairly low toxicity. *In vitro*, ansamycin inhibits HIV at levels which can be obtained *in vivo*. Phase I studies are underway.

Sodium fusidate is a steroidal antibiotic which inhibits protein synthesis. It has activity against HIV *in vitro*, (Faber et al, 1987); the mechanism may well be cytopathic rather than antiviral, i.e. it damages the cells in which the virus is dividing rather than the virus itself. Pilot studies of this drug in patients who have been unable to tolerate zidovudine have revealed a high incidence of skin rashes requiring cessation of therapy. Serum p24 data at the moment are inconclusive.

Dideoxycytidine is a dideoxynucleoside in the same family of drugs as zidovudine. *In vitro*, it appears to be more potent in its HIV inhibiting effect than zidovudine, it is relatively resistant to an enzyme which normally breaks down cytidine analogues, is absorbed orally and has relatively low animal toxicity. However, in phase I studies, there have been unwanted side effects in the form of neuropathy.

Group C

Tumour necrosis factor, another lymphokine, has also been demonstrated to have *in vitro* activity against HIV, and phase I studies are in progress in the United States. Sodium oxychlorosene has been shown to have *in vitro* activity against herpes simplex virus, vaccinia virus and HIV. A group of plant alkaloids which are glucosidase inhibitors, e.g. castanspermine, inhibit enzymes which trim glycosylated proteins before full glycosylation. These compounds have been shown to inhibit HIV *in vitro*. Finally, oligonucleotides with homology to the nucleotide sequences in the HIV genome have been shown to inhibit HIV replication *in vitro* and to act synergistically with the dideoxynucleosides. Acyclovir acts perhaps synergistically with zidovudine, and placebo controlled trials of this combination are underway. However, at a dose of 800 mg 6 hourly orally in six patients, acyclovir did not produce an alteration of serum p24 levels *in vivo*, nor did its combination in six patients with zidovudine produce any obvious benefit in terms of antigen suppression (De Wolf et al, 1988).

Dideoxynucleosides

This group of compounds was synthesised 20 years ago and shown to inhibit murine retroviruses 12 years ago. They act as DNA chain terminating inhibitors of reverse transcriptase (by blocking 3,5 phosphodiester linkages). Also they deplete intracellular pools of phosphorylated nucleotides. Zidovudine was shown to have *in vitro* activity against HIV, and then in a phase I study found to be well absorbed orally and to have 60% bioavailability. It is largely metabolised by being glucuronidated in the liver and excreted by the kidney. It has a half life in plasma of one hour. The phase I studies showed an increased T helper count, decrease in allergy, bone marrow toxicity and penetration of the CSF to a concentration of about half that of plasma. In addition, in these uncontrolled studies, six patients with HIV associated dementia, peripheral neuropathy or both had some improvement of symptoms and signs as assessed by clinical examination, neuropsychometric testing, nerve conduction studies, or brain scan (positron emission tomography) (Yarchoan et al, 1987).

A multi-centre controlled trial in patients with AIDS (recovery from first episode of *P. carinii)* and ARC was started in February 1986 with recruitment running through until June 1986. It was stopped in September 1986 at a time when over half of the patients had completed four months of therapy (Fischl et al, 1987). The dose was 250 mg four-hourly. There were no significant differences in the demographic features between the two groups, apart from a shorter time between pneumocystis and the start of therapy in the zidovudine group (10 days). There were significant reductions in mortality and incidence of opportunistic infections in the treatment group. There was no effect on the incidence of development of Kaposi's sarcoma in placebo or treatment group, but numbers were small (10 vs 6). In addition, Karnofsky performance was retained, there was significant weight gain, loss of fever and reduced AIDS related symptom scores. There were also significant increases in T helper cell counts, a decrease in allergy and approximately a 90% reduction in serum p24 levels (Jackson et al, 1988). Significant side effects were nausea, myalgia, insomnia and more severe headache. The most important toxicity occurred in the bone marrow with a megaloblastic macrocytic anaemia, leucopenia and neutropenia (Richman et al, 1987). Predictors of toxicity were a pre-existing low T helper cell count, neutropenia, anaemia and a low-normal serum B12. Sick patients developed worse toxicity, and paracetamol appeared to potentiate the neutropenia. 31% of the treated patients required transfusions and 21% required more than one (compared to 11% of the placebo patients requiring transfusions).

Since the release of zidovudine in the spring of 1987, it has been used widely by clinicians in the developed world for patients with symptomatic HIV disease in stage IV of the CDC classification of HIV infection, even though benefit was demonstrated only in patients with constitutional symptoms, certain clinical signs and laboratory parameters which signify a poor prognosis, and those who had recovered from a first episode of PCP. This extension of its use away from the groups enrolled in the controlled trial is both compassionate and logical if one considers the prognosis of patients in this group and the mode of action of the drug. Physicians are assuming that all patients that have recovered from an opportunistic infection might benefit, and that even if no effect has yet been demonstrated in Kaposi's sarcoma, such patients often succumb to an intervening opportunistic infection. The effects of the drug on miscellaneous

HIV related conditions, such as lymphoid interstitial pneumonitis and sclerosing cholangitis, are unknown, but it is likely that patients will be treated empirically.

Placebo controlled trials are now underway in (a) asymptomatic anti-HIV positive patients with laboratory markers, such as antigenaemia or low T helper counts, which are associated from prospective cohort studies with a more rapid development of symptomatic disease, and (b) anti-HIV positive patients with or without these markers; the trial population is being stratified for these variables on entry, so that patients with them are equally distributed between treatment and placebo groups.

More recently zidovudine, given orally 250 mg six-hourly, 500 mg six-hourly or 500 mg twice daily, has been shown to depress serum p24 levels in asymptomatic patients and, in one patient, CSF p24 levels (De Wolf et al, 1988). Although the demonstration of an antiviral effect cannot be extrapolated at this stage to an effect on disease outcome, it is likely that such a dose regimen will prove an attractive one to those embarking on placebo controlled trials in asymptomatic individuals.

ANTIVIRAL THERAPY - FUTURE

Future progress will require a close collaboration between basic scientists and pharmaceutical companies. At the end of last year, few companies had facilities for the in vitro assessment of antiviral drugs. As a result, Government funding in both the United States and the U.K. has allowed the establishment of centres which can screen a large number of compounds. Such screening of currently available drugs may well provide information quickly about other promising compounds. However, at the same time directed research programmes in both countries will bring together basic scientists, such as molecular biologists, immunologists and chemists. As a result, the recent advances in our knowledge with respect to the interaction of the virus with the cell and the replication of HIV will reveal a variety of potential future targets for antiviral therapy. The production of viral proteins, the development of antibodies to them and the characterisation of these proteins and enzymes will provide a more rational approach to specific inhibition of the virus (Table 2). The potential targets have been highlighted (Yarchoan et al, 1987) and include interference with the virus/receptor interaction by antibodies or synthetic ligands (peptides), interference with uncoating of the virus by

amantadine-like substances, inhibition of the reverse
transcriptase enzyme directly or indirectly via DNA chain
termination, inhibition of the RNAase enzyme which eliminates
the RNA strand from the DNA copy, and inhibition of integrase
function (a virally determined property which allows for
integration). Agents acting at any of these sites might prevent

TABLE 2. Targets for Antiviral Therapy

Target	Therapy
Virus receptor	Antibodies or ligands
Uncoating	Amantadine-like
Reverse transcriptase	Inhibitors/chain terminators
RNAase	Inhibitors
Integration	Viral "integrase" inhibitors
RNA translation	Tat-III or art-trs inhibitors "anti-sense constructs"
Viral protein synthesis and assembly	Enzyme inhibitors e.g.protease, glucosidase
Viral budding	Interferons, antibodies, ligands

infection of a cell. Potential targets, which would decrease viral
production from cells, might be interference with RNA
translation using inhibitors of the regulatory genes or their
products, such as oligodeoxynucleotides or anti-sense constructs.
In its assembly, the virus undergoes secondary processing by a
variety of enzymes, such as the protease enzyme which is virally
determined, and host glycosylating and myristylating enzymes.
Inhibitors of these functions may be found. Finally, the virus
buds from the cell. Antibodies and ligands which interfere with
virus entry may also act at this site. In addition, interferons may
act at a variety of sites of viral replication, including viral
budding.

REFERENCES

Carter W A, Strayer D R, Brodsky I (1987). Clinical, immunological and virological effects of Ampligen, a mismatched double-stranded RNA, in patients with AIDS or AIDS-related complex. Lancet i: 1286-1291.

Crumpacker C, Heagy W, Bubley G et al (1987). Ribavirin treatment of the acquired immunodeficiency synrome (AIDS) and the acquired immunodeficiency syndrome related complex (ARC). Ann Intern Med 107: 664-674.

De Wolf F, Lange J M A, Goudsmit J, Cload P, De Gans J, Schellekens P Th A, Coutinho R A, Fiddian A P, Van der Noordan J (1988). Effect of zidovudine on serum human immunodeficiency virus antigen levels in symptom free subjects. Lancet i: 373-376.

Faber V, Newell A, Dalgleish A G, Malkovsky M (1987). Inhibition of HIV replication in vitro by Fusidic acid. Lancet ii: 827-828.

Fischl M A, Richman D D, Grieco M H et al (1987). The efficacy of azidothymidine (AZT) in the treatment of patients with AIDS and AIDS-related complex. A double blind placebo controlled trial. New Engl J Med 317: 185-191.

Jackson G G, Paul D A, Falle L A, Ruberis M, Despotes C, Mack D, Knigge M, Emeson E E (1988). Human immunodeficiency virus (HIV) antigenaemia (p24) in the acquired immunodeficiency syndrome (AIDS) and the effect of treatment with zidovudine (AZT). Ann Inter Med 108: 175-180.

Richman D D, Fischl M A, Grieco M H et al (1987). The toxicity of azidothymidine (AZT) in the treatment of patients with AIDS and AIDS-related complex. N Eng J Med 317: 192-197.

Yarchoan R et al (1987). Response of human immunodeficiency virus associated neurological disease to 3'-azido-3' deoxythymidine. Lancet i: 132-135.

Yarchoan R, Broder S (1987). Development of antiretroviral therapy for the acquired immunodeficiency syndrome and related disorders. N Engl J Med 316: 557-564.

The Global Impact of AIDS, pages 397–402
© 1988 Alan R. Liss, Inc.

52.   THE TEN PARADOXES OF AIDS – SUMMING UP THE CONFERENCE

The Hon Justice Michael Kirby CMG

President, Court of Appeal, Supreme Court, Sydney, Australia

Oscar Wilde, whose spirit haunts the courtrooms of this city and reproaches us for earlier prejudice (1), once apologised for writing a long letter. He said he did not have time to write briefly. Yet that is what I must do now.

I can do no more - on your behalf - than to collect a number of the images and the paradoxes of what we have learned from the Conference and to offer, tentatively, a few conclusions, which are inescapably personal.

The first paradox arose out of the eminently sensible and well targeted speech of Minister Newton who opened the conference. Yet on the very eve of the conclusion of our meeting, this great liberal nation - the cradle of democracy - is considering legislation which, putting it at the lowest (if I can attempt a British understatement), will not help the public health campaign on AIDS (2). Ministers and top officials are often well informed. Legislators may not, in all their diversity, be so well informed and may be susceptible to transient pressures. The danger of the virus of Highly Inefficient Laws ("HIL") grows every day in all of our countries (3). It is most serious because we are in the exponential phase of this epidemic, as was repeatedly pointed out during the meeting.

Secondly, the social and economic data disclosed during the conference revealed the enormous and growing tide of the problem - particularly in Africa, Latin America and the Caribbean. In a sense, as Professor Frankenberg suggested (pp 191-199) the stigmatised groups in the developed countries have been the sentinels - bearing the first impact for all humankind. We should not forget their suffering. We should learn with them and, sadly, from their funerals.

Yet despite this toll, the indefatigable Dr Jonathan Mann (pp 3-7) and Dr Manuel Carballo (pp 81-93) and also Dr Koop (pp 307-311) and Dr Meyer (pp 329-334) found some reasons for hope in the "third epidemic of AIDS in society". Could we yet turn this calamity to long range human advantage - by intense international cooperation; by the symbiosis of world health and human rights; by the lessons for other curable diseases; and by a new approach to the very definition of what "health" is?

Thirdly, we learned of the importance of the exchange of information on the subject of life and death. It must be rapid and frank. Who would have thought five years ago that we would be here talking of condoms and anal sex? Yet many speakers cautioned about the need for sensitivity in the choice of language for fear of reinforcing stigmatisation and prejudice, even by subliminal or unintended messages. There are no specially "innocent victims" of AIDS. This is not just a problem of men in pin-striped suits. There are only patients and communities who are suffering and who demand an effective response.

Fourthly, we saw special attention to the "at risk groups" who have, in different lands, taken the first blows of AIDS. Yet if we have learned nothing else here it is that it is behaviour and activity that is risky. The danger of identifying groups, as such, is that we may reinforce stereotypes in a way that is entirely counterproductive. This point was vividly made by Dr Day with her brilliant work on prostitutes, who are typically infected by their boyfriends not their condomed clients (4). Surgeon General Koop also pointed out that there is always a cost/benefit equation in any response targeted at particular groups, whoever they may be (pp 307-311).

Fifthly, we saw new resolution in calculating the direct and indirect economic costs of AIDS in developed and developing countries. This is good. Dr Over suggested that this development may help mobilize investment in the cure, out of the realisation of the very dimension of what is at stake (pp 123-135). (One to $1\frac{1}{2}$ million infected in the USA, according to Dr Noble (pp 35-41). Annual cost of US $8.5 billion in that country by 1991, according to Mrs Scitovsky(pp 137-144).) Yet we have a long way to go. I sensed a certain frustration at the lack of adequate discussion, almost to the very end, about the cure and the vaccine and their possibilities. Was this silence ominous, in the long as well as the short run? There was certainly frustration at the typical lack of an effective response by traditional social security departments, mentioned by Professor Glennester in his summary of the fourth session; to say nothing of the frequent lack of emotional support, and the social and personal isolation of those who are ill and those who grieve. We should ponder on the private crises of the Tanzanian women with the Juliana T-shirts, distributed on the long trucking routes of Africa by infected travellers, leaving the virus behind (pp 233-239). We should remember that Zambian youth whose end was recounted by Dr Campbell (5). Unable to take his suffering any more, he set fire to his hut and died alone in that cruel way surrounded by his grieving, puzzled village.

Sixthly, we saw various models of the economic costs of AIDS - with the primary impact of the virus on the most productive years of the patient (pp 95-106). Yet no one can venture the value of a human life in purely economic terms. This was a point made (I hope facetiously) from the floor, when it was pointed out that the death of drug addicts in New York might actually **help** the American economy and that the death of the human mammal in Africa may help preserve other fauna and flora. For those who grieve, the value of a loved one lost to AIDS is beyond purely economic price. That is why there were many calls for more attention to the social and personal impacts of AIDS at any later conference of this kind.

Seventhly, when feeling overburdened by the size of the emerging problem and by its new facets, we could still take heart from the progress made: the screening of blood products in most countries (pp 271-276, 357-367), early evidence of changing sexual practices on a macro scale (pp 35-41, 307-311, 329-334) and needle exchanges, against all the odds, in societies concurrently engaged in a so called "war against drugs" (pp 313-316, 323-327, 369-373). There has also been international cooperation on the rarest scale.

Eighthly, we feel obsessed by the graphs showing the rapid rise of cases of AIDS. Yet we need the constant reminder of the necessity of retaining our sense of proportion. There are treatable diseases which we may be neglecting. Although AIDS has now overtaken suicide and motor car injuries in many developed countries (6), still the total of those infected does not even approach the deaths and suffering caused by the global yet still rising use of tobacco and alcohol. Adjustments to public health policies to address the challenge of AIDS must be made with careful attention to the requirements of concentrating resources where they can achieve the greatest human benefits.

Ninthly, we heard Jonathan Mann pay proper tribute to the media for bringing the AIDS virus so quickly to an unprecedented global knowledge, as the international Gallup surveys showed it has (pp 347-355). And yet many of those most at risk watch little TV. They may not even be able to read the vivid posters dutifully prepared by national AIDS committees (7). As well, we have seen even in London in recent days, how some of the popular press pander to outright prejudice. Is it any wonder that the myth of the mosquito and tale of the toilet seat still flourish? And as for the vaunted "free press" of the United States - not a single question was asked of President Reagan about AIDS for more than three years after it became a proper matter of national concern. I hope that Mr Bush and Governor Dukakis will not be so gently treated (8).

Tenthly, we heard in the audience an impatience for a new sense of urgency, which we certainly all share. But if it was a call for a single drum, there are many who will urge caution. That drum may lead, in one place, to a "sign" identifying those at risk, as one human ecologist urged should be introduced as a protection to the uninfected. We have already seen those signs earlier this century.

Alternatively, this drum may lead to the "island mentality". But with so many millions affected, there is just no place to go for the infected. There is not enough barbed wire. Not enough guards. Madagascar (9) and Australia (10) are not now available. So we must find the solutions by well targeted policies **within**, and not by resurrecting new Sachsenhausens (pp 317-322).

A thread of Ariadne ran through this diverse conference despite all the frustration expressed by the participants. It leads, in the end, to a principle for action. That principle requires that what we do about AIDS should be guided by efficiency and equity. Of course, we could catch a few more criminals if we had unlimited phone taps, spies in every street and if we returned to the thumbscrew. We do not do so because our sense of equity and respect for human rights restrain us. So with AIDS. We could possibly stop some infections by adopting draconian measures. But we hold back because there are other precious features of our societies which we must safeguard at the same time as we are dealing with the containment of AIDS.

This conference is not in the mood for more rhetoric or ringing perorations. Nearly 50 years ago in this city, faced with the virus of fascism in its two manifestations and in a dark hour, Churchill declared that humanity had reached not the end, nor even the beginning of the end but the end of the beginning. Much death and suffering lay ahead and also, as we know now, unprecedented and quite original scientific and technological innovation.

So that is where we are in London in March 1988. We now scatter to the four corners of the world, where AIDS is :-

* Judges to their benches, remembering that human rights matter most when they are hardest to accord;
* Religious people return to their ministry;
* Doctors and nurses to their patients' care;
* Educators to their pedagogy;
* Politicians, I hope, go back mainly to other things.

And, above all, at the "bottom line", scientists and technologists should return to their speculation and experiments which, more than words and laws and condoms and "AIDS talk" will, in the end, release us from this unprecedented human and global calamity.

REFERENCES

1. Ellman R (1987). Oscar Wilde. London, Hamish Hamilton, pp. 450: ff.

2. Clause 29 of the Local Government Bill which was then before the House of Commons. It would restrict "promotion" of homosexuality in British schools.

3. Kirby M D. The new AIDS virus - ineffective and unjust laws. Unpublished paper for the International Symposium on AIDS, Paris, 23 October 1987.

4. Day S, Ward H (1988). HIV and prostitute women in London. The First International Conference on the Global Impact of AIDS, London 8-10 March 1988. Abstracts, s4.6, p.37.

5. Campbell I D (1988). AIDS care and prevention in a Zambian rural community. **Ibid**, s4.8, p.37.

6.   Valleron A J, Flandre P (1988). Demographic consequences of mortality from AIDS in France in 1990: AIDS ahead of suicide and close to motor vehicle deaths. **Ibid,** S2.8, p.22.

7.   Reference to the many tabloid presentations in the posters displayed at the conference.

8.   Reference to the then current leading contenders in the campaign for election to the Presidency of the United States of America.

9.   Reference to Hitler's proposal to banish the Jews of Europe to Madagascar as part of the "Final Solution".

10. Reference to the First Fleet which brought the first British settlers to Australia in 1788.

APPENDIX

COUNCIL OF EUROPE
COMMITTEE OF MINISTERS

Recommendation No. R (87) 25

OF THE COMMITTEE OF MINISTERS TO MEMBER
STATES CONCERNING A COMMON EUROPEAN
PUBLIC HEALTH POLICY TO FIGHT THE
ACQUIRED IMMUNODEFICIENCY SYNDROME
(AIDS)

(Adopted by the Committee of Ministers on
26 November 1987 at its 81st Session)

The Committee of Ministers, under the terms of Article
15.b of the Statute of the Council of Europe,

Considering that the aim of the Council of Europe is to
achieve greater unity between its members and that this aim
may be pursued, *inter alia*, by the adoption of common action in
the health field;

Aware of the growing challenge for public health authorities
represented by a new and severe health hazard, the Human
Immunodeficiency Virus (HIV) infection, transmissible by sexual
intercourse, through the blood, during pregnancy and perinatally,
and which can induce a variety of conditions such as AIDS, Aids
Related Complex (ARC), various cancers, neurological and other
disorders, as well as some problems with respect to healthy
carriers;

Conscious that there is at present neither vaccine nor cure
for AIDS;

Considering that, under these circumstances, HIV infection
will dangerously increase and spread in the population if no
immediate and effective preventive action is taken;

Considering that such an epidemic will represent a very
heavy burden for health services and social security systems, and
will have serious economic consequences;

403

Considering that it may also pose ethical, legal and social problems in terms of stigmatisation and discrimination;

Bearing in mind the Convention for the Protection of Human Rights and Fundamental Freedoms;

Recalling its Recommendations No. R (83) 8 and No. R (85) 12 concerning the screening of blood donors for AIDS markers;

Judging that the implementation of a harmonised comprehensive preventive policy at European level may effectively limit the spread of the disease.

In the light of present knowledge, recommends the governments of member states to :

I.   declare the fight against AIDS an urgent national priority;

II.   carefully devise, in the light of socio-cultural contexts, the most appropriate public health policy for the prevention of AIDS by drawing up a comprehensive strategy consisting of programmes and measures which:

       - are scientifically justified and expedient to impede the spread of the infection with a view to the protection of the health of the citizens, and

       - do not interfere unnecessarily with their individual rights to objective information, freedom and private life;

III.   follow to this end the guidelines set out in the appendix to this recommendation;

IV.   intensify co-operation within Europe in pursuing studies on specific aspects of the control of AIDS with a view to:

       1. assisting national health administrations in continuously adjusting their public health policy to actual requirements;

       2. optimising the effectiveness of such policies by avoiding duplication of efforts through exchange of information, comparison and assessment of strategies;

       3. identifying common areas of research in the field of AIDS prevention, diagnosis and treatment, for which specific

funds should be allocated;

4. achieving a concerted harmonised European policy in the fight against AIDS.

Appendix to Recommendation No. R (87) 25

GUIDELINES FOR THE DRAWING UP OF A PUBLIC HEALTH POLICY TO FIGHT AIDS

1. Co-ordinating committees

Those governments which have not yet done so, should urgently set up co-ordinating committees as national, regional and local levels in keeping with the size and administrative structure of the country.

1.1 Task of the committees

The task of the national commitee should consist in the drawing up of a public health policy for the prevention of AIDS taking into account the complex implications at strategical level (for the essential elements of this policy, see Item 2 hereafter).

The appointment of regional and local committees should serve as a means of ensuring a regular flow of information and vertical and horizontal co-operation in the implementation of the policy and co-ordination of actions.

The national committee should monitor the implementation of the policy by instituting an appropriate feed-back system for permanent revision and adaptation of the policy.

Resources should be made available, both in terms of finance and personnel, to implement the nationally agreed policy at regional and local levels.

1.2 Membership of the committees

Membership of the national committee should include, for example, representatives of relevant governmental sectors: health, social affairs, social security, education, research etc.

The national committee should seek the advice of experts in various fields, interested parties, health staff, associations and organisations, whether public or private, whose work is relevant to AIDS prevention.

The membership of regional and local committees should include the same representatives at the corresponding level so as to reflect all concerned interests.

The committees whether national, regional or local, should be set up in such a way as to:

-   ensure a balanced approach integrating the various aspects and issues involved;

-   facilitate the drawing up of a consensus policy taking into account the various interests and allowing for an optimal use of scarce resources.

2. Formulation of a public health policy: essentials

The national AIDS committees should draw up a comprehensive policy based on an agreed strategy consisting of a series of co-ordinated and consistent programmes in a variety of complementary fields, combining:

- prevention:

-   health information programmes directed at the general public.
-   health education programmes targeted on groups at particular risk,
-   health promotion programmes;

- public health regulatory measures;

- strengthening of health care services;

- training of staff;

- evaluation and research.

2.1 Prevention: health information, education and promotion

National health administrations should concentrate their efforts on preventive measures aimed at behavioural change to control the epidemic since these are of singular importance as long as a vaccine and cure have not been found.

To this end, a health communication strategy should be devised at the national level taking account of the views of health education, mass communication and social science experts, professional advertisers etc; such a strategy should be based on the following programmes which will respectively bear short, medium and long-term effects:

- health information programmes directed at the general public with a view to maintaining awareness, avoiding panic reactions and preparing for targeted health educational activities;
- health education programmes directed at groups particularly at risk with a view to achieving behavioural change;
- health promotion programmes with a view to helping individuals in choosing healthy life-styles.

2.1.1 Health information programmes directed at the general public

The objective should consist in counteracting misinformation, prejudice and fear by raising the level of knowledge about the modes of transmission, the spread of the infection and the risk associated with behavioural patterns. The public should be informed of measures to prevent infection and, in particular, that sexual transmission may be prevented by careful selection of sexual partners, by avoiding casual sexual contact and by the use of condoms.

Special attention should be paid to the media whose role in shaping public opinion is crucial; a strategy should be adopted to favour responsible reporting on the subject; to this end dossiers should be regularly prepared and made available to the press.

2.1.2 Health education programmes targeted on groups particularly at risk

Such programmes should be planned on a medium-term basis, as their main objective, behavioural change, cannot be reached overnight.

Three overriding principles should permeate health education activities:

- behavioural change depends on the attitude of the individual;
- the individual is reponsible for the outcome of his behaviour towards himself, others and society;
- the individual must be treated with dignity and respect.

No health education programme (primary prevention) should be initiated if not backed up be secondary and tertiary prevention facilities (that is, sites for voluntary testing, counselling, treatment and psycho-social support services).

Target groups to be considered may vary in size from country to country and programmes and activities should reflect this variability; however, in view of the transmission modes, the following should in any case be taken into account;

- intravenous drug users,
- men with homosexual contacts,
- prostitutes,
- customers of prostitutes,
- "sex-tourists", coming from or travelling to areas where AIDS is endemic,
- haemophiliacs,
- people staying in or travelling to areas with a high prevalence of AIDS,
- the prison population,
- adolescents.

2.1.3 Health promotional programmes

Sex education should be integrated in a wider reflection on life-styles and human relationships. Such programmes should encourage individuals to assume responsibility for their health by becoming aware of risks and benefits inherent in various life-styles.

2.2 Public health regulatory measures

In the light of present knowledge, given the absence of curative treatment and in view of the complexity of spread of HIV infection.

2.2.1 Screening:

- systematic screening programmes should be fully implemented in respect of donations of blood, mothers' milk, organs, tissues, cells and, in particular, semen donation in compliance with the usual strict requirements of informed consent and regulations for confidentiality of data; for greater security, heat-treatment or other inactivation procedures of plasma products should continue to be enforced; self-exclusion from donation should continue to be strongly recommended to individuals with high-risk behaviour;

- there should be no compulsory screening of the general population nor of particular population groups;

- health authorities should instead invest resources in the setting up of sites - when these do not already exist - for voluntary testing fully respecting confidentiality regulations, and for arranging under the same conditions contact tracing of partners of seropositives;

- voluntary testing should be backed up by counselling services which should be readily accessible or even free of charge;

- the identification, where necessary, of groups to whom to recommend voluntary testing should be decided upon by health authorities in close co-operation with experts in the field; the identification on the basis of risk factors of cases to whom to recommend voluntary testing should be the task of medical staff;

- quality of testing should be ensured through the appointment of reference centres.

2.2.2   Other measures:

- public health regulatory measures such as health controls, restriction of movement or isolation of carriers, should as a general rule not be introduced on a compulsory basis;

- in the light of the present knowledge, discriminatory measures such as control at borders, exclusion of carriers from school, employment, housing, etc. should not be introduced as they are not justified either scientifically or ethically.

2.2.3   Information relating to seropositivity:

- individuals, whether donors or not, should be informed of a confirmed positive result of a blood test; they should be referred to competent medical and counselling services to be informed or precautions to be taken to protect their own health and to avoid spreading the infection to other individuals;

- if they take appropriate measures, health staff can usually avoid contamination; patients should, therefore, themselves be left to advise health staff of their seropositivity unless the patient has specifically authorised a doctor to pass on this information.

2.2.4   For the purposes of gaining insight into the epidemiology of HIV infection:

- the reporting of AIDS cases in strict compliance with confidentiality regulations is strongly recommended;

- where implemented, the reporting of seropositivity should also be carried out in strict compliance with confidentiality regulations;

- the setting up of epidemiological studies of representative samples or cohorts of the general population and groups with risk behaviour on a voluntary basis and in compliance with regulations of confidentiality and anonymity is to be considered essential in identifying risk factors associated with seropositivity and changing patterns of the disease.

2.3 Strengthening of health care services

Flexible plans consistent with the epidemiological projections and capable of efficiently meeting increasing needs should be drawn up; in this respect the responsible health authorities should:

- ensure adequate in-patient facilities or reinforce existing in-patient units for the treatment of AIDS and related conditions, staffing them with multidisciplinary teams;

- organise out-patient facilities supported by community care services allowing patients to maintain as much as possible a private and a social community-integrated life;

- organise psycho-social support services for in and out-patients as well as for asymptomatic carriers, their partners and families.

2.4 Training of staff

Appropriate training programmes should be organised for all categories of health staff, especially for those working in the field of diagnosis, treatment, control of transmission of infections, psychological support and terminal care.

Staff in the social services should be trained in the implementation of policies and regulations, as well as in patient and family assistance and psychological support.

Staff who may have occupational exposure to infected fluids and secretions should be kept informed of sensible hygienic precautions to be taken both for themselves and for their clients.

Training for teachers should be organised to allow them to integrate AIDS prevention in health education.

2.5 Evaluation and research

Development of research and co-operation at European level through the designation of reference centres in all AIDS-related fields is an urgent priority to combat AIDS, would be of great benefit both in terms of effectiveness of programmes and costs, and should therefore be strongly supported by national health administrations.

Index

413